T0226983

Editors

ASIF M. ILYAS
SHITAL N. PARIKH
SAQIB REHMAN
GILES R. SCUDERI
FELASFA M. WODAJO

ORTHOPEDIC CLINICS
OF NORTH AMERICA

www.orthopedic.theclinics.com

October 2013 • Volume 44 • Number 4

ELSEVIER

1600 John F. Kennedy Boulevard • Suite 1800 • Philadelphia, Pennsylvania, 19103-2899.

http://www.orthopedic.theclinics.com

ORTHOPEDIC CLINICS OF NORTH AMERICA Volume 44, Number 4
October 2013 ISSN 0030-5898, ISBN-13: 978-0-323-22729-2

Editor: Jennifer Flynn-Briggs

Orthopedic Clinics of North America (ISSN 0030-5898) is published quarterly by Elsevier Inc., 360 Park Avenue South, New York, NY 10010-1710. Months of issue are January, April, July, and October. Business and Editorial Offices: 1600 John F. Kennedy Blvd., Suite 1800, Philadelphia, PA 19103-2899. Customer Service Office: 3251 Riverport Lane, Maryland Heights, MO 63043. Periodicals postage paid at New York, NY and additional mailing offices. Subscription prices are $293.00 per year for (US individuals), $554.00 per year for (US institutions), $347.00 per year (Canadian individuals), $664.00 per year (Canadian institutions), $427.00 per year (international individuals), $689.00 per year (international institutions), $144.00 per year (US students), $208.00 per year (Canadian and international students). Foreign air speed delivery is included in all *Clinics* subscription prices. All prices are subject to change without notice. **POSTMASTER:** Send change of address to *Orthopedic Clinics of North America*, **Elsevier Health Sciences Division, Subscription Customer Service, 3251 Riverport Lane, Maryland Heights, MO 63043. Customer Service (orders, claims, online, change of address): Elsevier Health Sciences Division, Subscription Customer Service, 3251 Riverport Lane, Maryland Heights, MO 63043. Tel: 1-800-654-2452 (U.S. and Canada); 314-447-8871 (outside U.S. and Canada). Fax: 314-447-8029. E-mail: journalscustomerservice-usa@elsevier. com (for print support); journalsonlinesupport-usa@elsevier.com (for online support).**

Reprints. For copies of 100 or more, of articles in this publication, please contact the Commercial Reprints Department, Elsevier Inc., 360 Park Avenue South, New York, NY 10010-1710. Tel.: 212-633-3874; Fax: 212-633-3820; E-mail: reprints@elsevier. com.

Orthopedic Clinics of North America is covered in *MEDLINE/PubMed* (*Index Medicus*), *Cinahl, Excerpta Medica,* and *Cumulative Index to Nursing and Allied Health Literature.*

Printed and bound by CPI Group (UK) Ltd, Croydon, CR0 4YY

Transferred to digital print 2012

Contributors

EDITORS

ASIF M. ILYAS, MD - *Upper Extremity*
Program Fellowship, Director of Hand and
Upper Extremity Surgery, Rothman Institute,
Associate Professor of Orthopaedic Surgery,
Thomas Jefferson University, Philadelphia,
Pennsylvania

SHITAL N. PARIKH, MD, FACS - *Pediatrics*
Pediatric Orthopaedic Sports Medicine,
Associate Professor of Orthopaedic Surgery,
Cincinnati Children's Hospital Medical Center,
University of Cincinnati School of Medicine,
Cincinnati, Ohio

SAQIB REHMAN, MD - *Trauma*
Director of Orthopaedic Trauma, Associate
Professor of Orthopaedic Surgery, Department
of Orthopaedic Surgery and Sports Medicine,
School of Medicine, Temple University
Hospital, Temple University, Philadelphia,
Pennsylvania

GILES R. SCUDERI, MD - *Adult
Reconstruction*
Vice President, Orthopedic Service Line,
Northshore LIJ Health System; Director, ISK
Institute, New York, New York

FELASFA M. WODAJO, MD - *Musculoskeletal
Oncology*
Assistant Professor, Orthopedic Surgery,
Georgetown University Hospital, VCU School
of Medicine, Inova Campus, Virginia

AUTHORS

JOSEPH A. ABBOUD, MD
Rothman Institute, Thomas Jefferson
University, Philadelphia, Pennsylvania

REID A. ABRAMS, MD
Chief, Division of Hand and Microvascular
Surgery, Vice Chair, Department of Orthopedic
Surgery, Professor of Clinical Orthopedic
Surgery, Professor of Clinical Surgery,
University of California, San Diego School of
Medicine, San Diego, California

ABDO BACHOURA, MD
Research Fellow, The Philadelphia Hand
Center, Thomas Jefferson University Hospital,
Philadelphia, Pennsylvania

KEITH BALDWIN, MD, MPH, MSPT
Assistant Professor, Department of Orthopedic
Surgery, Hospital of the University of
Pennsylvania, Philadelphia, Pennsylvania

**SAMIK BANERJEE, MS (Orth), MRCS
(Glasg)**
Center for Joint Preservation and
Replacement, Rubin Institute for Advanced
Orthopedics; Department of Orthopaedic
Surgery, Sinai Hospital of Baltimore, Baltimore,
Maryland

TRACEY P. BASTROM, MA
Clinical Research Program Manager,
Orthopedic Research Department, Rady
Children's Hospital, San Diego, California

JEAN-CLAUDE G. D'ALLEYRAND, MD
Department of Orthopaedics, Walter Reed
National Military Medical Center, Bethesda;
Department of Orthopaedics, R Adams Cowley
Shock Trauma Center, University of Maryland
School of Medicine, Baltimore, Maryland

JESSE DASHE, MD
Resident Physician, University of California, San Diego, California

ERIC W. EDMONDS, MD
Director 360 Sports Medicine, Assistant Clinical Professor, Department of Orthopedics, Pediatric Orthopedic and Scoliosis Center, Rady Children's Hospital San Diego, University of California, San Diego, California

ORRIN I. FRANKO, MD
University of California San Diego School of Medicine, San Diego, California

VICTORIA GORDON, BA
Rothman Institute, Thomas Jefferson University, Philadelphia, Pennsylvania

JUSTIN M. HALLER, MD
Resident, Department of Orthopaedics, University of Utah, Salt Lake City, Utah

TIMOTHY E. HEWETT, PhD, FACSM
Director, Professor, The Sports Health and Performance Institute, The Ohio State University; Human Performance Lab, Division of Sports Medicine, Sports Medicine Biodynamics Center, Cincinnati Children's Hospital Medical Center, Cincinnati, Ohio; Department of Physiology and Cell Biology; Department of Orthopaedic Surgery; Department of Family Medicine; Department of Biomedical Engineering, The Ohio State University, Columbus, Ohio

JOHN G. HORNEFF, MD
Resident, Department of Orthopedic Surgery, Hospital of the University of Pennsylvania, Philadelphia, Pennsylvania

KIMONA ISSA, MD
Center for Joint Preservation and Replacement, Rubin Institute for Advanced Orthopedics; Department of Orthopaedic Surgery, Sinai Hospital of Baltimore, Baltimore, Maryland

PETER S. JOHNSTON, MD
Southern Maryland Orthopaedic and Sports Medicine, Leonardtown, Maryland

CHRISTOPHER H. JUDSON, MD
Orthopaedic Surgery Resident, Department of Orthopaedic Surgery, University of Connecticut Health Center, Farmington, Connecticut

ATUL F. KAMATH, MD
Fellow, Department of Orthopedic Surgery, Mayo Clinic, Rochester, Minnesota

BHAVEEN H. KAPADIA, MD
Center for Joint Preservation and Replacement, Rubin Institute for Advanced Orthopedics; Department of Orthopaedic Surgery, Sinai Hospital of Baltimore, Baltimore, Maryland

MARY ANN KEENAN, MD
Professor, Department of Orthopedic Surgery, Hospital of the University of Pennsylvania, Philadelphia, Pennsylvania

HARPAL S. KHANUJA, MD
Center for Joint Preservation and Replacement, Rubin Institute for Advanced Orthopedics; Department of Orthopaedic Surgery, Sinai Hospital of Baltimore, Baltimore, Maryland

MATTHEW J. KRAEUTLER, BS
Rothman Institute, Thomas Jefferson University, Philadelphia, Pennsylvania

ERIK N. KUBIAK, MD
Associate Professor, Department of Orthopaedics, University of Utah, Salt Lake City, Utah

DOMINIQUE LARON, MD
Resident, Department of Orthopedic Surgery, Children's Hospital and Research Center Oakland, University of California San Francisco, Oakland, California

DAVID G. LEWALLEN, MD
Professor, Department of Orthopedic Surgery, Mayo Clinic, Rochester, Minnesota

ROONGSAK LIMTHONGTHANG, MD
Clinical Instructor, Department of Orthopaedic Surgery, Faculty of Medicine Siriraj Hospital, Mahidol University, Bangkoknoi District, Bangkok, Thailand

TRAVIS H. MATHENEY, MD
Assistant Professor, Department of Orthopaedic Surgery, Boston Children's Hospital, Boston, Massachusetts

JOSEPH MCCARTHY, MD
Vice Chairman, Department of Orthopedic
Surgery, Massachusetts General Hospital,
Boston; Director, Kaplan Joint Replacement
Center, Newton Wellesley Hospital, Newton,
Massachusetts

SEAN MC MILLAN, DO
Chief of Orthopedics, Our Lady of Lourdes
Burlington Campus; Director of Orthopedic
Sports Medicine, Burlington, New Jersey

MICHAEL A. MONT, MD
Center for Joint Preservation and
Replacement, Rubin Institute for Advanced
Orthopedics; Department of Orthopaedic
Surgery, Sinai Hospital of Baltimore, Baltimore,
Maryland

GREGORY D. MYER, PhD, CSCS, FACSM
Director, Research and Human Performance
Lab, Division of Sports Medicine, Cincinnati
Children's Hospital Medical Center;
Department of Pediatrics and Orthopaedic
Surgery, University of Cincinnati College of
Medicine; Athletic Training Division, School of
Health and Rehabilitation Sciences, The Ohio
State University, Columbus, Ohio

SURENA NAMDARI, MD, MSc
Assistant Professor, Thomas Jefferson
University Hospital, Rothman Institute,
Philadelphia, Pennsylvania

A. LEE OSTERMAN, MD
Professor, The Philadelphia Hand Center,
Thomas Jefferson University Hospital,
Philadelphia, Pennsylvania

ROBERT V. O'TOOLE, MD
Associate Professor, Department of
Orthopaedics, R Adams Cowley Shock Trauma
Center, University of Maryland School of
Medicine, Baltimore, Maryland

NIRAV K. PANDYA, MD
Assistant Professor, Department of Orthopedic
Surgery, University of California San Francisco,
Oakland, California

MARK V. PATERNO, PT, PhD, SCS, ATC
Associate Professor, Division of Sports
Medicine, Sports Medicine Biodynamics
Center, Cincinnati Children's Hospital Medical
Center; Department of Pediatrics, University of

Cincinnati College of Medicine; Acting
Scientific Director, Division of Occupational
Therapy and Physical Therapy, Cincinnati
Children's Hospital Medical Center, Cincinnati,
Ohio

E. SCOTT PAXTON, MD
Rothman Institute, Thomas Jefferson
University, Philadelphia, Pennsylvania

MARC J. PHILIPPON, MD
The Steadman Philippon Research Institute,
Center for Outcomes-Based Orthopaedic
Research, Vail, Colorado

ROBERT PIVEC, MD
Center for Joint Preservation and
Replacement, Rubin Institute for Advanced
Orthopedics, Sinai Hospital of Baltimore,
Baltimore, Maryland

MICHAEL Q. POTTER, MD
Resident, Department of Orthopaedics,
University of Utah, Salt Lake City, Utah

HERNAN PRIETO, MD
Fellow, Department of Orthopedic Surgery,
Mayo Clinic, Rochester, Minnesota

SAQIB REHMAN, MD
Director of Orthopaedic Trauma, Associate
Professor of Orthopaedic Surgery, Department
of Orthopaedic Surgery and Sports Medicine,
School of Medicine, Temple University
Hospital, Temple University, Philadelphia,
Pennsylvania

JOANNA H. ROOCROFT, MA
Research Associate, Orthopedic Research
Department, Rady Children's Hospital,
San Diego, California

WUDBHAV N. SANKAR, MD
Assistant Professor, Division of Orthopaedic
Surgery, The Children's Hospital of
Philadelphia, Philadelphia, Pennsylvania

ROBERT L. SATCHER Jr, MD, PhD
Department of Orthopaedic Oncology, MD
Anderson Cancer Center, Houston, Texas

RACHEL J. SHAKKED, MD
Resident, Department of Orthopaedic Surgery,
NYU Hospital for Joint Diseases, New York,
New York

JACK G. SKENDZEL, MD
The Steadman Philippon Research Institute,
Center for Outcomes-Based Orthopaedic
Research, Vail, Colorado

PANUPAN SONGCHAROEN, MD
Professor, Department of Orthopaedic
Surgery, Faculty of Medicine Siriraj Hospital,
Mahidol University, Bangkoknoi District,
Bangkok, Thailand

JEFFERY A. TAYLOR-HAAS, PT, DPT, OCS, CSCS
Coordinator of Orthopaedic and Sports
Physical Therapy, Division of Occupational
Therapy and Physical Therapy, Cincinnati
Children's Hospital Medical Center; Human
Performance Lab, Division of Sports Medicine,
Sports Medicine Biodynamics Center,
Cincinnati Children's Hospital Medical Center,
Cincinnati, Ohio

NIRMAL C. TEJWANI, MD
Professor, Department of Orthopaedics,
New York University Medical Center,
New York, New York

MIHIR M. THACKER, MD
Department of Orthopedic Surgery,
Nemours - Alfred I duPont Hospital for
Children, Wilmington, Delaware; Assistant
Professor of Orthopedic Surgery, Thomas
Jefferson University, Philadelphia

RICK TOSTI, MD
Resident, Department of Orthopaedic Surgery
and Sports Medicine, School of Medicine,
Temple University, Philadelphia, Pennsylvania

GERALD R. WILLIAMS, MD
Rothman Institute, Thomas Jefferson
University, Philadelphia, Pennsylvania

JENNIFER MORIATIS WOLF, MD
Associate Professor, Department of
Orthopaedic Surgery, University of
Connecticut Health Center, Farmington,
Connecticut

IRA ZALTZ, MD
Clinical Associate Professor, Department of
Orthopaedic Surgery, William Beaumont
Hospital, Royal Oaks, Michigan

Contents

Adult Reconstruction

Trauma

This article summarizes the evolution of literature and practice related to fracture care in polytrauma patients. Particular emphasis is given to the management of femoral shaft fractures and the concept of damage control in these complex patients. The application of these guidelines in common clinical practice is also discussed.

Orthopedic surgeons frequently provide weight-bearing recommendations to guide patient recovery following lower extremity fractures. This article discusses the available literature regarding the effects of early weight bearing on fracture healing, patient compliance with weight bearing restrictions, and the effect of different weight bearing protocols following acetabular, tibial plateau, tibial plafond, ankle, and calcaneus fractures.

Talus fractures result from high-energy mechanisms and usually occur at the neck. Functional outcome after talar neck fracture worsens with increasing Hawkins grade. The mainstay of treatment for talar neck fractures is anatomic reduction and internal fixation. Prompt reduction of dislocations should be performed. Patients should be taken to the operating room as soon as stabilized. Dual incisions and a combination of minifragment plates and screws should be used. Talar body fractures have a high rate of ankle and subtalar arthritis. Lateral process fractures are frequently missed on radiographs. Complications after talus fractures include osteonecrosis, malunion, post-traumatic arthritis, and infection.

This article discusses contemporary management strategies for gunshot-related fractures with special attention paid to the initial evaluation, role of debridement, principles of fixation, need and duration of antibiotic therapy, and management of sequelae. Pertinent sequelae detailed are fractures associated with vascular injury, compartment syndrome, massive loss of soft tissue and bone, nerve injury, and lead toxicity.

Pediatrics

Upper Extremity

recovery and surgery may be needed. Detailed preoperative evaluation is recommended for localization of the lesions. The treatment of upper arm type injury comprises restoration of elbow flexion and shoulder control. Good functional results may be achieved after multiple nerve transfers. The treatment of total arm type includes hand function reconstruction, in addition to shoulder and elbow treatment. Current options for hand function reconstruction include functioning free muscle transfers and nerve transfers.

Musculoskeletal Oncology

ORTHOPEDIC CLINICS OF NORTH AMERICA

FORTHCOMING ISSUES

Beginning with the July 2013 issue, *Orthopedic Clinics of North America* will appear in this new format. Rather than focusing on a single topic, each issue will contain articles on key areas in orthopedics—adult reconstruction, upper extremity, trauma, paediatrics and oncology. Articles on sports medicine and foot and ankle will also be included on a regular basis. As the practice of orthopedics has become more specialized, the format of one topic per issue is no longer fulfilling our readers' needs. The new format is intended to address these changing needs.

Orthopedic Clinics of North America will continue to publish a print issue four times a year, in January, April, July, and October. However, it will also include online-only articles that will be published on a rolling basis (not in accordance with our quarterly publication dates). These articles, along with articles from our print issues, will be available on http://www.orthopedic.theclinics.com/.

RECENT ISSUES

April 2013
Osteoporosis and Fragility Fractures
Jason A. Lowe, and Gary E. Friedlaender, *Editors*

January 2013
Emerging Concepts in Upper Extremity Trauma
Michael P. Leslie, and Seth D. Dodds, *Editors*

DOWNLOAD Free App!

Review Articles
THE CLINICS

YOUR iPhone and iPad

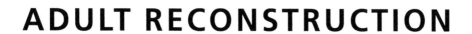

ADULT RECONSTRUCTION

Preface
Adult Reconstruction

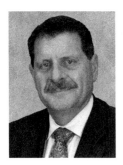

Giles R. Scuderi, MD
Editor

Recent advances in imaging and surgical techniques have led to an increased awareness of pathologic conditions around the hip joint affecting active patients. Conditions, such as labral tears, femoral acetabular impingement, dysplasia, osteoarthritis, and osteonecrosis, can cause significant disability, limiting not only participation in recreational activities but also all activities of daily living. The following articles focus on the management of such pathologic conditions affecting the hip that can impact this young patient population. It will become obvious that a successful outcome in treating these patients will be dependent on an accurate diagnosis with appropriate examination and imaging in order to formulate a thoughtful approach.

Hip arthroscopy has been an evolving procedure attracting a great deal of attention with recent advances in surgical techniques, such as repair of labral tears as opposed to debridement. Joint preservation procedures are admirable and often beneficial, but anomalies of the hip joint with associated dysplasia can alter hip kinematics, leading to premature development of hip osteoarthritis. As the osteoarthritis advances, total hip arthroplasty may be indicated with the intent to relieve the pain in these young active patients with a durable and predictable prosthesis. In an effort to increase the longevity of the prosthesis, alternate bearing surfaces, such as metal on metal, metal on ceramic, and metal on highly crosslinked polyethylene, have been introduced but the advantages and disadvantages of each device must be carefully considered.

It is my expectation that the following articles will address the above-mentioned issues and provide the insight into the accurate diagnosis and selection of an appropriate treatment plan.

Giles R. Scuderi, MD
Orthopedic Service Line
Northshore LIJ Health System
New York, NY, USA

ISK Institute
New York, NY, USA

E-mail address:
gscuderi@nshs.edu

Orthop Clin N Am 44 (2013) xiii
http://dx.doi.org/10.1016/j.ocl.2013.07.008
0030-5898/13/$ – see front matter © 2013 Published by Elsevier Inc.

Alternative Bearings in Total Hip Arthroplasty in the Young Patient

Atul F. Kamath, MD, Hernan Prieto, MD,
David G. Lewallen, MD*

KEYWORDS

- Total hip arthroplasty (replacement) • Alternative bearings • Young patient • Implant wear
- Ceramic • Metal on metal • Highly cross-linked polyethylene

KEY POINTS

- With modern implants, surgical technique, and cementless fixation methods, the durability of total hip arthroplasty may now be related to the wear properties of the bearing surfaces.
- Alternative bearing surfaces may offer a solution to the wear-associated problems that have limited traditional total hip articulations.
- Bearing alternatives to traditional metal-on-polyethylene couples include metal/ceramic on highly cross-linked polyethylene, ceramic on ceramic, metal on metal, and ceramic on metal.
- Articulation choice must be evaluated in terms of the advantages and disadvantages (risks) associated with each bearing couple.
- Metal-on-metal bearings must be used with caution given the evolving understanding of local adverse responses to metal particulate debris.
- Further study in large cohorts of patients with greater follow-up will clarify the usefulness and durability of alternative bearings in total hip arthroplasty in young patients.

INTRODUCTION

Several causes may lead to advanced hip arthritis in the young patient. These causes include avascular necrosis, juvenile idiopathic arthritis, prior infection, slipped capital femoral epiphysis, fracture, Legg-Calves-Perthes disease, developmental dysplasia, and femoroacetabular impingement. The common pathway of severe destructive changes within the hip joint may cause disabling symptoms in the young. For advanced hip arthritis, and when medical management and nonoperative strategies fail, total hip arthroplasty (THA) may be performed in this patient population for pain relief and to improve function.

The demands placed on the hip in the young patient, including activity level and repetitive loading, have led to accelerated failure of THA.[1] Increased loading cycles and higher activity[2] over an increased lifespan, rather than time from prosthetic implantation alone, leads to early implant failure in highly active individuals. The historically high failure rates[3] and poor longevity[4,5] may dissuade surgeons from offering THA as a treatment option to

Funding Sources: Institutional research support from DePuy, Smith & Nephew, Stryker, Wright Medical, Zimmer (D.G. Lewallen); nil (A.F. Kamath and H. Prieto).
Conflict of Interest: Royalties from Zimmer and consultant for Osteotech, Orthosonics, and Zimmer (D.G. Lewallen); nil (A.F. Kamath and H. Prieto).
Department of Orthopedic Surgery, Mayo Clinic, 200 First Street Southwest, Gonda 14, Rochester, MN 55905, USA
* Corresponding author.
E-mail address: lewallen.david@mayo.edu

Orthop Clin N Am 44 (2013) 451–462
http://dx.doi.org/10.1016/j.ocl.2013.06.001
0030-5898/13/$ – see front matter © 2013 Elsevier Inc. All rights reserved.

this young population. In light of these results in young patients, THA has traditionally been reserved for selected patients in whom alternative management strategies have failed.

Improvements in prosthetic design and cementless fixation methods have addressed many of the previous limitations in performing joint replacements in young patients.[6] Along with advances in operative techniques, instrumentation, and patient selection, THA is now a more favorable reconstructive option in active and young patients.[7–10] Early reports of primary uncemented THA showed adequate survivorship using first-generation implants,[11] and survival rates as high as 99% after 10 years have been reported in patients less than 50 years old using second-generation designs.[12] In the ultrayoung patient, THA has proved successful in series of early-term and midterm follow-up,[13,14] including those specifically studying the use of alternative bearings in cementless THA.[15]

Pooled femoral mechanical rates in a meta-analysis of cementless THA (mean age, 41.4 years) and hip resurfacing arthroplasty (mean age, 46.6 years) were 1.3% at a mean follow-up of 8.4 years after THA and a 2.6% rate of failure at a mean of 3.9 years after resurfacing.[16] Modern-generation cementless femoral fixation has proved dependable across multiple designs. On the acetabular side, cementless cup fixation has shown similar results, including a recent study of 9584 primary THAs implanted from 1984 to 2004[17]: no cases of aseptic loosening were seen with more recent three-dimensional highly porous metal surfaces.

With advances in fixation on the acetabular and femoral sides, the limiting factor in durability of joint replacements over the past 2 decades has been bearing surface wear. With the success of THA and its applications to the young, it is estimated that, by 2030, patients less than 65 years old will comprise 52% of primary THAs.[18] The demand in patients aged 45 to 54 years for primary THA in 2030 is projected to be nearly 6 times higher than in 2006. Alternative bearing surfaces may offer a solution to the wear-associated problems that have limited traditional total hip articulations. These new surfaces provide attractive tribologic solutions for the young patient with hip pain and advanced arthritis.

ALTERNATIVE BEARING OPTIONS

There is ongoing debate regarding the optimal bearing surface in young patients. Poor THA survivorship in young patients has been attributed to cemented fixation strategies, screw-in acetabular designs, and the wear properties of conventional polyethylene (PE). The osteolysis seen with conventional ultrahigh-molecular-weight PE wear in the active young patient has prompted the resurgence of alternative bearing surfaces. From the National Inpatient Sample database, 39% of primary THA in 2005 to 2006 had a unique modifier for the bearing surface.[19]

Bearing alternatives to traditional metal-on-conventional-PE couples include metal or ceramic heads on highly cross-linked PE, ceramic on ceramic (CoC), metal on metal (MoM), and ceramic on metal (CoM). Each of these bearing couples provides improved wear properties compared with metal on conventional PE (**Table 1**).[20] The Global Orthopedic Registry (GLORY),[21] incorporating 100 hospitals in 13 countries, provided a breakdown on the choice of bearing surfaces: conventional PE, 36%; highly cross-linked PE, 55%; MoM, 5%; and CoC, 4%. In the United States, 63% of primary THA received cross-linked PE, and 28% received conventional PE.

Highly Cross-linked Polyethylene

Mechanical loosening accounted for 19.7% of all revision THA in a 2005 to 2006 national sample.[19] Introduced in the late 1990s, the several processes of cross-linking PE seem to offer a promising answer to the issue of wear.[22] Articulations involving PE provide a less radical departure from traditional hard-on-soft bearing options. Furthermore, wear rates may be less sensitive to femoral head size or small changes in component positioning with highly cross-linked PE.[23–25]

In contrast with previous attempts to improve PE that have resulted in poor clinical results,[26] the lower wear rates with highly cross-linked PE in vivo at 10 years should theoretically lead to less osteolysis in the long term.[27] With these improvements, highly cross-linked PE has emerged as a viable choice for most patients having THA

Table 1 Wear rates according to bearing couple	
Bearing Articulation Materials	**Wear Rate (µm/y)**
Metal on conventional polyethylene	120–200
Ceramic on conventional polyethylene	80–100
Metal on highly cross-lined polyethylene	0–25
MoM	1–5
CoM	~1
CoC	<1

and may be used with either metal or ceramic head combinations. When cross-linked PE liners are used, surgeons have a wide array of intraoperative choices with regard to head size, orientation of elevation, and offset (eg, standard or lateral offset). As cost constraints emerge, it should be recognized that PE bearings are currently less expensive than comparable ceramic or metal bearings and will almost certainly remain so.

However, cross-linking leads to changes in other material properties besides wear, such as lower yield strength and ultimate tensile strength. There is also lower impact strength, elongation to failure, and resistance to crack propagation. Most of the property alterations are small to moderate, but must be carefully evaluated in light of their use in high-demand, young patients. Next-generation techniques to improve cross-linked PE have focused on improving wear resistance with less effect on the mechanical properties associated with postirradiation melting. Production of highly cross-linked PE uses methods to extinguish free radicals, such as vitamin E doping[28] or sequential application of radiation, with annealing after each dose.[29]

CoC

Ceramic-on-ceramic articulations were developed in the 1970s in Europe.[30] In the United States, Food and Drug Administration approval was granted in 2003. Ceramic-ceramic bearing surfaces provide several benefits with regard to wear reduction in vitro and in vivo,[31,32] making it a reasonable bearing surface in a young patient population. The hardness and resistance to third-body wear allows a low surface roughness over time. This low surface roughness, along with small grain size, creates a low coefficient of friction. Moreover, ceramics have excellent wettability, which leads to a reduction in adhesive wear and better lubrication properties.[33]

The wear rate of ceramic bearing surfaces can be 4000 times less than the traditional metal-on-PE bearing surfaces.[34] The wear debris from ceramic bearing surfaces is also well tolerated, and alumina particles are bioinert compared with metal and PE debris.[35] These decreased wear rates have correlated with lower amounts of osteolysis and better preservation of bone stock, which is an important consideration when performing THA in young patients with long life expectancy and the potential need for future revision surgery. The evolution of ceramic bearings continues with the use of Biolox Delta (CeramTec AG), an alumina matrix composite. Encouraging early results have been reported.[36]

MoM

MoM bearings have been in use for more than 6 decades and their use was first published more than 30 years ago.[37] Problems with early MoM designs included poor manufacturing tolerances and material selection, early impingement, and inadequate clearance. Next-generation MoM implants benefited from improved manufacturing methods and tolerances, which resulted in low wear rates in vitro.[38] A large European clinical experience, along with the ability to use large head sizes to reduce dislocation risk, made MoM implants an attractive option for the young, high-activity patient. In 2010, the National Joint Registry for England and Wales reported that 14% of patients less than 55 years old having hip arthroplasty underwent resurfacing procedures alone.[39] Advantages compared with other hard bearings include no head/liner fracture risk as with ceramics, and that scratches to the metal surfaces could self-heal. Recent concerns include adverse tissue reactions to metal debris generated by some surface replacement and MoM THA articulations, and corrosion at the head-neck junction of some MoM THA systems with large heads.

CoM

Ceramic-metal articulations were designed as another hard-on-hard bearing alternative. Several in vitro, as well as clinical, studies[40,41] have sought to explore the clinical usefulness and wear characteristics of this bearing couple. MacDonald and colleagues[42] reported on similar metal ion levels between CoM and MoM articulations in vivo.

CLINICAL DATA
Highly Cross-linked Polyethylene

Highly cross-linked PE has shown a substantial reduction in wear compared with conventional PE.[43] Reduction in wear of 85% to 90% has been seen with 28-mm and 32-mm femoral heads, respectively.[44] In a randomized study, Thomas and colleagues[45] reported that no patient with a highly cross-linked PE liner had a wear rate greater than the osteolysis threshold (0.1 mm/y). In the conventional PE study arm, 9% of patients went beyond this threshold.

D'Antonio and colleagues[46] found a 58% reduction in wear with second-generation, sequentially annealed, highly cross-linked PE compared with first-generation, annealed, highly cross-linked PE. No osteolysis was reported, and cup inclination did not affect linear wear. Although volumetric wear may be slightly higher with large femoral heads on cross-linked PE, there does not seem to be a difference in linear wear rates.[23,24] Compared with conventional PE, cross-linked PE has shown significantly lower wear rates against smooth and scratched surfaces.[47,48]

Ceramic on highly cross-linked polyethylene

Rajaee and colleagues[49] reported that the use of metal on PE increased from 21.6% patients in 2006 to 25.2% in 2009, whereas ceramic on PE (CoP) increased from 13.5% in 2007 to 25.7% in 2009. This trend may be explained by surgeons' attempts to minimize complications associated with hard-on-hard bearings. The increase in CoP bearings is likely related to a steady-state wear rate 40% lower than that of metal on PE.[50]

Studies of ceramic on conventional PE are mixed. Migaud and colleagues[51] reported a 46% rate of osteolysis. In contrast with this, Urban and colleagues[52] found no osteolysis about the femoral or the acetabular components after 18 years of follow-up, with mean linear wear rates between 0.03 and 0.1 mm/y. Data regarding ceramic heads against highly cross-linked PE are limited by short-term follow-up.[53] Garvin and colleagues,[54] in a 2-year follow-up study of CoP (oxidized zirconium femoral head with a highly cross-linked PE acetabular liner), reported that true linear wear was 4 μm per year, which corresponds with one of the lowest reports of in vivo wear in the literature.

CoC

Ceramics have had a long and successful history in Europe, with evidence of low clinical wear and osteolysis.[8–10] In a 2011 systematic review, Zywiel and colleagues[55] found that the 4 level I studies of CoC THA reported survival from 96% at 8 years up to 100% at a mean of 51 months. In a prospective multicenter study, 1709 alumina ceramic hips were reviewed and no cases of osteolysis were reported.[52] Other comparative studies report 1.7% of osteolysis in the CoC group versus 19.4% of the metal-on-PE group.[46] After 2 to 9 years of follow-up in 194 alumina THAs (average age, 49 years), Murphy and colleagues[56] reported that no patients had osteolysis, and survivorship at 9 years was 96%. For those hips without prior surgery, the survivorship was 99.3%. Lee and colleagues[31] reported 99% survivorship at 10 years in a group of patients with a mean age of 41 years. D'Antonio and colleagues[57] compared average 5-year follow-up data for CoC and metal-on-PE (328 total hips): the revision rates were 2.7% (CoC) and 7.5% (metal-on-PE) with no ceramic fractures. The rate of osteolysis was 1.4% for CoC and 14% for metal-on-PE. D'Antonio and colleagues[46] later presented that the 10-year

survivorship of CoC implants was significantly higher than that of the metal-on-PE implants (95.9% and 91.3%, respectively; $P = .0122$) and the 8-year rate of survivorship of the Trident implants (another ceramic group study) was 97.7%. Similar results have been seen in other reports.[47,52]

Survivorship analysis in a series from the Mayo Clinic showed promising short-term to midterm results (average follow-up 50 months) using CoC bearing surfaces in young patients (mean age, 16.4 years), with a 96% survival rate in 24 uncemented THAs.[58] Nikolaou and colleagues[59] presented the 5-year results of a randomized controlled trial comparing the clinical and radiological outcomes of 102 THAs in patients less than 65 years of age. The three arms were CoC, metal on conventional PE, and metal on highly cross-linked PE. Two hips had been revised, one for infection and one for periprosthetic fracture. At the final follow-up there were no significant differences between the groups for the mean Western Ontario and McMaster Universities osteoarthritis index, Short Form-12, or Harris hip scores. Radiological outcomes revealed no significant wear in the ceramic group. However, comparison of standard and highly cross-linked PE revealed an almost 3-fold difference in the mean annual linear wear rates (0.151 mm/y vs 0.059 mm/y, respectively; $P < .001$).

MoM

There are positive long-term studies on the clinical outcomes of MoM hip arthroplasty in young active patients,[60] and 84.4% survival at 20-year follow-up.[61] In a 2011 systematic review, Zywiel and colleagues[55] reported on the 4 level I or II second-generation stemmed MoM THA studies. These studies showed a 96% to 100% mean survival at 38 to 60 months' follow-up. The 2 level I hip resurfacing studies reported 94% and 98% mean survival at 56 and 33 months.

However, several meta-analysis and systematic reviews show no significant difference between MoM and conventional THA with regard to functional outcomes, as measured by Harris hip scores, and radiographic outcomes.[36,37] Patients with MoM THA showed up to a nearly 4 times greater complication rate in those series. Milosev and colleagues[62] presented survivorships of 69 MoM THAs (mean age, 60 years), 200 metal-on-PE THAs (mean age, 71 years), and 218 CoC THAs (mean age, 60 years). Survival at 10 years with regard to revision for any reason was 0.984, 0.956, and 0.879 for the metal-on-PE, CoC, and MoM groups, respectively. The survival for MoM articulations was significantly worse compared with that for metal on PE. With revision for aseptic loosening as an end point, survival at 10 years was 0.995, 0.990, and 0.894 for the metal-on-PE, CoC, and MoM groups, respectively. Again, with this end point, MoM survival was significantly worse than that for either the CoC or metal-on-PE groups.

CoM

Isaac and colleagues[41] found significantly lower chromium levels in CoM hips compared with MoM hips. Cobalt levels were lower, but the difference was not statistically significant. Explanted CoM components were tested in a wear simulator. The investigators reported that the CoM components showed higher bedding-in but then similar wear rates (although an order of magnitude less) than those of other studies testing MoM bearings. The clinical outliers were related to component malposition. In a double-blinded randomized controlled trial, Schouten and colleagues[40] compared CoM and MoM couplings. They found an equivalent increase in serum metal ion levels. The functional outcome scores up to 1 year after surgery were similar.

Ceramicized Metal on Polyethylene

Oxinium has been introduced as a means of having the low wear characteristics of a ceramic head, but without the risk of fracture. The clinical data that are currently available do not suggest decreased cross-linked PE wear with the use of an Oxinium head compared with a cobalt-chrome head.[63]

Bourne and colleagues[64] found that Oxinium femoral heads reduced wear even in clinically relevant roughened conditions. However, there is also conflicting evidence that surface damage of ceramicized femoral heads could accelerate wear.[65]

Registry Data

In the 2012 National Joint Replacement Registry (NJRR) Report, the Australian Orthopaedic Association presented 6 bearing surfaces with 11-year cumulative revision data: metal and ceramic on both nonmodified (conventional) and modified (cross-linked or vitamin E impregnated) PE, MoM, and CoC.[66] The report also included ceramicized metal on modified PE, with a follow-up of 8 years. The MoM articulation had the highest cumulative revision rate: at 11 years, revision for loosening/osteolysis (4.2%), metal sensitivity (3.8%), and infection (1.8%) were all greater than those rates for metal on PE (2.2%, 0%, and 0.7%, respectively). MoM articulations with head sizes greater than or equal to 36 mm had higher revision rates

than those with head sizes less than or equal to 32 mm. Patients less than 65 years of age with a head size greater than 32 mm had a higher rate of revision than patients 65 years or older with smaller head sizes. Modified PE had a lower rate of revision (5.1%) than nonmodified PE (9.1%), with a difference beginning at 6 months; no difference in revision rate with regard to head size was seen within the modified PE subgroup. For the first time, the registry was able to detect this lower rate of revision for all 3 combinations (ceramic, metal, and ceramicized metal on modified PE) versus nonmodified PE groups. The group with ceramicized metal on modified PE had the lowest revision rate; however, this bearing group had limited patient numbers. Also recorded in the registry were 300 ceramic head/metal bearing couples and 391 metal head/ceramic bearings. The metal head/ceramic bearing articulation had a higher rate of revision (at 5 years, 7.1% cumulate revision) compared with most other bearings, whereas the ceramic head/metal bearing revision rate (4.0% cumulative revision at 3 years) did not seem to be markedly different from other bearing couples.

The Australian Orthopaedic Association NJRR first identified an increased revision rate with regard to MoM prostheses in 2008, when the prostheses were used in conventional hip replacement.[67] A relationship to larger femoral head sizes was reported in 2009[68] and, more comprehensively, in 2010.[69] In the aggregate, larger MoM femoral heads were associated with more than 2 times the rate of revision as that associated with smaller MoM femoral heads (a revision rate of 4.5% for head sizes of ≤32 mm vs a revision rate of 9.4% for sizes of >32 mm). Although the revision rate attributed to dislocation was lower for larger femoral head sizes, the revision rate attributed to loosening, infection, and metal sensitivity was higher for larger sizes.

The 2012 Annual Report of the National Joint Registry for England and Wales highlighted the further decline of the use of stemmed MoM implants. From a peak of 9000 procedures in 2008 (an increase in use attributable to larger diameter heads, of 36 mm and larger), a progressive yearly decline was seen up until the latest data in the 2012 report. Revisions for aseptic loosening and pain (the most common reasons for revision of stemmed MoM prostheses in both men and women) were significantly higher in patients with MoM. A woman aged 60 years had a 5-year revision rate for an uncemented 46-mm MoM prosthesis of 6.1% compared with a revision rate of 1.6% for a hybrid 28-mm metal-on-PE articulation. Hip resurfacing resulted in similar implant survivorship to other surgical options only in men with large femoral heads; inferior implant survivorship was seen in other patient subgroups, particularly women.[70]

The themes of higher failure rates with large-head MoM prostheses, as well as higher failure rates in women with large-head MoM prostheses, had been shown previously in both the National Joint Registry for England and Wales[71] and the New Zealand Joint Registry[72]: at 5 years, the rate of revision of large femoral head MoM prostheses was at least twice that of all other cemented, hybrid, and conventional THAs. Women less than 55 years of age with large femoral head MoM prostheses had a higher rate of revision than older women with large femoral head MoM articulations.

COMPLICATIONS AND FAILURE MODES
Highly Cross-linked Polyethylene

Although highly cross-linked PE has shown encouraging results beyond a decade of clinical use, further long-term data are needed to assess bearing longevity and degree of clinically evident osteolysis. Furthermore, in vitro studies are needed to better understand PE wear mechanisms under more aggressive/realistic testing scenarios, such as scratched femoral heads and third-body abrasives.

The specific failure modes and material strength of PEs are manufacturer dependent, being caused by the degree of cross-linking, amount of free radical formation, method by which free radicals are quenched, and any treatments after cross-linking. The material's properties after cross-linking carry a risk of liner fracture,[73–75] and there is a risk of locking mechanism failure, especially with cup malposition. The minimum thickness for cross-linked liners is not known. Although there have been reports of catastrophic liner failure, it is unclear what contributions implant alignment and socket design may have had compared with the decreased mechanical properties of the material alone.

Adverse local tissue reactions can occur in patients with a metal-on-PE bearing secondary to corrosion at the modular femoral head-neck taper. The clinical presentation is similar to the adverse local tissue reactions seen in patients with MoM bearings.

CoC

Because of the brittleness of ceramics, there is a small risk of fracture. The risk of fracture with ceramic components has been reduced with modern technology and manufacturing quality, using smaller grain size, increased burst strength, and proof testing of each implant. From an estimated

fracture risk in 1974 of 1 in 300, the estimated fracture risk in 2000 was less than 1 in 2000 to 10,000. Fracture rates range from 0.005% to 0.02% for alumina bearing surfaces.[76] In a series of 500,000 femoral heads reported in 2000, Willmann[77] reported an estimated risk of 0.012%.

The cause of squeaking is unclear and likely multifactorial. The incidence of squeaking has generally been reported as between 2.7%[78] and 7%,[79] but higher incidences have been reported (up to 21%[80]). Squeaking may be related to ceramic-ceramic lubrication. Noise occurs when the fluid film between the two surfaces is disrupted, likely because of metal transfer, as shown by Trousdale and colleagues.[81] Edge loading can cause fluid film disruption, stripe wear, and an area of localized friction. The energy created through frictional forces may be transformed to a squeaking noise via vibration of the implant. Squeaking may be more commonly reported with certain designs, such as a TMZF femoral component with a V-40 neck diameter.[82] Wear debris generation may cause osteolysis, even in third-generation ceramic couples.[83]

Like other hard-hard bearings, ceramic components are sensitive to cup position. There is a risk of runaway wear with malposition and edge loading, and risks of impingement demand precise implantation of the prosthesis. Ceramics are also limited by reduced intraoperative flexibility related to cup size, neck lengths, and liner options. The failure modes associated with modular ceramic-metal junctions need to be better understood.

MoM

Several problems with MoM technology have manifested, and large registry cohorts, including the Australian NJRR, have identified higher failure rates with MoM articulations. Very high failure rates for certain prostheses, including the articular surface replacement,[84] have led to product withdrawal.

Toxicity from metal ions has raised concerns among surgeons, the public, and governmental agencies.[85,86] The constellation of findings, including metallosis, effusions/pseudotumor formation, and soft tissue damage (**Fig. 1**), has been termed adverse local tissue reactions.[87] On histologic analysis, aseptic lymphocytic vasculitis-associated lesions have been characterized as phenomena of MoM bearings.[88] The metallic wear debris and soft tissue responses may lead to early implant failure and soft tissue destruction, including damage of abductor musculature. Metal ions generated from metal-metal articulations may lead to increased serum ion concentrations

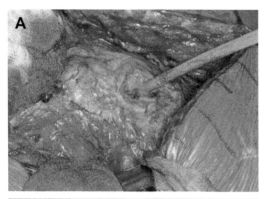

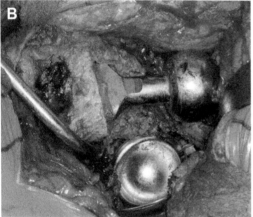

Fig. 1. (A, B) Soft tissue destruction, pseudotumor formation, and metallosis in a 60-year-old woman with persistent groin pain status post MoM THA.

of chromium and cobalt. The correlation between serum ion concentrations and bearing wear is being elucidated.[89,90] A study of 37 revised MoM hips, including resurfacing and THA across 5 implant manufacturers, included 65% women.[91] Ten of 37 patients had adverse tissue reaction. Studies measuring metal ion concentrations have found that patients receiving MoM articulations had significantly greater serum and urine metal ion concentrations compared with patients receiving conventional articulations.[92]

In addition to the head-cup articulation, another area of metal-metal ion generation is the femoral head-neck taper junction in modular femoral components. Tissue reactions can occur in patients with a metal-on-PE bearing secondary to corrosion at the trunnion or other modular parts of the femoral construct. A differential increase of serum cobalt levels with respect to chromium levels may inform a diagnosis of trunnionosis.[93]

MoM implants narrow the tolerances for successful THA. Cup malpositioning (eg, abduction angle greater than 55°), mismatch between femoral head size and neck trunnions, and particulars of

specific implant designs may all negatively contribute to the lubrication milieu, edge loading, and wear.[94,95] Deformation of the acetabular shell during insertion by edge impaction may also cause occult issues with MoM bearings. Femoral neck fracture is another complication unique to MoM bearings, particularly resurfacing arthroplasty. Like other hard-on-hard bearings, MoM bearings may cause audible mechanical symptoms like clicking and squeaking.

Close monitoring with radiographs and serum ion levels for MoM bearings should follow current recommendation guidelines.[96] For the painful arthroplasty, close examination, including advanced imaging studies, should be performed. Ultrasound is a useful screening method, but its sensitivity decreases with very obese patients and it is less effective than computed tomography or magnetic resonance imaging (MRI) at detection of medially located lesions. MRI has high sensitivity and is able to detect osteolysis.[97]

At present, MoM must be used with caution in young populations. Its use has declined markedly in the United States, with some centers still offering surface replacement to select patients, usually young men of large stature with high offset who challenge standard THA systems. Metal-metal THA has largely been abandoned in the United States. Although MoM wear characteristics are excellent, the full risks of metal hypersensitivity, extent and causes of local soft tissue destruction, and theoretic risks to other end-organ systems are still being elucidated.[98]

SUMMARY

THA has been well established in long-term studies in older patients as a reliable, reproducible, and durable treatment option for hip arthritis.[99,100] However, studies in younger patients have traditionally shown less promising results. The higher failure rate of THA in young patients has been attributed to high activity level and excessive demands on the prosthetic hip,[22] along with traditional techniques and cemented components.[21]

Emphasis on osseous integration and primary host fixation offers an attractive solution for long-term survivorship in the young.[39,40] Modern-generation uncemented THA has been shown to have an excellent outcome.[21,34–36] As surgical techniques are refined and advances are made in prosthetic component design and durability, THA offers an increasingly favorable option for the treatment of disabling hip arthritis. A key advance has been the introduction of modern acetabular and femoral arthroplasty components and alternative articulating bearing materials.

With a growing body of literature supporting cementless acetabular and femoral fixation in the young, improved bearing surfaces may offer the next key advancement. It now may be reasonable to ask whether alternative bearings can provide a long-term solution for the young and most active patients. Our preferred bearings according to particular age groups and activity level are shown in **Table 2**.

In interpreting the literature in the young, heterogeneity in underlying diagnosis, bearing surfaces used, and prior surgeries may confound results in small series. Moreover, the Harris hip score may not be an ideal scoring system for the adolescent patient undergoing THA[44] because of a ceiling effect. In contrast, certain subsets of young patients may not see dramatic improvements in Harris hip scores because of residual functional limitations from underlying, preoperative baseline functional status and systemic disease, and chronic/congenital compensatory mechanisms. For the ultrayoung, studies often do not stratify between middle-aged patients and those 30 years old or younger because of smaller numbers,[101–107] making it difficult to ascertain the clinical success of THA. More commonly, the combined results for THA across multiple age groups are reported, with a higher proportion of THAs performed in older patients.

The goal of bearing selection should be to optimize an already highly evolved and successful procedure,[108] considering that radically new designs or materials should not be introduced widely until validation via a stepwise process.[109] With the adoption of newer technologies, implants should be monitored via large arthroplasty registries, because registries provide important information that may not be captured through clinical trials or institutional series.

At early to intermediate follow-up, clinical and radiographic results are promising following modern, uncemented, alternative bearing THA in the young. Further study in large cohorts of patients with greater follow-up will clarify the usefulness and durability of alternative bearings in THA in young patients. Articulation choice must be evaluated in terms of the advantages and disadvantages (risks) associated with each bearing couple. Adequate patient preoperative education regarding the risks and benefits of each alternative bearing couple is essential. The cost of new technology should also be evaluated.[110] Although new implants are more costly, projections regarding cost savings with a theoretic reduction in future revision surgery should also be weighed. Alternative bearing materials offer hope for longevity of THA, but their clinical performance at the 15-year and 20-year time marks will determine the true usefulness. Based on the available evidence, metal or ceramic on highly cross-linked PE is used for most THAs in young patients at our institution.

REFERENCES

1. Puolakka TJ, Pajamaki KJ, Halonen PJ, et al. The Finnish Arthroplasty Register. Report of the hip register. Acta Orthop Scand 2001;72:433–41.
2. Schmalzried TP, Shepherd EF, Dorey FJ, et al. The John Charnley Award. Wear is a function of use, not time. Clin Orthop Relat Res 2000;(381):36–46.
3. Torchia ME, Klassen RA, Bianco AJ. Total hip arthroplasty with cement in patients less than twenty years old. Long-term results. J Bone Joint Surg Am 1996;78:995–1003.
4. Bessette BJ, Fassier F, Tanzer M, et al. Total hip arthroplasty in patients younger than 21 years: a minimum, 10-year follow-up. Can J Surg 2003;46:257–62.
5. Cage DJ, Granberry WM, Tullos HS. Long-term results of total arthroplasty in adolescents with debilitating polyarthropathy. Clin Orthop 1992;283:156–62.
6. Engh CA, Hopper RH Jr. Porous-coated total hip arthroplasty in the young. Orthopedics 1998;21(9):953–6.
7. Garino JP. Modern CoC total hip systems in the United States: early results. Clin Orthop 2000;379:41–7.
8. Hamadouche M, Boutin P, Daussange J, et al. Alumina-on-alumina total hip arthroplasty: a minimum 18.5-year follow-up study. J Bone Joint Surg Am 2002;84:69–77.

Table 2
Authors' preferred bearing selections based on age and patient characteristics

Age (y)	Bearing Couple Considerations
Ultrayoung (<30)	Consider ceramic-ceramic
30–60	Ceramic or metal on HCLPE
Small bones, young patient (40–55)	Ceramic-metal (off label)
>65	Metal on HCLPE
Selected elderly	Metal on polyethylene (cemented)

Abbreviation: HCLPE, highly cross-linked polyethylene.

9. Mittelmeier H, Heisel J. Sixteen-years' experience with ceramic hip prostheses. Clin Orthop 1992; 282:64–72.

10. Sedel L. Evolution of alumina-on-alumina implants: a review. Clin Orthop 2000;379:48–54.

11. Duffy GP, Berry DJ, Rowland C, et al. Primary uncemented total hip arthroplasty in patients <40 years old: 10- to 14-year results using first-generation proximally porous-coated implants. J Arthroplasty 2001;16(8 Suppl 1):140–4.

12. Kim YH, Oh SH, Kim JS. Primary total hip arthroplasty with a second-generation cementless total hip prosthesis in patients younger than fifty years of age. J Bone Joint Surg Am 2003;85(1):109–14.

13. Clohisy JC, Oryhon JM, Seyler TM, et al. Function and fixation of total hip arthroplasty in patients 25 years of age or younger. Clin Orthop Relat Res 2010;468:3207–13.

14. Restrepo C, Lettich T, Roberts N, et al. Uncemented total hip arthroplasty in patients less than twenty-years. Acta Orthop Belg 2008;74(5):615–22.

15. Kamath AF, Sheth NP, Hosalkar HH, et al. Modern total hip arthroplasty in patients younger than 21 years. J Arthroplasty 2012;27(3):402–8.

16. Springer BD, Connelly SE, Odum SM, et al. Cementless femoral components in young patients: review and meta-analysis of total hip arthroplasty and hip resurfacing. J Arthroplasty 2009; 24(Suppl 6):2–8.

17. Howard JL, Kremers HM, Loechler YA, et al. Comparative survival of uncemented acetabular components following primary total hip arthroplasty. J Bone Joint Surg Am 2011;93(17):1597–604.

18. Kurtz SM, Lau E, Ong K, et al. Future young patient demand for primary and revision joint replacement: national projections from 2010 to 2030. Clin Orthop Relat Res 2009;467(10):2606–12.

19. Bozic KJ, Kurtz S, Lau E, et al. The epidemiology of bearing surface usage in total hip arthroplasty in the United States. J Bone Joint Surg Am 2009; 91(7):1614–20.

20. Greenwald AS, Garino JP, American Academy of Orthopaedic Surgeons, Committee on Biomedical Engineering, American Academy of Orthopaedic Surgeons, Committee on Hip and Knee Arthritis. Alternative bearing surfaces: the good, the bad, and the ugly. J Bone Joint Surg Am 2001; 83(Suppl 2 Pt 2):68–72.

21. Anderson FA Jr. Overview of the GLOBAL orthopaedic registry (GLORY). Am J Orthop (Belle Mead NJ) 2010;39(Suppl 9):2–4.

22. Muratoglu OK, Bragdon CR, O'Connor DO, et al. A novel method of cross-linking ultra-high-molecular-weight polyethylene to improve wear, reduce oxidation, and retain mechanical properties. Recipient of the 1999 HAP Paul Award. J Arthroplasty 2001;16(2):149–60.

23. Hammerberg EM, Wan Z, Dastane M, et al. Wear and range of motion of different femoral head sizes. J Arthroplasty 2010;25(6):839–43.

24. Lachiewicz PF, Heckman DS, Soileau ES, et al. Femoral head size and wear of highly cross-linked polyethylene at 5 to 8 years. Clin Orthop Relat Res 2009;467(12):3290–6.

25. Muratoglu OK, Bragdon CR, O'Connor D, et al. Larger diameter femoral heads used in conjunction with a highly cross-linked ultrahigh molecular weight polyethylene: a new concept. J Arthroplasty 2001; 16(8 Suppl 1):24–30.

26. Livingston BJ, Chmell MJ, Spector M, et al. Complications of total hip arthroplasty associated with the use of an acetabular component with a Hylamer liner. J Bone Joint Surg Am 1997;79:1529–38.

27. Bragdon CR, Doerner M, Martell J, Multicenter Study Group. The 2012 John Charnley Award: clinical multicenter studies of the wear performance of highly crosslinked remelted polyethylene in THA. Clin Orthop Relat Res 2013;471(2):393–402.

28. Oral E, Wannomae KK, Hawkins N, et al. Alpha-tocopherol-doped irradiated UHMWPE for high fatigue resistance and low wear. Biomaterials 2004; 25:5515–22.

29. Dumbleton JH, D'Antonio JA, Manley MT, et al. The basis for a second-generation highly cross-linked UHMWPE. Clin Orthop Relat Res 2006;453:265–71.

30. Boutin P. Total arthroplasty of the hip by fritted aluminum prosthesis. Experimental study and 1st clinical applications. Rev Chir Orthop Reparatrice Appar Mot 1972;58(3):229–46.

31. Lee YK, Ha YC, Yoo JJ, et al. Alumina-on-alumina total hip arthroplasty: a concise follow-up, at a minimum of ten years, of a previous report. J Bone Joint Surg Am 2010;92:1715–9.

32. Petsatodis GE, Papadopoulos PP, Papavasiliou KA, et al. Primary cementless total hip arthroplasty with an alumina ceramic-on-ceramic bearing: results after a minimum of twenty years of follow-up. J Bone Joint Surg Am 2010;92(3):639–44.

33. Skinner HB. Ceramic bearing surfaces. Clin Orthop Relat Res 1999;369:83.

34. Dorlot JM, Christel P, Meunier A. Wear analysis of retrieved alumina heads and sockets of hip prosthesis. J Biomed Mater Res 1989;23(Suppl A3): 299.

35. Christel PS. Biocompatibility of surgical-grade dense polycrystalline alumina. Clin Orthop Relat Res 1992;282:10.

36. Hamilton WG, McAuley JP, Dennis DA, et al. THA with delta ceramic on ceramic: results of a multicenter investigational device exemption trial. Clin Orthop Relat Res 2010;468(2):358–66.

37. McKee GK, Watson-Farrar J. Replacement of arthritic hips by the McKee-Farrar prosthesis. J Bone Joint Surg Br 1966;48:245.

38. Clarke IC, Good V, Williams P, et al. Ultra-low wear rates for rigid-on-rigid bearings in total hip replacements. Proc Inst Mech Eng H 2000;214:331.

39. National Joint Registry for England and Wales. 8th Annual Report 2011. Available at: http://www.hqip.org.uk/assets/NCAPOP-Library/NJR-8th-Annual-Report-2011.pdf. Accessed July 26, 2013.

40. Schouten R, Malone AA, Tiffen C, et al. A prospective, randomised controlled trial comparing ceramic-on-metal and metal-on-metal bearing surfaces in total hip replacement. J Bone Joint Surg Br 2012;94(11):1462–7.

41. Isaac GH, Brockett C, Breckon A, et al. Ceramic-on-metal bearings in total hip replacement: whole blood metal ion levels and analysis of retrieved components. J Bone Joint Surg Br 2009;91(9):1134–41.

42. MacDonald SJ, Engh CA, Naudie D, et al. Ceramic on metal versus metal on metal clinical and metal ion results of a prospective FDA RCT. Paper 005. Presented at the Annual Meeting of the American Academy of Orthopaedic Surgeons. New Orleans, March 9–13, 2010.

43. Callaghan JJ, Cuckler JM, Huddleston JI, et al, Implant Wear Symposium 2007 Clinical Work Group. How have alternative bearings (such as metal-on-metal, highly cross-linked polyethylene, and ceramic-on-ceramic) affected the prevention and treatment of osteolysis? J Am Acad Orthop Surg 2008;16(Suppl 1):S33–8.

44. Hermida JC, Bergula A, Chen P, et al. Comparison of the wear rates of twenty-eight and thirty-two-millimeter femoral heads on crosslinked polyethylene acetabular cups in a wear simulator. J Bone Joint Surg Am 2003;85:2325–31.

45. Thomas GE, Simpson DJ, Mehmood S, et al. The seven-year wear of highly cross-linked polyethylene in total hip arthroplasty: a double-blind, randomized controlled trial using radiostereometric analysis. J Bone Joint Surg Am 2011;93(8):716–22.

46. D'Antonio JA, Capello WN, Ramakrishnan R. Second-generation annealed highly cross-linked polyethylene exhibits low wear. Clin Orthop Relat Res 2012;470(6):1696–704.

47. Galvin A, Kang L, Tipper J, et al. Wear of cross-linked polyethylene under different tribological conditions. J Mater Sci Mater Med 2006;17(3):235–43.

48. Bragdon CR, Jasty M, Muratoglu OK, et al. Third-body wear of highly cross-linked polyethylene in a hip simulator. J Arthroplasty 2003;18(5):553–61.

49. Rajaee SS, Trofa D, Matzkin E, et al. National trends in primary total hip arthroplasty in extremely young patients: a focus on bearing surface usage. J Arthroplasty 2012;27:1870–8.

50. Galvin AL, Jennings LM, Tipper JL, et al. Wear and creep of highly crosslinked polyethylene against cobalt chrome and ceramic femoral heads. Proc Inst Mech Eng H 2010;224(10):1175–83.

51. Migaud H, Putman S, Krantz N, et al. Cementless metal-on-metal versus ceramic-on-polyethylene hip arthroplasty in patients less than fifty years of age: a comparative study with twelve to fourteen-year follow-up. J Bone Joint Surg Am 2011;93(Suppl 2):137–42.

52. Urban JA, Garvin KL, Boese CK, et al. Ceramic-on-polyethylene bearing surfaces in total hip arthroplasty: seventeen to twenty-one-year results. J Bone Joint Surg Am 2001;83(11):1688–94.

53. Meftah M, Ebrahimpour PB, He C, et al. Preliminary clinical and radiographic results of large ceramic heads on highly cross-linked polyethylene. Orthopedics 2011;34(6):e133–7.

54. Garvin KL, Hartman CW, Mangla J, et al. Wear analysis in THA utilizing oxidized zirconium and crosslinked polyethylene. Clin Orthop Relat Res 2009;467(1):141–5.

55. Zywiel MG, Sayeed SA, Johnson AJ, et al. Survival of hard-on-hard bearings in total hip arthroplasty: a systematic review. Clin Orthop Relat Res 2011;469(6):1536–46.

56. Murphy SB, Ecker TM, Tannast M. Two- to 9-year clinical results of alumina CoC THA. Clin Orthop Relat Res 2006;453:97–102.

57. D'Antonio J, Capello W, Manley M, et al. Alumina ceramic bearings for total hip arthroplasty: five-year results of a prospective randomized study. Clin Orthop Relat Res 2005;(436):164–71.

58. Finkbone PR, Severson EP, Cabanela ME, et al. Ceramic-on-ceramic total hip arthroplasty in patients younger than 20 years. J Arthroplasty 2012;27(2):213–9.

59. Nikolaou VS, Edwards MR, Bogoch E, et al. A prospective randomised controlled trial comparing three alternative bearing surfaces in primary total hip replacement. J Bone Joint Surg Br 2012;94(4):459–65.

60. Eswaramoorthy V, Moonot P, Kalairajah Y, et al. The Metasul metal-on-metal articulation in primary total hip replacement: clinical and radiological results at ten years. J Bone Joint Surg Br 2008;90:1278.

61. Vendittoli PA, Amzica T, Roy AG, et al. Metal ion release with large-diameter metal-on-metal hip arthroplasty. J Arthroplasty 2011;26:282–8.

62. Milošev I, Kovač S, Trebše R, et al. Comparison of ten-year survivorship of hip prostheses with use of conventional polyethylene, metal-on-metal, or ceramic-on-ceramic bearings. J Bone Joint Surg Am 2012;94(19):1756–63.

63. Kawate K, Ohmura T, Kawahara I, et al. Differences in highly cross-linked polyethylene wear between zirconia and cobalt-chromium femoral heads in Japanese patients: a prospective, randomized study. J Arthroplasty 2009;24(8):1221–4.

64. Bourne RB, Barrack R, Rorabeck CH, et al. Arthroplasty options for the young patient: Oxinium on cross-linked polyethylene. Clin Orthop Relat Res 2005;441:159–67.

65. Lee R, Essner A, Wang A, et al. Scratch and wear performance of prosthetic femoral head components against crosslinked UHMWPE sockets. Wear 2009;267(11):1915–21.

66. Australian Orthopaedic Association National Joint Replacement Registry. Annual report 2012. Available at: https://aoanjrr.dmac.adelaide.edu.au/en. Accessed July 26, 2013.

67. Australian Orthopaedic Association National Joint Replacement Registry. Annual report 2008. Available at: https://aoanjrr.dmac.adelaide.edu.au/en. Accessed July 26, 2013.

68. Australian Orthopaedic Association National Joint Replacement Registry. Annual report 2009. Available at: https://aoanjrr.dmac.adelaide.edu.au/en. Accessed July 26, 2013.

69. Australian Orthopaedic Association National Joint Replacement Registry. Annual report 2010. Available at: https://aoanjrr.dmac.adelaide.edu.au/en. Accessed July 26, 2013.

70. Smith AJ, Dieppe P, Howard PW, et al, National Joint Registry for England and Wales. Failure rates of metal-on-metal hip resurfacings: analysis of data from the National Joint Registry for England and Wales. Lancet 2012;380(9855):1759–66.

71. National Joint Registry for England and Wales. 7th Annual Report 2010. Available at: http://www.njrcentre.org.uk/njrcentre/portals/0/njr%207th%20annual%20report%202010.pdf. Accessed July 26, 2013.

72. New Zealand Orthopaedic Association. The New Zealand Joint Registry: eleven year report: January 1999 to December 2009. 2010 Oct. Available at: http://nzoa.org.nz/system/files/NJR%2011%20Year%20Report%20Jan%2099%20-%20Dec%2009.pdf. Accessed July 26, 2013.

73. Bradford L, Kurland R, Sankaran M, et al. Early failure due to osteolysis associated with contemporary highly cross-linked ultra-high molecular weight polyethylene. A case report. J Bone Joint Surg Am 2004;86(5):1051–6.

74. Tower SS, Currier JH, Currier BH, et al. Rim cracking of the cross-linked longevity polyethylene acetabular liner after total hip arthroplasty. J Bone Joint Surg Am 2007;89(10):2212–7.

75. Furmanski J, Anderson M, Bal S, et al. Clinical fracture of cross-linked UHMWPE acetabular liners. Biomaterials 2009;30(29):5572–82.

76. Hannouche D, Nich C, Bizot P, et al. Fractures of ceramic bearings: history and present status. Clin Orthop Relat Res 2003;417:19–26.

77. Willmann G. Ceramic femoral head retrieval data. Clin Orthop Relat Res 2000;379:22–8.

78. Restrepo C, Parvizi J, Kurtz SM, et al. The noisy ceramic hip: is component malpositioning the cause? J Arthroplasty 2008;23:643.

79. Ranawat AS, Ranawat CS. The squeaking hip: a cause for concern—agrees. Orthopedics 2007;30(738):743.

80. Keurentjes JC, Kuipers RM, Wever DJ, et al. High incidence of squeaking in THAs with alumina ceramic-on-ceramic bearings. Clin Orthop Relat Res 2008;466(6):1438–43.

81. Chevillotte C, Trousdale RT, Chen Q, et al. The 2009 Frank Stinchfield Award: "Hip squeaking": a biomechanical study of ceramic-on-ceramic bearing surfaces. Clin Orthop Relat Res 2010;468(2):345–50.

82. Restrepo C, Post ZD, Kai B, et al. The effect of stem design on the prevalence of squeaking following ceramic-on-ceramic bearing total hip arthroplasty. J Bone Joint Surg Am 2010;92(3):550–7.

83. Murali R, Bonar SF, Kirsh G, et al. Osteolysis in third-generation alumina ceramic-on-ceramic hip bearings with severe impingement and titanium metallosis. J Arthroplasty 2008;23(8):1240.e13–9.

84. de Steiger RN, Hang JR, Miller LN, et al. Five-year results of the ASR X-large Acetabular System and the ASR Hip Resurfacing System: an analysis from the Australian Orthopaedic Association National Joint Replacement Registry. J Bone Joint Surg Am 2011;93:2287–93.

85. United States Food and Drug Administration. Meeting Materials of the Orthopaedic and Rehabilitation Devices Panel. 2012. Available at: http://www.fda.gov/AdvisoryCommittees/CommitteesMeetingMaterials/MedicalDevices/MedicalDevicesAdvisoryCommittee/OrthopaedicandRehabilitationDevicesPanel/ucm309184.htm. Accessed February 17, 2013.

86. Medicines and Healthcare Products Regulatory Agency. Medical device alert: all metal-on-metal (MoM) hip replacements. 2010. Available at: http://www.mhra.gov.uk/home/groups/dts-bs/documents/medicaldevicealert/con079162.pdf. Accessed February 17, 2013.

87. Schmalzried TP. Metal-metal bearing surfaces in hip arthroplasty. Orthopedics 2009;32:661.

88. Davies AP, Willert HG, Campbell PA, et al. An unusual lymphocytic perivascular infiltration in tissues around contemporary metal-on-metal joint replacements. J Bone Joint Surg Am 2005;87(1):18–27.

89. De Smet K, De Haan R, Calistri A, et al. Metal ion measurement as a diagnostic tool to identify problems with metal-on-metal hip resurfacing. J Bone Joint Surg Am 2008;90(Suppl 4):202–8.

90. Jacobs JJ, Skipor AK, Campbell PA, et al. Can metal levels be used to monitor metal-on-metal hip arthroplasties? J Arthroplasty 2004;19(Suppl 3):59–65.

91. Browne JA, Bechtold CD, Berry DJ, et al. Failed metal-on-metal hip arthroplasties: a spectrum of

clinical presentations and operative findings. Clin Orthop Relat Res 2010;468(9):2313–20.

92. Zijlstra WP, Van Raay JJ, Bulstra SK, et al. No superiority of cemented metal-on-metal over metal-on-polyethylene THA in a randomized controlled trial at 10-year follow-up. Orthopedics 2010;33:154.

93. Cooper HJ, Della Valle CJ, Berger RA, et al. Corrosion at the head-neck taper as a cause for adverse local tissue reactions after total hip arthroplasty. J Bone Joint Surg Am 2012;94:1655–61.

94. Ebramzadeh E, Campbell PA, Takamura KM, et al. Failure modes of 433 metal-on-metal hip implants: how, why, and wear. Orthop Clin North Am 2011; 42:241–50.

95. De Haan R, Pattyn C, Gill HS, et al. Correlation between inclination of the acetabular component and metal ion levels in metal-on-metal hip resurfacing replacement. J Bone Joint Surg Br 2008;90:1291–7.

96. Lombardi AV Jr, Barrack RL, Berend KR, et al. The Hip Society: algorithmic approach to diagnosis and management of metal-on-metal arthroplasty. J Bone Joint Surg Br 2012;94(11 Suppl A):14–8.

97. Hayter CL, Gold SL, Koff MF, et al. MRI findings in painful metal-on-metal hip arthroplasty. AJR Am J Roentgenol 2012;199(4):884–93.

98. Keegan GM, Learmonth ID, Case CP. Orthopaedic metals and their potential toxicity in the arthroplasty patient: a review of current knowledge and future strategies [review]. J Bone Joint Surg Br 2007; 89(5):567–73.

99. Kavanagh BF, Dewitz MA, Ilstrup DM, et al. Charnley total hip arthroplasty with cement. Fifteen-year results. J Bone Joint Surg Am 1989;71:1496–503.

100. Kim YH, Oh SH, Kim JS, et al. Contemporary total hip arthroplasty with and without cement in patients with osteonecrosis of the femoral head. J Bone Joint Surg Am 2003;85:675–81.

101. Bsila RS, Inglis AE, Ranawat CS. Joint replacement surgery in patients under thirty. J Bone Joint Surg Am 1976;58:1098–104.

102. Callaghan JJ, Forest EE, Sporer SM, et al. Total hip arthroplasty in the young adult. Clin Orthop 1997; 344:257–62.

103. Collis DK. Long-term (twelve to eighteen-year) follow-up of cemented total hip replacements in patients who were less than fifty years old. A follow-up note. J Bone Joint Surg Am 1991;73:593–7.

104. Cornell CN, Ranawat CS. Survivorship analysis of total hip replacements. Results in a series of active patients who were less than fifty-five years old. J Bone Joint Surg Am 1986;68:1430–4.

105. Dorr LD, Luckett M, Conaty JP. Total hip arthroplasties in patients younger than 45 years. A nine-to ten-year follow-up study. Clin Orthop 1990;260: 215–9.

106. Kerboull L, Hamadouche M, Courpied JP, et al. Long-term results of Charnley-Kerboull hip arthroplasty in patients younger than 50 years. Clin Orthop 2004;418:112–8.

107. McAuley JP, Szuszczewicz ES, Young A, et al. Total hip arthroplasty in patients 50 years and younger. Clin Orthop 2004;418:119–25.

108. Anand R, Graves SE, de Steiger RN, et al. What is the benefit of introducing new hip and knee prostheses? J Bone Joint Surg Am 2011;93(Suppl 3): 51–4.

109. Malchau H. Introducing new technology: a stepwise algorithm. Spine (Phila Pa 1976) 2000;25: 285.

110. Bozic KJ, Morshed S, Silverstein MD, et al. Use of cost-effectiveness analysis to evaluate new technologies in orthopaedics. The case of alternative bearing surfaces in total hip arthroplasty. J Bone Joint Surg Am 2006;88(4):706–14.

Osteonecrosis of the Hip
Treatment Options and Outcomes

Samik Banerjee, MS (Orth), MRCS (Glasg), Kimona Issa, MD,
Robert Pivec, MD, Bhaveen H. Kapadia, MD,
Harpal S. Khanuja, MD, Michael A. Mont, MD*

KEYWORDS

- Osteonecrosis • Avascular necrosis • Treatment • Outcomes

KEY POINTS

- A multitude of medical treatment options have been described for the treatment of early stage osteonecrosis.
- Mesenchymal stem cell–based therapies with conventional methods of treatment have shown early promise in the treatment of the precollapse stage of osteonecrosis.
- Prospective randomized multicenter trials comparing pharmacotherapy with core decompression and stem cell–based therapies are needed in future.
- Cementless total hip arthroplasty with highly cross-linked polyethylene and new generation of ceramic bearings have shown excellent results at short-term to midterm follow-up.

INTRODUCTION

Osteonecrosis (ON) of the hip, with its varied causes and poorly understood pathogenesis, is an incapacitating disease primarily affecting the active population in the third and fourth decades of life.[1–6] Management of ON has continued to remain a dilemma despite improvements in both medical and surgical treatment of this disease.[7] The goal of management is to diagnose ON early in the precollapse stage and prevent subsequent progression to collapse and end-stage arthritis (**Fig. 1**). Treatment has typically been based on the staging of ON (**Table 1**); however, various other factors, such as the extent of the lesion, location, and causes, are often also taken into account when planning treatment. Although numerous studies reporting on a variety of operative and nonoperative methods have been published in the literature, there has been no consensus with regard to the ideal treatment of the precollapse stage of these lesions. Moreover, encouraging clinical outcomes following recent advances in short stem designs, porous biomaterials for cementless fixation, and ceramic or highly cross-linked polyethylene bearings have led to debate about the optimal implant for hip arthroplasty in patients with end-stage ON. This article presents a review of the current evidence regarding the outcomes of various nonoperative and operative treatment options for ON.

NONOPERATIVE TREATMENT

A variety of pharmacologic and biophysical treatments have recently been suggested for

Disclosures: Michael A. Mont receives royalties from Stryker; is a consultant for Janssen, Sage Products, Inc, Salient Surgical, Stryker, OCSI, Tissue Gene; receives institutional support from Stryker; and is on the Speakers Bureau for Sage Products, Inc; Harpal S. Khanuja is a paid consultant for Ethicon, Johnson & Johnson; the remaining authors have no disclosures to make. No Funding was received in support of this work.
Center for Joint Preservation and Replacement, Rubin Institute for Advanced Orthopedics, Sinai Hospital of Baltimore, 2401 West Belvedere Avenue, Baltimore, MD 21215, USA
* Corresponding author.
E-mail addresses: mmont@lifebridgehealth.org; rhondamont@aol.com

Orthop Clin N Am 44 (2013) 463–476
http://dx.doi.org/10.1016/j.ocl.2013.07.004
0030-5898/13/$ – see front matter © 2013 Elsevier Inc. All rights reserved.

orthopedic.theclinics.com

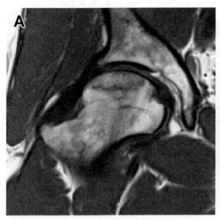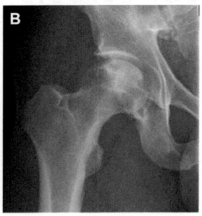

Fig. 1. Magnetic resonance imaging (*A*) and anteroposterior radiograph (*B*) of a 39-year-old woman with Ficat and Arlet grade III ON of the right femur and acetabulum.

prevention of disease progression following ON.[1] These treatment modalities have been proposed to favorably affect various points in the purported etiopathogenic pathway of ON. The goal of medical treatment in the precollapse stage is to improve function and provide pain relief, prevent radiographic progression to subchondral fracture and collapse, and allow healing of the necrotic

Table 1
Overview of commonly used staging systems for ON of the hip

Ficat and Arlet		University of Pennsylvania		ARCO		Japanese Orthopedic Association	
Stage	Findings	Stage	Findings	Stage	Findings	Stage	Findings
I	Normal radiograph	0	Normal hip	0	Normal hip	1	Demarcation line
II a	Diffuse cystic/ sclerotic lesions	I	MRI findings only	1	MRI findings only	2	Early femoral head flattening
II b	Crescent sign (subchondral fracture)	II	Diffuse cystic/ sclerotic lesions	2	Focal osteoporosis, cystic lesions, sclerosis	3	Cystic lesions
III	Presence of sequestrum in radiograph; femoral head collapse	III	Subchondral step-off	3	Crescent sign (subchondral fracture)	—	—
IV	Loss of articular cartilage and osteoarthritis with a deformed femoral head	IV	Femoral head flattening	4	Acetabular involvement	—	—
—	—	V	Acetabular involvement or joint space narrowing	—	—	—	—
—	—	VI	Advanced joint degeneration	—	—	—	—

Abbreviations: ARCO, Association Research Circulation Osseous; MRI, magnetic resonance imaging.

lesions. The following nonsurgical modalities have shown promise in the treatment of the precollapse stage of ON.

Non–Weight Bearing

Although non–weight bearing has been proposed as a treatment option for early stage ON (stage I and II, Ficat and Arlet), Mont and colleagues,[8] in a meta-analysis of 819 patients, reported poor clinical outcomes in more than 80% of the patients at a mean follow-up of 34 months (range, 1.6–10 years) following nonoperative treatment. No difference in outcomes was seen between full, partial, and non–weight-bearing regimens in their study. In a recent systematic review with level II evidence the same author reported that 59% (394 of 664 hips) of asymptomatic hips had onset of symptoms or progressed to collapse at a mean follow-up of 7 years (range, 0.2–20 years).[9] The investigators also reported that the incidence of progression to collapse was highest in patients who had sickle cell disease (73%; 29 of 40 hips) in contrast with patients who had systemic lupus erythematosus, who had the lowest rate of progression to collapse at 17% (10 of 59 hips). One-hundred and forty-nine hips (32%) with small or medium-sized lesions (<50% of head involvement) progressed to symptoms or collapse, whereas large lesions (>50%) had an 84% rate of progression.

Bisphosphonates

Progression of early stage ON to subchondral fracture and collapse is known to be related to the increased osteoclastic bone resorption around the necrotic region, which occurs as a result of the physiologic healing process.[10,11] Bisphosphonates reduce osteoclastic activity and inhibit bone turnover, and have been proposed in the treatment of early stage ON.[12–16] The improvement in bone mineral density in the femoral head following their long-term use may thus prevent, or at least delay, the development of collapse.

Agarwala and colleagues,[15] in their report of 395 hips at a mean follow-up of 4 years (range, 1–8 years), reported a radiographic progression to collapse in 12.6% (27 of 215 hips) in stage I and 55.8% (72 of 129 hips) in stage II (Ficat and Arlet staging) following treatment with alendronate 10 mg daily for 3 years. The mean time to collapse was 3.5 years (range, 3–6 years) in stage I and 2.9 years (range, 2–5 years) in stage II hips. The same author in a recent publication of 53 hips at 10-year follow-up reported a 29% collapse rate in the precollapse stage of ON (10 of 34 hips) following 3 years of continuous alendronate use

at 70 mg weekly.[14] The investigators thus concluded that the natural history of untreated ON with more than 70% collapse rate was favorably altered with alendronate use.[17]

Lai and colleagues,[12] in a prospective randomized study of 54 hips in Steinberg stage II and III ON, reported a significant decrease in the rate of radiographic progression to collapse in patients treated with 70 mg of alendronate (2 of 29 hips) weekly for 1 year compared with the placebo group (19 of 25 hips; P<.001) at 2-year (range, 2–2.3 years) follow-up. Moreover, 14% (4 of 29 hips) of patients in the treatment of group had radiographic progression of 1 stage or more during the observation period compared with 80% (20 of 25 hips) in the placebo group.

However, Chen and colleagues[18] reported conflicting evidence in a recent prospective, randomized, double-blinded, placebo-controlled trial (level I evidence) with 65 hips in stage IIC and IIIC (University of Pennsylvania classification). They reported no significant difference in radiographic disease progression, quality-of-life improvement, and prevention of total hip arthroplasty between the alendronate and the placebo cohorts at the final follow-up at 2 years. However, the investigators thought that the study was underpowered to detect statistical significance despite a numerical reduction in the rate of disease progression (61% vs 66%) and total hip arthroplasty conversion (12.5% vs 15.2%) in the alendronate group.

Anticoagulants

Hypofibrinolysis and thrombophilia leading to venous outflow obstruction and increased intraosseous pressure have been reported by various researchers to be a pathogenic factor in the development of ON.[19] Thus, conceptually systemic anticoagulation may delay or may even reverse the process of ischemic ON by preventing clot propagation and enhancing clot lysis. Glueck and colleagues,[20] in a prospective study of 25 patients (35 hips) with known thrombophilia and Ficat stage I or II ON of the hip, reported that 95% of hips (19 of 20 hips) with primary ON and 20% (3 of 15 hips) of patients with secondary ON (secondary to corticosteroid use) had no progression of disease at a minimum follow-up of 2 years (mean, 3 years; range, 2–4 years) following enoxaparin therapy (60 mg/d for 3 months).

Hypolipidemics

Corticosteroids have been reported in multiple studies to be associated with the development of ON.[21–24] These pharmacologic agents induce differentiation of pluripotent marrow stem cells into the adipocyte lineage by stimulating expression of adipocyte-specific genes 422(aP2) and PPARγ2 while decreasing expression of Cbfa1/Runx2 and osteocalcin promoter, which normally promotes differentiation into an osteocyte lineage.[25,26] In addition, corticosteroids increase angiogenic sensitivity to vasospastic agents like endothelin-1 and decrease response of blood vessels to vasodilators such as bradykinin.[27,28] Statins have been reported to counteract this abnormal adipocyte differentiation by promoting osteoblastic differentiation and may prevent the development of corticosteroid-induced ON.[29]

In a retrospective analysis of 284 patients receiving high-dose corticosteroids, Pritchett[30] reported that 3 patients (1%) developed ON following statin treatment at a mean follow-up of 7.5 years (range, 5–11 years). However, Ajmal and colleagues[31] reported that statin therapy did not significantly reduce the risk of ON in their series of 338 renal transplant patients receiving high-dose corticosteroids at a mean follow-up of 7.5 years compared with patients who did not receive statins (range, 3.5–19 years; $P = .8$).

Extracorporeal Shock Wave Therapy

Incidental finding of increased pelvic bone mineral density seen after extracorporeal shock wave therapy for renal stones stimulated interest in its use in orthopedics. Although the mechanism through which extracorporeal shock wave therapy exerts its beneficial effects in ON is currently unknown, it seems that extracorporeal shock wave therapy causes stimulation of neovascularization through increased expression of angiogenic growth factors.[32] Ludwig and colleagues,[33] in a prospective study of 21 patients, reported improvement in pain, mobility, and Harris hip scores in 66.6% (14 patients) at 1-year final follow-up. Follow-up magnetic resonance imaging (MRI) revealed either a decrease in size of the necrotic regions (6 patients) or healing of the lesions (4 patients), whereas the area of poor circulation remained unchanged in the remaining 4 patients.

Wang and colleagues,[34] in a randomized trial of 57 hips at a mean follow-up of 2 years (range, 2–3.3 years) comparing extracorporeal shock wave therapy with bone grafting, reported significant improvement in pain and Harris hip scores, and decreased need for total hip arthroplasty in the extracorporeal shock wave therapy group ($P<.001$). Seventy-nine percent of patients improved (≥50% reduction in hip pain and ≥50% improvement in hip function), whereas 20%

remained unchanged or became worse following extracorporeal shock wave therapy. In the bone grafting cohort, 29% of patients improved, whereas 72% deteriorated or remained unchanged. More recently, the same investigators in a long-term follow-up study (mean, 8.5 years; range, 7.7–8.8 years) of these 57 hips reported that patients with extracorporeal shock wave therapy had significantly better clinical outcomes (76% vs 21% good or fair; $P<.001$) and decreased need for total hip arthroplasty (24% vs 64%; $P = .002$) compared with the bone grafting cohort.

Hsu and colleagues,[35] in a prospective randomized study of 98 hips comparing extracorporeal shock wave therapy and a cocktail regimen of extracorporeal shock wave therapy, hyperbaric oxygen, and alendronate, reported similar improvement in clinical outcomes in both cohorts at mean 2-year follow-up (range, 1.5–4 years). The size of the lesion either remained unchanged or improved in 90% of patients in both groups at final follow-up. Wang and colleagues,[36] in a randomized trial of 55 hips with stage I to III ON (Association Research Circulation Osseous classification) reported no significant difference in the pain control ($P = .4$), hip function ($P = .1$), and the need for total hip arthroplasty ($P = .8$) with extracorporeal shock wave therapy (6000 impulses at 28 kV at each session) in patients with systemic lupus erythematosus (SLE) and a non-SLE control group at minimum of 2 years' follow-up.

Pulsed Electromagnetic Therapy

Pulsed electromagnetic therapy is thought to favorably affect early stage ON through stimulation of osteogenesis and angiogenesis similar to extracorporeal shock wave therapy. Massari and colleagues,[37] in their retrospective analysis of 76 hips treated with electromagnetic field stimulation in Ficat stage I to III, reported that the 94% of hips in stage I and II avoided the need for total hip arthroplasty with a significantly higher proportion of hips in stage III progressing to total hip arthroplasty at a mean follow-up of 2 years. At present, evidence in favor of electromagnetic stimulation is limited and further research is needed to explore its potential role in early stage ON.

Hyperbaric Oxygen

Hyperbaric oxygen therapy, by increasing extracellular oxygen concentration, reduces cellular ischemia, and is also known to reduce edema by inducing vasoconstriction. Reis and colleagues[38] reported radiographic improvement in 81% of their patients (n = 25) with Steinberg stage I ON following 100 days of daily hyperbaric oxygen therapy. Camporesi and colleagues[39] also reported improvement in pain and range-of-motion at final follow-up of 7 years in a study of 19 patients randomized to receive 30 treatment doses of either hyperbaric oxygen or hyperbaric air for a total period of 6 weeks. None of the patients in the hyperbaric oxygen group required total hip arthroplasty for disease progression at the time of final follow-up.

Vasodilators

Vasodilators from prostacyclin I2 derivatives (eg, iloprost) are known to improve blood flow in the terminal vessels and until recently their potential efficacy was only defined in the treatment of vasospastic conditions like vasculitis, pulmonary hypertension, SLE, Raynaud phenomenon, and sickle cell crisis.

Based on promising early evidence that iloprost may have a role in bone regeneration at the cellular level, Jager and colleagues[40] conducted a prospective study on 50 patients (98 joints) to explore the analgesic and curative potential of iloprost in the treatment of bone marrow edema (BME) and early stage ON. They reported significant improvement in pain, quality of life, Knee Society scores and Harris hip scores, and radiographic decrease (56% showing complete disappearance of BME) in the extent of BME in bones with Association Research Circulation Osseous (ARCO) stage I and II following a 5-day infusion protocol of intravenous iloprost at 6 months' follow-up. However, no improvement was seen in the advanced stages of ON despite showing an analgesic effect in some patients. Disch and colleagues[41] also reported significant improvement in pain, hip function, and BME in 33 patients (n = 16 with BME and n = 17

with ON) at mean 2 years' (range, 1–3 years) follow-up. At present, randomized controlled trials and further long-term data are needed before prostacyclin analogues can be recommended for routine use in early stage ON.

OPERATIVE TREATMENT
Core Decompression/Multiple Percutaneous Drilling

Core decompression has been used in the treatment of ON for more than 4 decades (**Fig. 2**). It is the most commonly performed procedure and is thought to decrease intraosseous pressure and improve blood flow to the necrotic area. This effect in turn may facilitate deposition of new bone in the diseased region. However, despite its continued use as a treatment option in early stage ON, there has been considerable debate about its role and efficacy in various causes of ON and in the presence of a variety of radiographic factors (eg, size, location, or collapse of the lesion). The overall success rate as defined by the need for further surgery has varied between 40% and 80% across multiple studies at 2-year to 7-year follow-up.[8,42] In a systematic review, Marker and colleagues[43] reported that recent techniques of core decompression resulted in significantly better clinical and radiographic outcomes, and lower rates of additional surgery (n = 1268; mean, 30%; range, 39%–100%) compared with studies before 1992 (n = 1337; mean, 41%; range, 29%–85%) ($P<.05$). However, there were fewer patients with Ficat stage III ON ($P<.001$) in the studies after 1992, which may have accounted for the improvement in the observed results. Based on the review, the investigators also reported that patients with Ficat stage III ON were more likely to have higher clinical

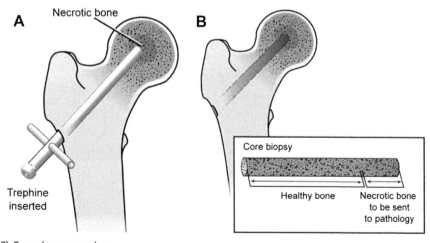

Fig. 2. (*A*, *B*) Core decompression.

failures, increased rate of radiographic progression, and additional surgeries, and thus may not be ideal candidates for core decompression.

Over the past decade many researchers have used multiple drilling as an alternative to core decompression because of its simplicity, ability to reach the anterior portion of the femoral head more easily than conventional core decompression, and low rate of potential complications (eg, subtrochanteric fractures or inadvertent head penetration).[44–46] Mont and colleagues,[44] in their study of 45 hips with Ficat stage I and II ON, reported an overall 71% (32 of 45 hips) successful outcome following a multiple-drilling (2–3 perforations) procedure using a 3-mm Steinman pin at a mean follow-up of 2 years (range, 1.7–3.3 years). Small to medium-sized lesions (<50%) and stage I hips had a higher success rate (24 of 30 hips) following the procedure compared with large lesions (>50%) and stage II hips (57%; 8 of 15 patients).

Song and colleagues,[45] in their retrospective study of 163 hips using multiple drilling as a treatment option for Ficat stage I to III ON, reported that 88% (52 of 59 hips) of small to medium-sized lesions required no additional surgical procedure at a mean follow-up of 7.2 years (range, 5–11.2 years). They also reported that 79% (31 of 39 hips) of stage I hips and 77% (62 of 81 hips) of stage II hips were considered as clinically successful (Harris hip score >75 points and no additional surgery needed).

In a study of 75 hips, in ARCO stage I to III ON, Lee and colleagues[46] recently reported that following multiple drilling (mean, 8.6; range, 5–11 perforations), increased preoperative intraosseous pressure reduced significantly from a mean 57 mm Hg (standard deviation 25 mm Hg) to near normal pressure (mean, 16 ± 9 mm Hg) after surgery. They further noted that hips that had an unsuccessful outcome (44%; 33 hips) following multiple drilling had significantly higher intertrochanteric intraosseous pressure (mean, 45 ± 25 mm Hg) or had a combined necrotic angle of more than 200°. The investigators concluded that the raised intertrochanteric pressure may have represented a general disturbance of circulation in the proximal femoral marrow that increases in severity with disease progression.

Nonvascularized Bone Grafting

Nonvascularized bone grafting involves thorough curettage and decompression of the necrotic region followed by packing of the cavity with bone grafts (eg, allogeneic, autogeneic, and bone graft substitute). The bone grafts have osteoinductive and osteoconductive properties and have been known to aid in healing of the affected region. Nonvascularized bone grafting is usually indicated for small to medium-sized lesions (Ficat stage I and II) and those with failed core decompression. The presence of collapse of more than 2 mm, acetabular involvement, or delamination of the cartilage are risk factors for poor results following nonvascularized bone grafting. Bone grafting is either performed through the core decompression tract (Phemister technique) or through a window in the articular cartilage (trapdoor procedure; **Fig. 3**) or a window through the femoral neck (light bulb procedure; **Fig. 4**).

The results of the Phemister technique vary greatly in the literature, with various studies reporting successful results in 36% to 90% of patients at 2 to 7 years' follow-up.[47–49] Varying success between 73% to 90% has been reported in multiple

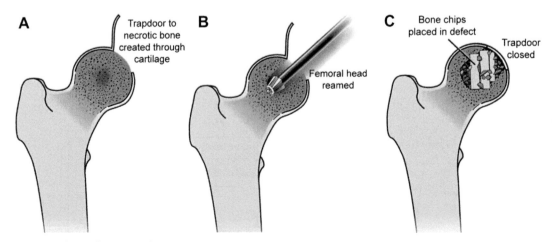

A Trapdoor to necrotic bone created through cartilage

B Femoral head reamed

C Bone chips placed in defect Trapdoor closed

Fig. 3. (*A–C*) Trapdoor procedure.

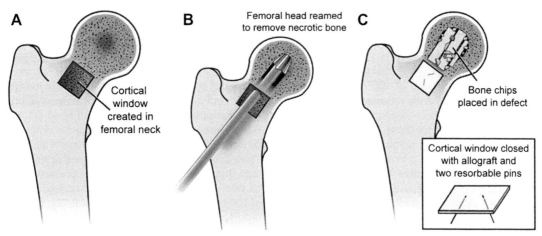

Fig. 4. (*A–C*) Light bulb procedure.

studies using this procedure at 2 to 15 years' follow-up. Seyler and colleagues,[50] in a study of 39 hips using the light bulb procedure, reported 83% survivorship in stage I and II ON and 78% survivorship at a minimum follow-up of 2 years (range, 2–4.2 years).

Vascularized Bone Grafting

Vascularized bone grafting has generally been recommended for Ficat stage I to III ON (**Fig. 5**). The vascularized bone graft provides a viable structural support (eg, vascularized fibula graft) to prevent articular cartilage collapse. Because of its intact blood supply and osteogenic potential (eg, vascularized iliac crest graft) it improves healing of the necrotic area. However, less successful outcomes have been reported with large lesions involving more than 50% of the femoral head or with more than 2 mm of collapse. Patients with prior history of heavy smoking, alcoholism, or other risk factors that could potentially affect the healing of the vascular anastomosis need to be carefully screened before the procedure. Moreover, patients with peripheral vascular disease may need to be excluded from this procedure.

Urbaniak and colleagues,[51] in their study of 103 hips treated with vascularized fibula grafting,

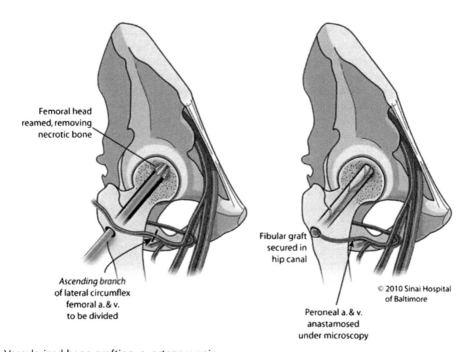

Fig. 5. Vascularized bone grafting. a, artery; v, vein.

reported 91% survivorship in stage II and 77% survivorship in stage III at a final follow-up of 5 years. Yoo and colleagues[52] also reported excellent results, with 89% survivorship in 124 hips in stage II and III at a minimum of 10 years' follow-up (mean, 13.9 years; range 10–23.7 years). Edward and colleagues[53] recently reported the long-term follow-up data (mean, 14.4 years; 10.5–26 years) on 65 hips with precollapse-stage ON treated with vascularized fibula grafting; 75% of the hips survived without the need for total hip arthroplasty at a minimum 10-year follow-up. The investigators noted that demographic and radiographic factors were not associated with changes in graft survivorship.

Bone Morphogenetic Proteins

Bone morphogenetic proteins (BMPs) have been proposed in the treatment of ON to aid the healing process following core decompression. Lieberman and colleagues[54] reported successful clinical results in 82% (14 of 17 hips) of patients treated with nonvascularized bone grafting and purified human BMP at a mean follow-up of 4.4 years (range, 2.2–7.8 years). Although available short-term data seem promising, further research is needed to explore the role of BMPs in ON.

Bone Marrow Instillation and Mesenchymal Stem Cell Therapy

The inadequate amount of creeping substitution and bone remodeling in the necrotic area has led researchers to use biologic augmentation of the repair process in the form of stem cells, demineralized bone matrix, BMPs, and bone marrow instillation into the defect after core decompression.[55–57] Bone marrow stromal cells are thought to secrete angiogenic growth factors that cause increased angiogenesis, which ultimately results in improvement in osteogenesis.

Ganji and colleagues,[58] in a prospective, randomized, double-blinded trial comparing the outcomes between core decompression and autologous bone marrow implantation in 24 hips at ARCO stages I and II, reported a significant improvement in pain and a lower rate of radiographic progression to collapse (stage III) in the bone marrow group (23%; 3 of 13 hips) than in the core decompression cohort (73%; 8 of 11 hips) at a final follow-up of 5 years. Bone marrow implantation did not significantly delay the need for total hip arthroplasty (15% vs 27%) or improve total Western Ontario and McMaster University (WOMAC) scores compared with core decompression.

Liu and colleagues,[59] in a retrospective analysis of 53 hips comparing the outcomes of core decompression and hydroxyapatite/polyamide implantation with or without bone marrow mesenchymal stem cells, also reported significantly higher radiographic and clinical success (Harris hip scores and pain scores) at a mean follow-up of 2 years (range, 1–3.3 years). The bone marrow group had a lower incidence of radiographic progression of collapse of the femoral head (21.4%; 6 of 28 hips) compared with the non–bone marrow group (59.3%; 16 of 27 hips) at final follow-up. Zhao and colleagues,[60] in a prospective randomized trial comparing core decompression with ex vivo cultured bone marrow mesenchymal cells in 104 hips with ARCO stage I and II ON, similarly reported significantly lower radiographic progression to collapse in the bone marrow group (23%; 10 of 44 hips) than in the core decompression group (4%; 2 of 53 hips) at 5-year final follow-up. Moreover, for each stage, significant improvement in the Harris hip scores and radiographic evidence of remaining necrotic volume was reported in the bone marrow group compared with the core decompression group ($P<.05$).

Sen and colleagues,[61] in a recent randomized control trial of 51 hips with ARCO stage I and II ON comparing core decompression with bone marrow mononuclear cell instillation, reported significant improvement in pain, deformity, and hip survival in the bone marrow cohort ($P<.05$) at final follow-up of 2 years. However, there was no significant difference in improvement in the MRI features between the two cohorts at final follow-up.

Proximal Femoral Osteotomies

The rationale behind proximal femoral osteotomies is to rotate the necrotic region away from the load-bearing area and replace it with the uninvolved portion of the head. A variety of intertrochanteric and rotational osteotomies have been described for ON of the hip, with reported success up to 93%.[62–65] However, despite their reported success in multiple single-surgeon series with level IV evidence, few prospective randomized trials comparing the outcomes of trochanteric osteotomies with other surgical treatments such as core decompression or bone grafting are currently unavailable.[62,64–69]

Zhao and colleagues,[68] in their study of 73 hips at a mean follow-up of 12.4 years (range, 5–31 years), reported that 91.8% (67 of 73 hips) of the hips remained intact and did not need conversion to a total hip arthroplasty following curved transtrochanteric varus osteotomy. There was significant improvement in Harris hip scores after surgery and the mean postoperative intact ratio was 57.2% (range, 27%–100%). To prevent progressive collapse they reported that the cutoff for the postoperative intact ratio was 33.6% (sensitivity 82.9% and specificity 100%; P = .001). Moreover, to prevent collapse and joint space narrowing, the cutoff intact ratio was reported to be 41.9% (sensitivity, 88.9%; specificity, 92.1%; P = .001).

Sakano and colleagues[70] similarly reported that, in their series of 20 hips, 90% (18 hips) did not collapse or require conversion to a total hip arthroplasty following transtrochanteric varus osteotomy at a mean follow-up of 4 years (range, 0.7–4.1 years). The mean postoperative intact ratio was 61% and the reported mean elevation of the greater trochanteric was 1.2 cm (range, 0.5–2 cm). Ito and colleagues[63] recently reported the long-term results of varus half wedge osteotomy in 34 hips at a mean follow-up of 18.1 years (range, 10.5–26 years). Overall, 74% (25 hips) had satisfactory results with a mean Harris hip score of more than 80 points despite having a mean limb length discrepancy of 19 mm (range, 8–36 mm). The investigators concluded that varus osteotomy of the proximal femur provides favorable long-term outcomes in the presence of more than one-third of normal superolateral bone.

Hip Arthroplasty

Total hip arthroplasty is usually reserved for unsalvageable end-stage ON or when other treatment modalities have failed **(Fig. 6)**.[71–73] Because of the young age of the patients and the high demands placed on the hip from increased activity, there have been concerns regarding the long-term outcomes of total hip arthroplasty in patients with ON, with some investigators reporting a high rate of aseptic loosening (between 8% and 37%).[74–78] Polyethylene wear and osteolysis has thus remained a challenge when treating patients with ON. However, recent advances in porous biomaterials, highly cross-linked polyethylene, and third-generation ceramic bearings may reduce the rate osteolysis and polyethylene wear and provide durable long-term fixation.[79,80] At present, total hip arthroplasty is indicated for patients with femoral head collapse of more than 2 mm (Ficat stage III) and in the presence of end-stage arthritis (Ficat stage IV). However, patients with multiple failed procedures may also be candidates for total hip arthroplasty.

Bipolar arthroplasty

Although bipolar arthroplasty has been mentioned in a few studies, high rates of loosening, migration and osteolysis, and need for subsequent total hip arthroplasty have reduced its use as a treatment option in ON. Tsumura and colleagues,[81] reporting long-term results (mean, 7.7 years; range, 5–15 years) after bipolar hemiarthroplasty for ON, reported a revision rate of 13.9% at final follow-up. Muraki and colleagues[82] also reported osteolysis and superomedial migration leading to revision surgery in 27.6% (21 of 76 hips) of patients at a mean follow-up period of 13.7 years (range, 5.9–24.9 years) following bipolar hemiarthroplasty for idiopathic ON. At present, there are few data to support continued use of bipolar arthroplasty in ON.

Resurfacing arthroplasty

The role of resurfacing arthroplasty in ON has been a matter of debate because it involves cementing the implant into a bed of dead bone **(Fig. 7)**.[83,84] However, Nakasone and colleagues[85] reported, in a recent study on 39 hips, that the extent of ON in the femoral head before and after machining and implantation had no significant correlation with survival of resurfacing implant at a mean follow-up of 8 years (range, 2–13 years). Multiple clinical studies have also reported excellent survivorship at short-term to-midterm follow-up.[84,86–88] Aulakh and colleagues,[86] in a multicenter study comparing resurfacing implant survivorship between 202 osteonecrotic and osteoarthritic hips, reported no difference in survivorship between the two cohorts at a mean follow-up of 7.5 years (range, 2.9–10 years).

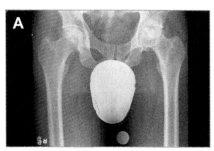 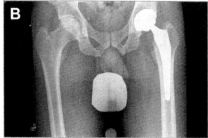

Fig. 6. Anteroposterior radiographs of a 43-year-old man with bilateral hip ON, showing (*A*) the Ficat and Arlet stage IV lesion in the left femoral head treated with a (*B*) total hip arthroplasty.

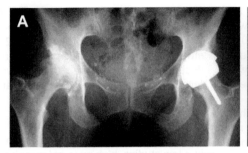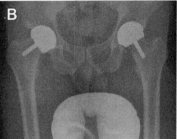

Fig. 7. (A, B) Resurfacing arthroplasty for end-stage ON.

In a matched-pair study of 40 hips in patients younger than 25 years of age, Sayeed and colleagues reported 100% survivorship following resurfacing arthroplasty for ON at a mean follow-up of 5 years (range, 2.8–7.3 years). Mont and colleagues,[89] in a matched pair study between osteoarthritic and osteonecrotic hips, also reported excellent clinical results in 93% of 42 osteonecrotic hips following resurfacing arthroplasty at a minimum of 2 years' follow-up (range, 2–6 years). The overall survival was similar between the two cohorts at final follow-up.

Total hip arthroplasty

Johansson and colleagues,[90] in a recent meta-analysis of 3277 hips, reported significantly higher rates of aseptic loosening following total hip arthroplasty in patients with ON following sickle cell disease, Gaucher disease, or after renal transplantation, whereas low rates of revision were seen in patients with SLE, idiopathic disease, and in heart transplant recipients. The rate of revision surgery following total hip arthroplasty in ON significantly decreased for those operated on after 1990, suggesting that ON does not lead to inferior outcomes with modern techniques of total hip arthroplasty. Min and colleagues,[80] in their evaluation of 162 hips with ON, reported 100% aseptic survivorship with no radiographic evidence of osteolysis at a mean follow-up of 7.2 years (range, 5–10.6 years) using highly cross-linked polyethylene bearings. The mean linear wear reported was 0.037 mm/y (range 0–0.099 mm/y) with none of the hips showing the osteolysis threshold of 0.01 mm/y. Kim and colleagues also reported 100% aseptic survivorship in 73 hips at a mean follow-up of 8.5 years (range, 7–9 years) in patients with ON who were younger than 50 years using alumina on highly cross-linked polyethylene bearings. The mean linear penetration was 0.05 ± 0.02 mm/y, with none of the patients needing component revision for polyethylene wear or osteolysis.

In a long-term follow-up study (mean, 17.3 years; range, 16–18 years) comparing cementless with hybrid fixation in ON, Kim and colleagues[91] reported 98% stem survivorship (cemented and cementless) and 85% cementless cup survivorship at final follow-up. The investigators concluded that polyethylene wear was the most common reason for revision in their study and was possibly related to the young age of the patients, excessive inclination of the acetabular cups more than 50°, and use of a 22-mm femoral head.

In summary, knowledge of the medical management of ON has expanded greatly in the past decade. Multicenter, prospective, randomized trials are needed to explore the efficacy of some of these options. With the advent of mesenchymal stem cell therapy a new era of operative treatment of the precollapse stage of ON is beginning. Moreover, with the introduction of highly porous fixation interfaces, new-generation ceramic bearings, and highly cross-linked polyethylene bearings, arthroplasty options for management of end-stage arthritis following ON seem promising.

DISCLOSURE

HSK is a paid consultant for Ethicon, Johnson & Johnson and is in the Editorial/Governing board Journal of Arthroplasty; board member in the AAOS and American Association of Hip and Knee Surgeons.

MAM receives royalties from Stryker; Wright Medical Technology, Inc; is a paid consultant for Biocomposites; DJ Orthopaedics; Janssen; Joint Active Systems; Medtronic; Sage Products, Inc; Stryker; TissueGene; Wright Medical Technology, Inc; has received research support from DJ Orthopaedics; Joint Active Systems; National Institutes of Health (NIAMS & NICHD); Sage Products, Inc; Stryker; Tissue Gene; Wright Medical Technology, Inc; is in editorial/governing board American Journal of Orthopedics; Journal of Arthroplasty; Journal of Bone and Joint Surgery - American; Journal of Knee Surgery; Surgical Techniques International; and is a board member for AAOS.

BHK is on the speaker bureau and is a consultant for Sage Products Inc.

RP, KI and SB have no disclosures.

REFERENCES

1. Rajpura A, Wright AC, Board TN. Medical management of osteonecrosis of the hip: a review. Hip international: the journal of clinical and experimental research on hip pathology and therapy 2011;21:385–92.
2. Malizos KN, Karantanas AH, Varitimidis SE, et al. Osteonecrosis of the femoral head: etiology, imaging and treatment. European journal of radiology 2007;63:16–28.
3. Jones LC, Hungerford DS. Osteonecrosis: etiology, diagnosis, and treatment. Current opinion in rheumatology 2004;16:443–9.
4. Jones JP Jr. Concepts of etiology and early pathogenesis of osteonecrosis. Instructional course lectures 1994;43:499–512.
5. Kenzora JE, Glimcher MJ. Accumulative cell stress: the multifactorial etiology of idiopathic osteonecrosis. The Orthopedic clinics of North America 1985;16:669–79.
6. Mont MA, Hungerford DS. Non-traumatic avascular necrosis of the femoral head. The Journal of bone and joint surgery American volume 1995;77:459–74.
7. Petrigliano FA, Lieberman JR. Osteonecrosis of the hip: novel approaches to evaluation and treatment. Clinical orthopaedics and related research 2007;465:53–62.
8. Mont MA, Carbone JJ, Fairbank AC. Core decompression versus nonoperative management for osteonecrosis of the hip. Clinical orthopaedics and related research 1996;169–78.
9. Mont MA, Zywiel MG, Marker DR, et al. The natural history of untreated asymptomatic osteonecrosis of the femoral head: a systematic literature review. The Journal of bone and joint surgery American volume 2010;92:2165–70.
10. Plenk H Jr, Gstettner M, Grossschmidt K, et al. Magnetic resonance imaging and histology of repair in femoral head osteonecrosis. Clinical orthopaedics and related research 2001;42–53.
11. Glimcher MJ, Kenzora JE. The biology of osteonecrosis of the human femoral head and its clinical implications. III. Discussion of the etiology and genesis of the pathological sequelae; commments on treatment. Clinical orthopaedics and related research 1979;273–312.
12. Lai KA, Shen WJ, Yang CY, et al. The use of alendronate to prevent early collapse of the femoral head in patients with nontraumatic osteonecrosis. A randomized clinical study. The Journal of bone and joint surgery American volume 2005;87:2155–9.
13. Agarwala S, Jain D, Joshi VR, et al. Efficacy of alendronate, a bisphosphonate, in the treatment of AVN of the hip. A prospective open-label study. Rheumatology (Oxford) 2005;44:352–9.
14. Agarwala S, Shah SB. Ten-year follow-up of avascular necrosis of femoral head treated with alendronate for 3 years. The Journal of arthroplasty 2011;26:1128–34.
15. Agarwala S, Shah S, Joshi VR. The use of alendronate in the treatment of avascular necrosis of the femoral head: follow-up to eight years. The Journal of bone and joint surgery British volume 2009;91:1013–8.
16. Rodan GA, Fleisch HA. Bisphosphonates: mechanisms of action. The Journal of clinical investigation 1996;97:2692–6.
17. Hernigou P, Poignard A, Nogier A, et al. Fate of very small asymptomatic stage-I osteonecrotic lesions of the hip. The Journal of bone and joint surgery American volume 2004;86-A:2589–93.
18. Chen CH, Chang JK, Lai KA, et al. Alendronate in the prevention of collapse of the femoral head in nontraumatic osteonecrosis: a two-year multicenter, prospective, randomized, double-blind, placebo-controlled study. Arthritis and rheumatism 2012;64:1572–8.
19. Glueck CJ, Freiberg RA, Wang P. Role of thrombosis in osteonecrosis. Current hematology reports 2003;2:417–22.
20. Glueck CJ, Freiberg RA, Sieve L, et al. Enoxaparin prevents progression of stages I and II osteonecrosis of the hip. Clinical orthopaedics and related research 2005;164–70.
21. Zhao FC, Li ZR, Guo KJ. Clinical analysis of osteonecrosis of the femoral head induced by steroids. Orthopaedic surgery 2012;4:28–34.
22. Wolverton SE. Can short courses of systemic corticosteroids truly cause osteonecrosis? Dermatologic therapy 2009;22:458–64.
23. Weldon D. The effects of corticosteroids on bone: osteonecrosis (avascular necrosis of the bone). Annals of allergy, asthma & immunology: official publication of the American College of Allergy, Asthma, & Immunology 2009;103:91–7 [quiz 7-100], 33.
24. Weinstein RS. Glucocorticoid-induced osteonecrosis. Endocrine 2012;41:183–90.
25. Cui Q, Wang GJ, Balian G. Steroid-induced adipogenesis in a pluripotential cell line from bone marrow. The Journal of bone and joint surgery American volume 1997;79:1054–63.
26. Li X, Jin L, Cui Q, et al. Steroid effects on osteogenesis through mesenchymal cell gene expression. Osteoporosis international: a journal established as result of cooperation between the European Foundation for Osteoporosis and the National Osteoporosis Foundation of the USA 2005;16:101–8.

27. Drescher W, Weigert KP, Bunger MH, et al. Femoral head blood flow reduction and hypercoagulability under 24 h megadose steroid treatment in pigs. Journal of orthopaedic research: official publication of the Orthopaedic Research Society 2004; 22:501–8.

28. Drescher W, Bunger MH, Weigert K, et al. Methylprednisolone enhances contraction of porcine femoral head epiphyseal arteries. Clinical orthopaedics and related research 2004;112–7.

29. Wang GJ, Cui Q, Balian G. The Nicolas Andry award. The pathogenesis and prevention of steroid-induced osteonecrosis. Clinical orthopaedics and related research 2000;295–310.

30. Pritchett JW. Statin therapy decreases the risk of osteonecrosis in patients receiving steroids. Clinical orthopaedics and related research 2001; 173–8.

31. Ajmal M, Matas AJ, Kuskowski M, et al. Does statin usage reduce the risk of corticosteroid-related osteonecrosis in renal transplant population? The Orthopedic clinics of North America 2009;40: 235–9.

32. Alves EM, Angrisani AT, Santiago MB. The use of extracorporeal shock waves in the treatment of osteonecrosis of the femoral head: a systematic review. Clinical rheumatology 2009;28:1247–51.

33. Ludwig J, Lauber S, Lauber HJ, et al. High-energy shock wave treatment of femoral head necrosis in adults. Clinical orthopaedics and related research 2001;119–26.

34. Wang CJ, Huang CC, Wang JW, et al. Long-term results of extracorporeal shockwave therapy and core decompression in osteonecrosis of the femoral head with eight- to nine-year follow-up. Biomedical journal 2012;35:481–5.

35. Hsu SL, Wang CJ, Lee MS, et al. Cocktail therapy for femoral head necrosis of the hip. Archives of orthopaedic and trauma surgery 2010;130:23–9.

36. Wang CJ, Ko JY, Chan YS, et al. Extracorporeal shockwave for hip necrosis in systemic lupus erythematosus. Lupus 2009;18:1082–6.

37. Massari L, Fini M, Cadossi R, et al. Biophysical stimulation with pulsed electromagnetic fields in osteonecrosis of the femoral head. The Journal of bone and joint surgery American volume 2006; 88(Suppl 3):56–60.

38. Reis ND, Schwartz O, Militianu D, et al. Hyperbaric oxygen therapy as a treatment for stage-I avascular necrosis of the femoral head. The Journal of bone and joint surgery British volume 2003;85: 371–5.

39. Camporesi EM, Vezzani G, Bosco G, et al. Hyperbaric oxygen therapy in femoral head necrosis. The Journal of arthroplasty 2010;25:118–23.

40. Jager M, Tillmann FP, Thornhill TS, et al. Rationale for prostaglandin I2 in bone marrow oedema–from theory to application. Arthritis research & therapy 2008;10:R120.

41. Disch AC, Matziolis G, Perka C. The management of necrosis-associated and idiopathic bone-marrow oedema of the proximal femur by intravenous iloprost. The Journal of bone and joint surgery British volume 2005;87:560–4.

42. Lavernia CJ, Sierra RJ. Core decompression in atraumatic osteonecrosis of the hip. The Journal of arthroplasty 2000;15:171–8.

43. Marker DR, Seyler TM, Ulrich SD, et al. Do modern techniques improve core decompression outcomes for hip osteonecrosis? Clinical orthopaedics and related research 2008;466:1093–103.

44. Mont MA, Ragland PS, Etienne G. Core decompression of the femoral head for osteonecrosis using percutaneous multiple small-diameter drilling. Clinical orthopaedics and related research 2004; 131–8.

45. Song WS, Yoo JJ, Kim YM, et al. Results of multiple drilling compared with those of conventional methods of core decompression. Clinical orthopaedics and related research 2007;454:139–46.

46. Lee MS, Hsieh PH, Chang YH, et al. Elevated intraosseous pressure in the intertrochanteric region is associated with poorer results in osteonecrosis of the femoral head treated by multiple drilling. The Journal of bone and joint surgery British volume 2008;90:852–7.

47. Buckley PD, Gearen PF, Petty RW. Structural bone-grafting for early atraumatic avascular necrosis of the femoral head. The Journal of bone and joint surgery American volume 1991;73: 1357–64.

48. Israelite C, Nelson CL, Ziarani CF, et al. Bilateral core decompression for osteonecrosis of the femoral head. Clinical orthopaedics and related research 2005;441:285–90.

49. Plakseychuk AY, Kim SY, Park BC, et al. Vascularized compared with nonvascularized fibular grafting for the treatment of osteonecrosis of the femoral head. The Journal of bone and joint surgery American volume 2003;85-A:589–96.

50. Seyler TM, Marker DR, Ulrich SD, et al. Nonvascularized bone grafting defers joint arthroplasty in hip osteonecrosis. Clinical orthopaedics and related research 2008;466:1125–32.

51. Urbaniak JR, Coogan PG, Gunneson EB, et al. Treatment of osteonecrosis of the femoral head with free vascularized fibular grafting. A long-term follow-up study of one hundred and three hips. The Journal of bone and joint surgery American volume 1995;77:681–94.

52. Yoo MC, Kim KI, Hahn CS, et al. Long-term followup of vascularized fibular grafting for femoral head necrosis. Clinical orthopaedics and related research 2008;466:1133–40.

53. Eward WC, Rineer CA, Urbaniak JR, et al. The vascularized fibular graft in precollapse osteonecrosis: is long-term hip preservation possible? Clinical orthopaedics and related research 2012;470: 2819-26.

54. Lieberman JR, Conduah A, Urist MR. Treatment of osteonecrosis of the femoral head with core decompression and human bone morphogenetic protein. Clinical orthopaedics and related research 2004;139-45.

55. Hernigou P, Poignard A, Zilber S, et al. Cell therapy of hip osteonecrosis with autologous bone marrow grafting. Indian journal of orthopaedics 2009;43: 40-5.

56. Hernigou P, Daltro G, Filippini P, et al. Percutaneous implantation of autologous bone marrow osteoprogenitor cells as treatment of bone avascular necrosis related to sickle cell disease. The open orthopaedics journal 2008;2:62-5.

57. Hernigou P, Poignard A, Manicom O, et al. The use of percutaneous autologous bone marrow transplantation in nonunion and avascular necrosis of bone. The Journal of bone and joint surgery British volume 2005;87:896-902.

58. Gangji V, De Maertelaer V, Hauzeur JP. Autologous bone marrow cell implantation in the treatment of non-traumatic osteonecrosis of the femoral head: Five year follow-up of a prospective controlled study. Bone 2011;49:1005-9.

59. Liu Y, Liu S, Su X. Core decompression and implantation of bone marrow mononuclear cells with porous hydroxylapatite composite filler for the treatment of osteonecrosis of the femoral head. Archives of orthopaedic and trauma surgery 2013; 133:125-33.

60. Zhao D, Cui D, Wang B, et al. Treatment of early stage osteonecrosis of the femoral head with autologous implantation of bone marrow-derived and cultured mesenchymal stem cells. Bone 2012;50: 325-30.

61. Sen RK, Tripathy SK, Aggarwal S, et al. Early results of core decompression and autologous bone marrow mononuclear cells instillation in femoral head osteonecrosis: a randomized control study. The Journal of arthroplasty 2012;27:679-86.

62. Sugioka Y, Hotokebuchi T, Tsutsui H. Transtrochanteric anterior rotational osteotomy for idiopathic and steroid-induced necrosis of the femoral head. Indications and long-term results. Clinical orthopaedics and related research 1992;111-20.

63. Ito H, Tanino H, Yamanaka Y, et al. Long-term results of conventional varus half-wedge proximal femoral osteotomy for the treatment of osteonecrosis of the femoral head. The Journal of bone and joint surgery British volume 2012;94:308-14.

64. Sugioka Y, Katsuki I, Hotokebuchi T. Transtrochanteric rotational osteotomy of the femoral head for

the treatment of osteonecrosis. Follow-up statistics. Clinical orthopaedics and related research 1982; 115-26.

65. Sugioka Y. Transtrochanteric anterior rotational osteotomy of the femoral head in the treatment of osteonecrosis affecting the hip: a new osteotomy operation. Clinical orthopaedics and related research 1978;191-201.

66. Hasegawa Y, Sakano S, Iwase T, et al. Pedicle bone grafting versus transtrochanteric rotational osteotomy for avascular necrosis of the femoral head. The Journal of bone and joint surgery British volume 2003;85:191-8.

67. Zhao G, Yamamoto T, Ikemura S, et al. Clinico-radiological factors affecting the joint space narrowing after transtrochanteric anterior rotational osteotomy for osteonecrosis of the femoral head. Journal of orthopaedic science: official journal of the Japanese Orthopaedic Association 2012;17: 390-6.

68. Zhao G, Yamamoto T, Ikemura S, et al. Radiological outcome analysis of transtrochanteric curved varus osteotomy for osteonecrosis of the femoral head at a mean follow-up of 12.4 years. The Journal of bone and joint surgery British volume 2010;92: 781-6.

69. Zhao G, Yamamoto T, Motomura G, et al. Radiological outcome analyses of transtrochanteric posterior rotational osteotomy for osteonecrosis of the femoral head at a mean follow-up of 11 years. Journal of orthopaedic science: official journal of the Japanese Orthopaedic Association 2013.

70. Sakano S, Hasegawa Y, Torii Y, et al. Curved intertrochanteric varus osteotomy for osteonecrosis of the femoral head. The Journal of bone and joint surgery British volume 2004;86:359-65.

71. Issa K, Naziri Q, Rasquinha VJ, et al. Outcomes of Primary Total Hip Arthroplasty in Systemic Lupus Erythematosus With a Proximally-Coated Cementless Stem. The Journal of arthroplasty 2013.

72. Issa K, Johnson AJ, Naziri Q, et al. Hip Osteonecrosis: Does Prior Hip Surgery Alter Outcomes Compared to an Initial Primary Total Hip Arthroplasty? The Journal of arthroplasty 2013.

73. Issa K, Naziri Q, Maheshwari AV, et al. Excellent Results and Minimal Complications of Total Hip Arthroplasty in Sickle Cell Hemoglobinopathy at Mid-Term Follow-Up Using Cementless Prosthetic Components. The Journal of arthroplasty 2013.

74. Brinker MR, Rosenberg AG, Kull L, et al. Primary total hip arthroplasty using noncemented porous-coated femoral components in patients with osteonecrosis of the femoral head. The Journal of arthroplasty 1994;9:457-68.

75. Piston RW, Engh CA, De Carvalho PI, et al. Osteonecrosis of the femoral head treated with total hip arthroplasty without cement. The Journal of bone

and joint surgery American volume 1994;76: 202–14.

76. Kim YH, Oh JH, Oh SH. Cementless total hip arthroplasty in patients with osteonecrosis of the femoral head. Clinical orthopaedics and related research 1995;73–84.

77. Salvati EA, Cornell CN. Long-term follow-up of total hip replacement in patients with avascular necrosis. Instructional course lectures 1988;37:67–73.

78. Taylor AH, Shannon M, Whitehouse SL, et al. Harris Galante cementless acetabular replacement in avascular necrosis. The Journal of bone and joint surgery British volume 2001;83:177–82.

79. Kim YH, Choi Y, Kim JS. Cementless total hip arthroplasty with ceramic-on-ceramic bearing in patients younger than 45 years with femoral-head osteonecrosis. International orthopaedics 2010; 34:1123–7.

80. Min BW, Lee KJ, Song KS, et al. Highly cross-linked polyethylene in total hip arthroplasty for osteonecrosis of the femoral head: a minimum 5-year follow-up study. The Journal of arthroplasty 2013;28:526–30.

81. Tsumura H, Torisu T, Kaku N, et al. Five- to fifteen-year clinical results and the radiographic evaluation of acetabular changes after bipolar hip arthroplasty for femoral head osteonecrosis. The Journal of arthroplasty 2005;20:892–7.

82. Muraki M, Sudo A, Hasegawa M, et al. Long-term results of bipolar hemiarthroplasty for osteoarthritis of the hip and idiopathic osteonecrosis of the femoral head. Journal of orthopaedic science: official journal of the Japanese Orthopaedic Association 2008;13:313–7.

83. Gross TP, Liu F. Comparative study between patients with osteonecrosis and osteoarthritis after hip resurfacing arthroplasty. Acta orthopaedica Belgica 2012;78:735–44.

84. Kabata T, Maeda T, Tanaka K, et al. Hemi-resurfacing versus total resurfacing for osteonecrosis of the femoral head. J Orthop Surg (Hong Kong) 2011;19: 177–80.

85. Nakasone S, Takao M, Sakai T, et al. Does the Extent of Osteonecrosis Affect the Survival of Hip Resurfacing? Clinical orthopaedics and related research 2013.

86. Aulakh TS, Rao C, Kuiper JH, et al. Hip resurfacing and osteonecrosis: results from an independent hip resurfacing register. Archives of orthopaedic and trauma surgery 2010;130:841–5.

87. Sayeed SA, Johnson AJ, Stroh DA, et al. Hip resurfacing in patients who have osteonecrosis and are 25 years or under. Clinical orthopaedics and related research 2011;469:1582–8.

88. Stulberg BN, Fitts SM, Zadzilka JD, et al. Resurfacing arthroplasty for patients with osteonecrosis. Bulletin of the NYU hospital for joint diseases 2009;67:138–41.

89. Mont MA, Seyler TM, Marker DR, et al. Use of metal-on-metal total hip resurfacing for the treatment of osteonecrosis of the femoral head. The Journal of bone and joint surgery American volume 2006;88(Suppl 3):90–7.

90. Johannson HR, Zywiel MG, Marker DR, et al. Osteonecrosis is not a predictor of poor outcomes in primary total hip arthroplasty: a systematic literature review. International orthopaedics 2011;35: 465–73.

91. Kim YH, Kim JS, Park JW, et al. Contemporary total hip arthroplasty with and without cement in patients with osteonecrosis of the femoral head: a concise follow-up, at an average of seventeen years, of a previous report. The Journal of bone and joint surgery American volume 2011;93: 1806–10.

Management of Labral Tears of the Hip in Young Patients

Jack G. Skendzel, MD, Marc J. Philippon, MD*

KEYWORDS

- Acetabular labrum • Femoroacetabular impingement • Labral tear • Labral repair
- Labral reconstruction

KEY POINTS

- Acetabular labral tears are an important cause of hip pain in young, athletic individuals.
- The labrum functions to enhance joint stability, maintain the "suction-seal" effect, and distribute pressure more evenly between the articulation of the femoral head and acetabulum.
- All areas of bony impingement must be addressed surgically to improve the mechanical environment and prevent further damage to the labrum and articular cartilage. A common cause of revision hip arthroscopy is a failure to address all areas of impingement.
- Surgical refixation of acetabular labral tears is an effective treatment option, with superior results in comparison with labral debridement.
- Caution must be used when placing suture anchors in the anterior acetabular rim to prevent iatrogenic damage to the articular cartilage.
- Labral reconstruction is an option in patients with a damaged labrum that cannot be debrided or repaired. Short-term follow-up of this technique shows encouraging results.

INTRODUCTION

Acetabular labral tears are recognized as an important cause of hip pain in young, athletic individuals. Acetabular labral tears were first described by Paterson[1] in 1957 after traumatic posterior hip dislocations, with a resulting bucket-handle labral tear serving as a block to a concentric reduction. Until recently, labral tears were thought to be relatively uncommon. However, advances in imaging and surgical techniques, as well as an improved understanding of hip pain, have led to increased awareness regarding labral tears and other pathologic conditions around the hip joint. The prevalence of labral tears in painful hips has been reported to be 22% to 55%,[2–4] and Register and colleagues[5] recently identified labral tears present in 69% of asymptomatic hips. Historically, treatment of labral lesions consisted of nonoperative measures or a partial excision performed through an anterior arthrotomy.[6] Although Harris and colleagues[7] suggested that an "intra-acetabular labrum" with degenerative labral changes could lead to the development of hip osteoarthritis, it was not until much later that Ganz and colleagues[8,9] described femoroacetabular impingement (FAI), and the relationship of bony abnormalities of the acetabular rim and femoral head-neck junction with labral tears

---

Disclosures: Dr M.J. Philippon receives consulting/royalty payments from Smith & Nephew, Arthrosurface, HIPCO, MIS, Bledose, DonJoy, and Slack, and research and other financial support from Smith & Nephew, Ossur, Arthrex, and Siemens. Dr J.G. Skendzel has no conflicts of interest.
Relationships: There are no commercial companies that have a direct financial interest in the subject matter or materials discussed in the article.
The Steadman Philippon Research Institute, Center for Outcomes-Based Orthopaedic Research, 181 West Meadow Drive, Suite 1000, Vail, CO 81657, USA
* Corresponding author.
E-mail address: drphilippon@sprivail.org

Orthop Clin N Am 44 (2013) 477–487
http://dx.doi.org/10.1016/j.ocl.2013.06.003
0030-5898/13/$ – see front matter © 2013 Elsevier Inc. All rights reserved.

and hip osteoarthritis. The investigators theorized that repetitive bony impingement causes damage to both the acetabular labrum and articular cartilage. McCarthy and colleagues[4] described a possible sequence of events that leads to joint degeneration, including excessive loading of the labrum through traction or impingement, fraying of the anterior margin of the labrum, articular cartilage delamination adjacent to the labrum lesion, and more global degenerative changes that occur in both the labrum and articular cartilage. The purpose of this article is to review the anatomy of the acetabular labrum, discuss the pathogenesis of labral tears, and discuss the various treatment options available, including arthroscopic labral repair and reconstruction.

ANATOMY AND FUNCTION OF THE ACETABULAR LABRUM

The hip is a ball-and-socket joint that is inherently stable, owing to highly constrained osseous anatomy. The labrum is a fibrocartilage structure that runs circumferentially around the margin of the acetabular rim and is attached to the transverse acetabular ligament both anteriorly and posteriorly. It has numerous functions, including maintenance of joint lubrication and the "suction-seal" effect, enhancement of joint stability, and protection of articular cartilage through improved distribution of pressure across the articulation between the femoral head and acetabulum.[10] The labrum increases the effective depth of the bony acetabulum and provides stability to the femoral head while increasing the effective amount of femoral-head coverage. It contributes, on average, up to 22% of the acetabular surface area that articulates with the femoral head, and increases the volume of the acetabulum by up to 33%.[11,12] The labrum, however, has limited healing capabilities. Kelly and colleagues[13] studied the vascular supply of the labrum in a cadaveric study, showing that it is a relatively avascular structure with most vessels originating from the capsular periphery, with few reaching the more central articular-sided region. Furthermore, the distribution of vessels is not homogeneous through the labrum.[14] The presence of free nerve endings has also been reported by Kim and Azuma,[15] suggesting proprioceptive and nociceptive properties.

The labrum contributes to the suction-seal effect to improve fluid-film lubrication and maintain negative intra-articular pressure within the central compartment.[16,17] A recent cadaveric study by Cadet and colleagues[18] demonstrated significant efflux of fluid from the hip joint in the presence of a labral tear, suggesting disruption of the fluid seal effect. Although labral repair decreased the outflow of fluid from the hip joint, a repaired labrum was not shown to be as effective as the labrum-intact condition. The hip labrum has also been identified as an important secondary stabilizer in cases of simulated disruption of iliofemoral ligament, and large tensile forces have been measured in the anterior acetabular labrum during hip external rotation and abduction movements.[19,20] Smith and colleagues[21] showed that even a damaged labrum continues to provide hip stability and resist femoral-head dislocation after the creation of circumferential tears less than 3 cm in length or after creation of a 1-cm labrectomy.

LABRAL PATHOLOGY

Labral tears are most common in the presence of a structural hip abnormality such as FAI or hip dysplasia.[22–24] Recent retrospective studies have shown that between 49% and 87% of all patients with a labral tear have osseous changes consistent with FAI.[22,25,26] In addition, although labral abnormality most commonly affects the anterosuperior labrum, the pattern of injury is highly dependent on the unique morphologic "fingerprint" present in the acetabulum and proximal femur, including the external mechanical loads and the arc of motion applied to the hip.[27,28] In cases of pincer-type FAI with acetabular overcoverage, there is repetitive contact between the femoral neck and the acetabular rim, with compression of the labrum that leads to degeneration early in the process. The articular cartilage is relatively uninvolved, with chondral injury limited to a narrow margin along the acetabular rim.[28] Eventually there is ossification of the labrum and further appositional bone formation that can exacerbate the magnitude of impingement, in addition to contre-coup lesions of the posteroinferior acetabular articular cartilage and the posteromedial aspect of the femoral head.[28,29]

In cam-type FAI with loss of femoral head-neck offset, there is early damage to the articular cartilage, in contrast to the pattern seen with pincer-type FAI. During hip motion, the cam deformity is rotated into the acetabular socket with a shearing-type injury pattern and delamination of the articular cartilage. The damage is localized to the corresponding location where the abnormal head-neck junction (**Fig. 1**) and acetabular rim make contact. Eventually there is separation of the labrum from the underlying subchondral bone, occurring at the transitional zone between the labrum and hyaline cartilage (**Fig. 2**).[8,28,30] Johnston and colleagues[31] reported an association between the lack of femoral head-neck

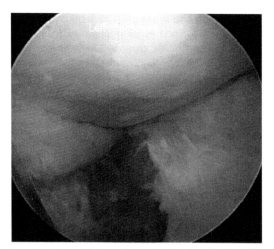

Fig. 1. View of the femoral head-neck junction showing a typical cam deformity with loss of offset.

sphericity and the size of the cam lesion with the extent of acetabular chondral damage and delamination. The investigators noted more intra-articular damage in patients with a higher α angle, including detachment of the labrum and full-thickness delamination of the articular cartilage.

Acetabular dysplasia is also responsible for pathologic changes to the labrum. The dysplastic hip is characterized by a shallow acetabulum with anterior and lateral acetabular undercoverage. In these cases, there is a shift in the normal center of contact between the femoral head and acetabulum to a more posterosuperior location, leading to pressure overload of the labrum and articular cartilage.[32,33] This shift has been associated with the premature development of osteoarthritis[34] as well as pathologic changes to the labrum, including hypertrophy, myxoid degeneration, and detachment from the acetabular rim.[27,35]

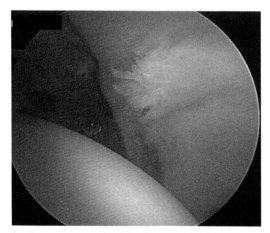

Fig. 2. Anterosuperior labral tear with delamination of the articular cartilage at the transition zone.

Lage and colleagues[36] described an arthroscopic classification for labral tears. Tears were divided into 4 categories based on the etiology: traumatic, degenerative, idiopathic, and congenital. In addition, 4 morphologic categories were used to classify labral tears: radial flap, radial fibrillated, longitudinal peripheral, and unstable. Seldes and colleagues[11] also described 2 different histologic types of labral tears, include Type 1 tears whereby there is detachment of the labrum from the articular surface at the transition zone between labrum and articular cartilage, and Type 2 tears whereby there are 1 or more cleavage planes within the substance of the labrum. Capsular laxity and psoas impingement can also lead to the development of labral tears. It is important to understand the cause of the labral tearing and ensure that all pathologic aspects are properly addressed, as poor clinical outcomes can result from a failure to adequately decompress all bony impingement at the time of surgery.[37] A summary of the various types of labral tears and the associated conditions is summarized in **Table 1**.

PATIENT HISTORY AND CLINICAL EVALUATION

A thorough history is important in making the correct diagnosis and determining the cause of the complaint. Most commonly, patients with labral tears will present with groin pain that is exacerbated by hip flexion. The exact location of the pain and any exacerbating or relieving factors is important in helping to narrow the differential diagnosis. A characteristic sign in patients with labral tears and hip impingement is the "C sign," whereby the patient holds his or her hand in the shape of a C proximal to the greater trochanter with the thumb directed posteriorly and the fingers pointing anteriorly toward the groin. This sign often indicates pain deep within the hip joint. The clinician must determine if there is a history of trauma that may have caused labral injury, or if the

Table 1
Classification of labral tears

Type	Underlying Condition
1. Morphologic alterations	A. Femoroacetabular impingement (cam, pincer, or mixed type) B. Dysplasia
2. Functional alterations	A. Instability B. Iliopsoas impingement
3. Trauma	Traumatic
4. Degeneration	Degenerative joint disease

symptoms are insidious in nature. Young athletes may also complain of mechanical symptoms such as locking, catching, or clicking. Certain sporting activities are highly associated with labral tearing, including football, hockey, skiing, bicycling, and dancing.[38,39] Pain may also be present with activities of daily living, such as putting on shoes and socks or getting in and out of a car. Radicular symptoms can also be confused with groin pain from a labral tear, and disorders of the gastrointestinal, genitourinary, and vascular systems can all cause referred pain to the hip and groin.[40] Pain over the lateral aspect of the hip suggests greater trochanteric bursitis and possible tightness of the iliotibial band. The clinician must also recognize that in patients with hip laxity there is greater reliance on the surrounding hip musculature to act as secondary stabilizers; therefore, these structures may become overused and tender or weakened on physical examination.

In young patients with a suspected labral tear, the clinical examination should focus on evaluation of gait and posture, active and passive range of motion of the lower extremities, and an assessment of the neurovascular structures. In the standing position, the presence of a Trendelenburg gait indicates weakness of the hip abductor muscles. A shortened stance phase indicates an antalgic gait caused by a painful extremity. Range of motion and strength testing should be performed in the bilateral extremities, and any differences noted. Mechanical symptoms including catching, clicking, or popping suggest intra-articular abnormality, such as damage to the articular cartilage, labral damage, or a loose body. In addition, a snapping iliotibial band over the greater trochanter or the iliopsoas tendon over the pelvic brim can cause a popping sensation with a circumduction motion of the hip. Several special tests have been described for evaluation of the hip in the supine position, including the FADDIR test, whereby the hip is moved into flexion, adduction, and internal rotation to recreate the patient's pain and to measure the amount of flexion and internal rotation; the Thomas test for psoas tightness; and the Patrick or FABER test to differentiate sacroiliac/lumbar spine abnormality from hip problems. Capsular laxity is assessed with the hip dial test, performed in the supine position.[41,42] All patients should also be examined for signs of systemic ligamentous laxity according to the criteria of Beighton and colleagues.[43] A thorough physical examination with provocative testing to recreate the location and intensity of the patient's pain is critical in understanding the underlying abnormality, including labral tears and any associated injuries to the surrounding structures.

A thorough and systematic radiographic examination is performed in all patients with hip pain and suspected labral disorder, including anteroposterior (AP) pelvis, cross-table lateral, and false-profile plain radiographic views of the involved hip. The AP pelvis is evaluated for the outline of the acetabular lines, and any pathologic features such as the presence of a crossover sign, whereby the outlines of the anterior and posterior acetabular wall cross to form a figure-of-8 pattern. This sign indicates relative anterior acetabular overcoverage. Global acetabular overcoverage, as seen in coxa profunda and coxa protrusio deformities, is suspected when the floor of the acetabular fossa touches or passes medially to the ilioischial line. On the cross-table lateral view, the α angle is measured to evaluate for cam-type FAI and any loss of femoral head-neck offset.[44] Anterior acetabular overcoverage or undercoverage and joint-space narrowing in the posteroinferior acetabular are assessed on the false-profile view. Magnetic resonance imaging (MRI) or magnetic resonance arthrography is often used in young patients with a painful hip to evaluate the acetabular labrum, joint capsule, articular cartilage, and periarticular structures.[45–47]

NONOPERATIVE TREATMENT

There is a paucity of evidence to support the nonoperative treatment of acetabular labral tears in young patients.[48] Philippon and colleagues[49] reported that early intervention for labral abnormality may lead to improved results, as shown in a cohort of professional hockey players where those who underwent intervention within 1 year from the time of injury returned to play earlier than those who waited. Simple measures such as activity modification and preventing provocative positions such as hip flexion and interior rotation can improve pain and prevent further episodes of impingement. Focused physical therapy and nonsteroidal anti-inflammatory drugs (NSAIDs) can be used initially, and can be combined with physical therapy for 10 to 12 weeks.[2] Greater trochanteric bursitis and a snapping iliopsoas are managed with rest/activity modification, NSAIDs, and stretching. Corticosteroid injections into the bursa can be administered if needed.[50,51] Intra-articular steroid injections may also be beneficial, especially in patients who have pain that is not responsive to nonoperative treatments.

Physical therapy can be used in patients with hip pain and labral tears to decrease pain and improve function. Casartelli and colleagues[52] compared hip-muscle strength testing and hip-flexor electromyography in 22 patients with FAI and compared the results with those of healthy, age-matched controls during active hip flexion. Whereas there was significant weakness in the FAI group when compared with the healthy controls, in particular of the abductions, adductors, hip flexors, and external rotators, there was no significant difference in the strength of hip internal rotators and extensors. Although the weakness observed could be due to many factors (eg, atrophy, reduced muscle activation, pain), these results may aid in the development of specific rehabilitation and therapy protocols to improve strength in those with FAI. Yazbek[48] described a nonsurgical therapy program used in 4 patients with clinical and MRI findings consistent with a labral tear. The rehabilitation protocol emphasized stabilization of the hip and lumbopelvic regions with correction of muscular imbalance, biomechanical control, and sport-specific functional progression. All patients showed an overall decrease in pain and an increase in function, correction of muscular imbalances, and improved muscle strength of the hip flexors, abductors, and extensors. Patients who fail to improve after a trial of nonoperative treatment are candidates for arthroscopic treatment.

OPERATIVE TREATMENT

There are several surgical treatment options available for the young patient with FAI. Both open surgical dislocation[53–55] and arthroscopic procedures[56–60] have demonstrated excellent short-term and mid-term results, including the ability to return to sports. It is critical that the clinician perform a thorough history and physical examination, and obtain the necessary imaging studies to identify not only labral abnormality but also osseous abnormalities such as FAI or dysplasia, in addition to damage to the articular cartilage, the ligamentum teres, and surrounding soft-tissue structures. The concomitant pathologic features must be addressed to achieve a successful outcome.[37] The goal of arthroscopic surgery is to correct the labral abnormality and relieve mechanical impingement, as well as address associated intra-articular abnormality.

There are several surgical options available to address labral lesions, including debridement, repair, or reconstruction. Improved clinical outcomes have been reported after either open or arthroscopic labral debridement.[61–64] Encouraging results for labral refixation have also been published. Espinosa and colleagues[54] retrospectively reported the results after labral resection or labral refixation in a series of patients who underwent open surgical dislocation for symptomatic FAI. Patients treated with labral refixation recovered

earlier and had superior clinical and radiographic outcomes when compared with the patients who had resection of the torn acetabular labrum. In 2009, Larson and Giveans[60] performed a similar study to compare the outcomes after arthroscopic labral debridement with those after labral repair. At the 1-year follow-up visit the investigators demonstrated improved subjective outcomes in both groups, although the modified Harris Hip Scores (mHHS) were superior in those with refixation when compared with the debridement group. The percentage of good to excellent results was also significantly improved in the labral repair group. More recently, Larson and colleagues[65] reported results of arthroscopic labral repair at a mean 3.5 years' follow-up. While the subjective scores improved for both the repair and debridement groups, the mHHS and visual analog scale (VAS) for pain were significantly better for the refixation group at all time points, with good to excellent results noted in 92% of patients in the refixation group. In addition, Philippon and colleagues[66] performed an experimental study in an ovine model, and showed that labral repairs are capable of healing through a fibrovascular scar that originates from the joint capsule or the exposed bony attachment of the labrum. The investigators noted, however, that labral healing was incomplete in all specimens, and degenerative changes were present in 89% of the hips after 24 weeks.

Labral reconstruction is another technique that may be used to treat patients with extensive labral damage that is not amenable to debridement or repair. Techniques using autologous iliotibial (IT) band and ligamentum teres grafts have been described.[67,68] Early results on the use of labral reconstruction to improve both the mechanical environment of the hip and clinical outcomes are promising.[67,69]

Surgical Technique: Labral Repair

The senior author (M.J.P.) performs hip arthroscopy in the modified supine position, although it may also be performed in the lateral position as described by Glick and colleagues.[70] A combined spinal-epidural is used routinely for anesthesia and postoperative analgesia. All prominences are well padded, and a wide perineal post is used to distribute pressure during traction and prevent iatrogenic injury. The hip is then placed in a position of 10° flexion, 15° internal rotation, 10° of lateral tilt, and neutral abduction. Traction is then applied to the operative leg on the magnitude of 25 to 50 lb (11.3–22.7 kg), with gentle countertraction being applied to the nonoperative extremity. After traction is applied, the operative leg is slightly adducted to force the femoral head laterally. The leg is internally rotated to align the femoral neck parallel to the floor. Fluoroscopy is used to confirm a "vacuum sign" and approximately 8 to 10 mm of distraction. Anatomic landmarks are identified, including the outline of the greater trochanter and the anterior inferior iliac spine (AIIS). The portals are then marked, and the hip area prepped and draped.

It is important to create arthroscopic portals in a reliable and safe fashion to avoid injury to nerves and blood vessels, in addition to the labrum and articular cartilage. Improper placement can also compromise adequate visualization during the procedure. The senior author uses 2 arthroscopic portals routinely, the anterolateral and mid-anterior portals. The anterolateral portal is established 1 cm proximal and 1 cm anterior to the tip of the greater trochanter. The mid-anterior portal is established 6 to 7 cm distal to the anterolateral portal at a 45° to 60° angle with respect to the longitudinal line passing through the anterolateral portal. The anterolateral portal is established first, followed by the mid-anterior portal, under direct arthroscopic visualization using a 70° arthroscope.

An interportal capsulotomy is performed next to improve passage of instruments and mobility within the joint. Care is taken to limit the medial extension of the capsulotomy to preserve the integrity of the iliofemoral ligament and prevent destabilization of the joint. The nature of the labral tear and the quality of the tissue are then assessed. Nonviable tissue can be removed with an arthroscopic shaver to improve visualization; often, a previously unrecognized flap or area of chondral delamination becomes visible. A treatment decision is then made (**Table 2**) based on the intraoperative findings. In all cases, as much labral tissue as possible is preserved. Isolated labral debridement is used only in cases of a small peripheral tear where enough tissue can be retained to preserve normal labral function.

The acetabular rim is then prepared and trimmed with the use of a motorized burr until a bleeding bed is visible. The labrum can be detached with a Beaver blade from the acetabular rim, or the surgeon may elect to leave the chondrolabral junction intact and work behind the labrum to remove the pincer lesion. Any unstable areas created by removal of the bony overhang (pincer lesion) can be treated with placement of a suture anchor. For each patient, the center edge angle is measured preoperatively so that the surgeon can resect the proper amount of bone and prevent iatrogenic instability. The cam lesion is addressed with an osteochondroplasty of the head-neck junction and is performed in the peripheral compartment.

The labrum is reattached to the rim using suture anchors that are placed into pilot holes drilled approximately 2 to 3 mm below the articular cartilage surface under direct visualization (**Fig. 3**). For most patients, 2.3-mm bioabsorbable anchors (**Fig. 4**) are placed for every 1 cm of labral detachment, on average. The most anterior portion of the labral tear is addressed first, and anchors are sequentially placed moving posteriorly. For labral tears extending anteriorly (to the 3-o'clock or 9-o'clock position), a small cut is made in the iliofemoral ligament to access the acetabular rim, instead of extending the existing capsulotomy and disrupting the fibers of the iliofemoral ligament. Care is taken to prevent penetration of the articular cartilage with the drill, especially when working in the anterosuperior aspect of the acetabulum.[71] When drilling the path for the anchor, the articular surface must be visualized to ensure there is no iatrogenic damage; if there is bubbling on the surface the drill is removed and redirected. When repairing anterior labral tears, most anchors are delivered through the mid-anterior portal, whereas posterior tears are accessed through the anterolateral portal. Fluoroscopy can be used to ensure optimal anchor placement. Again, when the anchor is placed the articular surface is visualized to verify it has not been damaged.

Once the anchors are placed, the sutures are tied for refixation of the labrum to the acetabular rim. A clear 8.25-mm cannula is placed through the working portal, and the sutures are drawn

Table 2
Treatment algorithm for acetabular labral tears

Size of Labrum	Detached	Degenerated	Bruised	Torn
Large labrum	Repair	Debride if enough tissue	Rim trimming and labral refixation	Repair or debride if enough tissue
Small labrum	Repair and reconstruct	Rim trimming and labral reconstruction	Osteoplasty for treatment of cam lesion	Repair and reconstruct

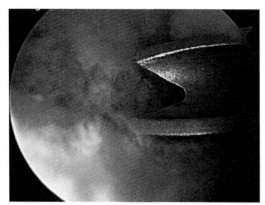

Fig. 3. A guide is placed through the anterolateral portal onto the acetabular rim below the articular surface.

through the cannula to ensure there is no entrapment of soft tissue. The sutures can be looped around the labrum or passed through it in a pierced fashion. This decision is based on the tissue quality and the desired final position of the labrum. In every case, the labrum should not be significantly everted to maintain a proper suction-seal effect with the femoral head. As a general guide, looped sutures will evert the labrum and pierced sutures will invert the labrum. If the labrum is hypotrophic, looped sutures are typically used to prevent tearing through the labrum with the arthroscopic suture penetrator. The suture limb closest to the labrum is passed between the labrum and acetabular rim with a suture passer. This suture is then either retrieved over the labrum for a looped-type repair, or retrieved through the labrum with a suture penetrator placed in its mid-substance in an outside-in fashion for a pierced-type repair. To prevent iatrogenic injury to the cartilage, the knots are

tied and placed on the capsular side of the labrum using standard arthroscopic knot-tying techniques (**Fig. 5**). The traction can be let down if necessary to evaluate the seal of the labrum on the femoral head (**Fig. 6**).

Surgical Technique: Labral Reconstruction

When the labrum cannot be repaired, an arthroscopic labral reconstruction using an IT band autograft, developed by the senior author (M.J.P.), may be performed to restore the labral seal and preserve physiologic hip function.[67] Indications for labral reconstruction includes cases of hypotrophic labrum (width less than 5 mm) caused by an anatomic variant or previous debridement, complex tears that completely disrupt the longitudinal fibers, and any circumstance whereby there is not enough tissue for labral repair.

A stable rim must be present to accommodate the graft (**Fig. 7**). Any residual bony overhang is removed with a motorized burr, and a bleeding cancellous bed is created for refixation of the graft and to allow for healing of the graft to the bone. The amount of labral deficiency is measured using the tip of the 5.5-mm motorized burr as a reference; this determines the size of the graft to be harvested. The hip is let out of traction and with the leg straight and internally rotated, a longitudinal incision is made just distal to the anterolateral portal over the greater trochanter. Sharp dissection is carried down until the IT band is exposed. The graft is harvested from the junction of the anterior two-thirds and posterior one-third of the IT band in the shape of a rectangle. The graft is typically 15 to 20 mm in width, and the longitudinal axis of the graft should be 130% to 140% of the intra-articular distance measured. The graft is brought to the back table and prepared. The

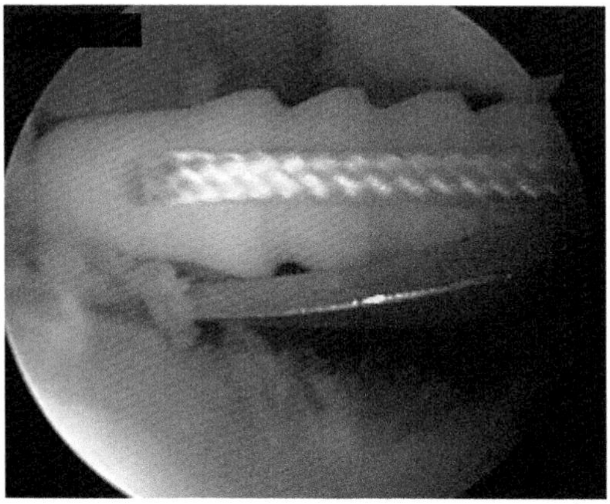

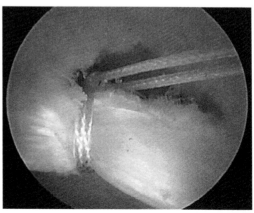

Fig. 4. After a pilot hole is drilled through the guide, a bioabsorbable anchor is impacted into place.

Fig. 5. An arthroscopic knot is tied on the capsular side of the labrum.

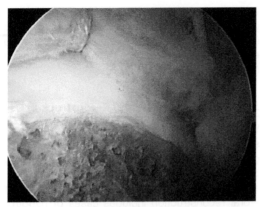

Fig. 6. After anchor placement, the traction is let down and the seal effect of the labrum on the femoral head is assessed.

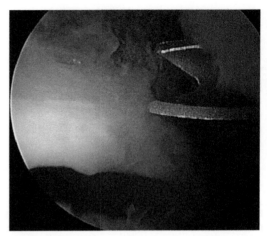

Fig. 8. The first suture anchor is placed at the anterior edge of the prepared surface to anchor the tubularized graft in place.

defect in the IT band is closed, and if indicated at this time a trochanteric bursectomy can be performed. All muscular and fatty tissue is removed, and sutures are placed at each end of the graft to capture it and allow for tensioning. The graft is tubularized with sutures, and a loop of suture is placed at the thickest lateral edge of the graft to maneuver the graft into the correct position. The graft is then bathed in platelet-rich plasma to enhance healing potential.

The leg is again placed in traction, and a suture anchor is placed at the anterior edge of the labral defect on the acetabular rim (**Fig. 8**). One limb of this suture is then placed through the graft outside of the joint using a free needle. A knot is then tied and pushed along with the graft using an arthroscopic knot pusher through an 8.25-mm clear cannula placed through the mid-anterior portal. A

second suture anchor is then placed at the posterior aspect of the defect through the anterolateral portal. The graft is fixed posteriorly using the previously placed looped suture at the proximal end of the IT band graft (**Fig. 9**). The other suture limb can be used to pierce the native edge of the intact labrum to create a side-to-side repair. Additional anchors are placed 1 cm apart around the acetabular rim until stable fixation is achieved. Traction is released and the sealing effect of the labrum tested during a dynamic examination. A flexible radiofrequency device can be used to remove frayed edges and ensure a smooth graft.

Rehabilitation After Labral Treatment

A standard rehabilitation protocol is used for all patients after labral repair or reconstruction.

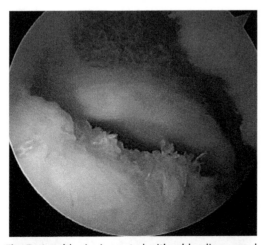

Fig. 7. A stable rim is created with a bleeding cancellous bed to accommodate the graft and allow for healing.

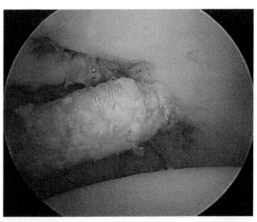

Fig. 9. A second suture anchor is placed posteriorly and is fixed to the suture loop at the proximal end of the graft.

Patients are encouraged to ride a stationary bike with no resistance, postoperatively on the day of surgery. Patients are restricted to 20 lb (9 kg) flat-foot weight bearing for 2 weeks, and this time is increased to 8 weeks if a microfracture is performed. Continuous passive motion is used for 4 hours per day for the first 2 weeks. An antirotation bolster is used to prevent external rotation of the hip while sleeping, and a hip brace is worn during the day to restrict external rotation and extension for 14 to 21 days after surgery. Circumduction exercises are performed to prevent adhesions. Endurance strengthening is started only after full motion is achieved.

SUMMARY

Recent advances in imaging and surgical techniques, as well as an improved understanding of hip pain, have led to increased awareness regarding labral tears and other pathologic conditions around the hip joint. Successful outcomes in patients with labral tears require a thoughtful approach by the clinician, including recognition of any bony impingement or dysplasia, understanding the characteristics and pattern of the labral tear, and the technical capability of performing a labral repair or reconstruction if indicated. Labral tissue should be preserved whenever possible through repair, and labral reconstruction should be used when sufficient labral tissue for repair is absent. The goal in all cases is to recreate the suction-seal effect, improve the intra-articular environment, reduce pain, and return the patients to daily activities and sport.

REFERENCES

1. Paterson I. The torn acetabular labrum. J Bone Joint Surg Br 1957;39:306–9.
2. Groh MM, Herrera J. A comprehensive review of hip labral tears. Curr Rev Musculoskelet Med 2009;2(2):105–17.
3. Narvani AA, Tsiridis E, Kendall S, et al. A preliminary report on prevalence of acetabular labrum tears in sports patients with groin pain. Knee Surg Sports Traumatol Arthrosc 2003;11(6): 403–8.
4. McCarthy JC, Noble PC, Schuck MR, et al. The Otto E. Aufranc Award: the role of labral lesions to development of early degenerative hip disease. Clin Orthop Relat Res 2001;393:25–37.
5. Register B, Pennock AT, Ho CP, et al. Prevalence of abnormal hip findings in asymptomatic participants: a prospective, blinded study. Am J Sports Med 2012;40(12):2720–4.
6. Altenberg AR. Acetabular labrum tears: a cause of hip pain and degenerative arthritis. South Med J 1977;70:174–5.
7. Harris WH, Bourne RB, Oh I. Intra-articular acetabular labrum: a possible etiological factor in certain cases of osteoarthritis of the hip. J Bone Joint Surg Am 1979;61(4):510–4.
8. Ganz R, Parvizi J, Beck M, et al. Femoroacetabular impingement: a cause for osteoarthritis of the hip. Clin Orthop Relat Res 2003;417:112–20.
9. Ganz R, Leunig M, Leunig-Ganz K, et al. The etiology of osteoarthritis of the hip. Clin Orthop Relat Res 2008;466:264–72.
10. Crawford MJ, Dy CJ, Alexander JW, et al. The 2007 Frank Stinchfield Award. The biomechanics of the hip labrum and the stability of the hip. Clin Orthop Relat Res 2007;465:16–22.
11. Seldes RM, Tan V, Hunt J, et al. Anatomy, histologic features, and vascularity of the adult acetabular labrum. Clin Orthop Relat Res 2001;382:232–40.
12. Tan V, Seldes RM, Katz MA, et al. Contribution of acetabular labrum to articulating surface area and femoral head coverage in adult hip joints: an anatomic study in cadavera. Am J Orthop 2001; 30:809–12.
13. Kelly BT, Shapiro GS, DiGiovanni CW, et al. Vascularity of the hip labrum: a cadaveric investigation. Arthroscopy 2005;21:3–11.
14. Petersen W, Petersen F, Tillmann B. Structure and vascularization of the acetabular labrum with regard to the pathogenesis and healing of labral lesions. Arch Orthop Trauma Surg 2003;123:283–8.
15. Kim YT, Azuma H. The nerve endings of the acetabular labrum. Clin Orthop Relat Res 1995; 320:176–81.
16. Ferguson SJ, Bryant JT, Ganz R, et al. The acetabular labrum seal: a poroelastic finite element model. Clin Biomech (Bristol, Avon) 2000;15:463–8.
17. Ferguson SJ, Bryant JT, Ganz R, et al. The influence of the acetabular labrum on hip joint cartilage consolidation: a poroelastic finite element model. J Biomech 2000;33:953–60.
18. Cadet ER, Chan AK, Vorys GC, et al. Investigation of the preservation of the fluid seal effect in the repaired, partially resected, and reconstructed acetabular labrum in a cadaveric hip model. Am J Sports Med 2012;40:2218–23.
19. Myers CA, Register BC, Lertwanich P, et al. Role of the acetabular labrum and the iliofemoral ligament in hip stability: an in vitro biplane fluoroscopy study. Am J Sports Med 2011;39:85S–91S.
20. Dy CJ, Thompson MT, Crawford MJ, et al. Tensile strain in the anterior part of the acetabular labrum during provocative maneuvering of the normal hip. J Bone Joint Surg Am 2008;90:1464–72.
21. Smith MV, Panchal HB, Ruberte Thiele RA, et al. Effect of acetabular labrum tears on hip stability and

labral strain in a joint compression model. Am J Sports Med 2011;39:103S–10S.

22. Wenger DE, Kendell KR, Miner MR, et al. Acetabular labral tears rarely occur in the absence of bony abnormalities. Clin Orthop Relat Res 2004; 426:145–50.

23. Dolan MM, Heyworth BE, Bedi A, et al. CT reveals a high incidence of osseous abnormalities in hips with labral tears. Clin Orthop Relat Res 2010;469:831–8.

24. Bedi A, Dolan M, Leunig M, et al. Static and dynamic mechanical causes of hip pain. Arthroscopy 2011;27:235–51.

25. Peelle MW, Rocca Della GJ, Maloney WJ. Acetabular and femoral radiographic abnormalities associated with labral tears. Clin Orthop Relat Res 2005;441:327–33.

26. Guevara CJ, Pietrobon R, Carothers JT. Comprehensive morphologic evaluation of the hip in patients with symptomatic labral tear. Clin Orthop Relat Res 2006;453:277–85.

27. Leunig M, Werlen S, Ungersböck A, et al. Evaluation of the acetabular labrum by MR arthrography. J Bone Joint Surg Br 1997;79:230–4.

28. Beck M, Kalhor M, Leunig M, et al. Hip morphology influences the pattern of damage to the acetabular cartilage: femoroacetabular impingement as a cause of early osteoarthritis of the hip. J Bone Joint Surg Br 2005;87:1012–8.

29. Corten K, Ganz R, Chosa E, et al. Bone apposition of the acetabular rim in deep hips: a distinct finding of global pincer impingement. J Bone Joint Surg Am 2011;93:10–6.

30. Tannast M, Goricki D, Beck M, et al. Hip damage occurs at the zone of femoroacetabular impingement. Clin Orthop Relat Res 2008;466:273–80.

31. Johnston TL, Schenker ML, Briggs KK, et al. Relationship between offset angle alpha and hip chondral injury in femoroacetabular impingement. Arthroscopy 2008;24:669–75.

32. Hipp JA, Sugano N, Millis MB, et al. Planning acetabular redirection osteotomies based on joint contact pressures. Clin Orthop Relat Res 1999; 364:134–43.

33. Russell ME, Shivanna KH, Grosland NM, et al. Cartilage contact pressure elevation in dysplastic hips: a chronic overload model. J Orthop Surg Res 2006;1:6.

34. Mavcic B, Iglic A, Kralj-Iglic V, et al. Cumulative hip contact stress predicts osteoarthritis in DDH. Clin Orthop Relat Res 2008;466:884–91.

35. Klaue K, Durnin CW, Ganz R. The acetabular rim syndrome. J Bone Joint Surg Br 1991;73:423–9.

36. Lage LA, Patel JV, Villar RN. The acetabular labral tear: an arthroscopic classification. Arthroscopy 1996;12:269–72.

37. Philippon MJ, Schenker ML, Briggs KK, et al. Revision hip arthroscopy. Am J Sports Med 2007;35: 1918–21.

38. Philippon MJ, Kuppersmith DA, Wolff AB, et al. Arthroscopic findings following traumatic hip dislocation in 14 professional athletes. Arthroscopy 2009;25:169–74.

39. Mitchell JC, Giannoudis PV, Millner PA, et al. A rare fracture-dislocation of the hip in a gymnast and review of the literature. Br J Sports Med 1999;33: 283–4.

40. Hass J, Hass R. Arthrochalasis multiplex congenita; congenital flaccidity of the joints. J Bone Joint Surg Am 1958;40:663–74.

41. Philippon MJ, Shenker ML, Briggs KK. The log roll test for assessing hip capsular laxity. Presented at the 12th European Society for Sports Traumatology, Knee Surgery and Arthroscopy 2000 Congress. Innsbruck, May 24–27, 2006.

42. Philippon MJ, Zehms CT, Briggs KK. Hip instability in the athlete. Oper Tech Sports Med 2007;15:189–94.

43. Beighton P, Solomon L, Soskolne CL. Articular mobility in an African population. Ann Rheum Dis 1973;32:413–8.

44. Notzli HP, Wyss TF, Stoecklin CH, et al. The contour of the femoral head-neck junction as a predictor for the risk of anterior impingement. J Bone Joint Surg Br 2002;84:556–60.

45. Rakhra KS. Magnetic resonance imaging of acetabular labral tears. J Bone Joint Surg Am 2011;93:28–34.

46. Kramer J, Recht MP. MR arthrography of the lower extremity. Radiol Clin North Am 2002;40:1121–32.

47. Mintz DN, Hooper T, Connell D, et al. Magnetic resonance imaging of the hip: detection of labral and chondral abnormalities using noncontrast imaging. Arthroscopy 2005;21:385–93.

48. Yazbek PM. Non-surgical treatment of acetabular labrum tears: a case series. J Orthop Sports Phys Ther 2011;41:346–53.

49. Philippon MJ, Weiss DR, Kuppersmith DA, et al. Arthroscopic labral repair and treatment of femoroacetabular impingement in professional hockey players. Am J Sports Med 2010;38:99–104.

50. Farr D, Selesnick H, Janecki C, et al. Arthroscopic bursectomy with concomitant iliotibial band release for the treatment of recalcitrant trochanteric bursitis. Arthroscopy 2007;23:905.e1–5.

51. Lustenberger DP, Ng VY, Best TM, et al. Efficacy of treatment of trochanteric bursitis: a systematic review. Clin J Sport Med 2011;21:447.

52. Casartelli NC, Maffiuletti NA, Item-Glatthorn JF, et al. Hip muscle weakness in patients with symptomatic femoroacetabular impingement. Osteoarthr Cartil 2011;19:816–21.

53. Bizzini M, Notzli HP, Maffiuletti NA. Femoroacetabular impingement in professional ice hockey players: a case series of 5 athletes after open surgical decompression of the hip. Am J Sports Med 2007;35:1955–9.

54. Espinosa N, Rothenfluh DA, Beck M, et al. Treatment of femoro-acetabular impingement: preliminary results of labral refixation. J Bone Joint Surg Am 2006;88:925–35.

55. Naal FD, Miozzari HH, Wyss TF, et al. Surgical hip dislocation for the treatment of femoroacetabular impingement in high-level athletes. Am J Sports Med 2011;39:544–50.

56. Philippon M, Schenker M, Briggs K, et al. Femoroacetabular impingement in 45 professional athletes: associated pathologies and return to sport following arthroscopic decompression. Knee Surg Sports Traumatol Arthrosc 2007;15:908–14.

57. Nho SJ, Magennis EM, Singh CK, et al. Outcomes after the arthroscopic treatment of femoroacetabular impingement in a mixed group of high-level athletes. Am J Sports Med 2011;39:14S–9S.

58. Byrd JW, Jones KS. Arthroscopic management of femoroacetabular impingement in athletes. Am J Sports Med 2011;39:7S–13S.

59. Byrd JW, Jones KS. Hip arthroscopy in athletes: 10-year follow-up. Am J Sports Med 2009;37:2140–3.

60. Larson CM, Giveans MR. Arthroscopic debridement versus refixation of the acetabular labrum associated with femoroacetabular impingement. Arthroscopy 2009;25:369–76.

61. Byrd JW, Jones KS. Hip arthroscopy for labral pathology: prospective analysis with 10-year follow-up. Arthroscopy 2009;25:365–8.

62. Farjo LA, Glick JM, Sampson TG. Hip arthroscopy for acetabular labral tears. Arthroscopy 1999;15:132–7.

63. Haviv B, O'Donnell J. Arthroscopic treatment for acetabular labral tears of the hip without bony dysmorphism. Am J Sports Med 2011;39:79S–84S.

64. Santori N, Villar RN. Acetabular labral tears: result of arthroscopic partial limbectomy. Arthroscopy 2000;16:11–5.

65. Larson CM, Giveans MR, Stone RM. Arthroscopic debridement versus refixation of the acetabular labrum associated with femoroacetabular impingement: mean 3.5-year follow-up. Am J Sports Med 2012;40:1015–21.

66. Philippon MJ, Arnoczky SP, Torrie A. Arthroscopic repair of the acetabular labrum: a histologic assessment of healing in an ovine model. Arthroscopy 2007;23:376–80.

67. Philippon MJ, Briggs KK, Hay CJ, et al. Arthroscopic labral reconstruction in the hip using iliotibial band autograft: technique and early outcomes. Arthroscopy 2010;26:750–6.

68. Sierra RJ, Trousdale RT. Labral reconstruction using the ligamentum teres capitis: report of a new technique. Clin Orthop Relat Res 2008;467:753–9.

69. Walker JA, Pagnotto M, Trousdale RT, et al. Preliminary pain and function after labral reconstruction during femoroacetabular impingement surgery. Clin Orthop Relat Res 2012;470:3414–20.

70. Glick JM, Sampson TG, Gordon RB, et al. Hip arthroscopy by the lateral approach. Arthroscopy 1987;3:4–12.

71. Lertwanich P, Ejnisman L, Torry MR, et al. Defining a safety margin for labral suture anchor insertion using the acetabular rim angle. Am J Sports Med 2011;39:111S–6S.

Arthroscopy of the Hip
Factors Affecting Outcome

Joseph McCarthy, MD[a], Sean Mc Millan, DO[b],*

KEYWORDS

- Hip arthroscopy • Survivorship • Osteoarthritis • Labral tear • Femoral acetabular impingement

KEY POINTS

- The presence of preoperative osteoarthritis is the biggest predictor of failed survivorship after hip arthroscopy.
- Preservation of labral function via repair seems to have a positive effect on survivorship.
- Failure to treat underlying femoroacetabular impingement may have negatively impacted the survivorship data of early hip arthroscopy.
- Improved chondral evaluation is needed to identify underlying lesions that may lead to poor survivorship not identifiable by conventional radiographs and magnetic resonance imaging.
- Gender and age do not seem to independently affect survivorship after hip arthroscopy.
- Symptoms persisting greater than 1 year before surgery resulted in poorer outcomes.

INTRODUCTION

Hip arthroscopy is a rapidly evolving procedure that has seen an exponential increase in the number of cases performed yearly. With hip arthroscopy still in its infancy in relation to knee and shoulder arthroscopy, there are still many questions yet to be answered. Axioms that were once thought to be true regarding the indications and treatment of hip arthroscopy are continually being revised. As with the knee and shoulder before it, the hip is now graduating into treatment that was otherwise thought to only be possible through an open surgical procedure.

Within this review, the authors set out to explore factors affecting the long-term survivorship of hip arthroscopy. As currently indicated, hip arthroscopy is generally reserved for relatively young patients; its goal should be to reduce pain, return function, and prevent or stave off the definite end point of hip arthroplasty. Advances in diagnostic imaging, arthroscopic devices and instruments, as well as the ability to now begin to retrospectively look back on our previous outcomes in hip arthroscopy all provide the window for viewing into the future of this evolving frontier.

INDICATIONS OF HIP ARTHROSCOPY

When hip arthroscopy was initially begun, treatment indications were extremely limited. Reasons for these limitations, included a lack of understanding of underlying cause as well as shortcomings due to inadequate instrumentation. However, hip arthroscopy indications have expanded to include both intra-articular and extra-articular pathology; these include acetabular labral tears, femoroacetabular impingement, chondral lesions, osteochondritis dissecans, hip capsule laxity and instability, ligamentum teres injuries, infection, snapping hip syndrome, iliopsoas bursitis, and loose bodies (**Table 1**).[1] Looser indications include management of symptomatic osteoarthritis of the hip joint.[2] Despite these expanding indications, it is still imperative that the correct diagnosis be made as to the root of the problem. As has been noted, hip pathology is a spectrum, often with numerous associations that must be identified,

[a] Massachusetts General Hospital, Newton Wellesley Hospital, 55 Fruit Street, Yawkey 3B, Boston, MA 02114, USA; [b] Our Lady of Lourdes Hospital, Professional Orthopedics at Lourdes Medical Associates, 2103 Burlington-Mount Holly Road, Burlington, NJ 08016, USA
* Corresponding author.
E-mail address: mcmillansean@hotmail.com

Orthop Clin N Am 44 (2013) 489–498
http://dx.doi.org/10.1016/j.ocl.2013.06.002

Table 1
Indications for hip arthroscopy by compartment

Intra-articular	Extra-articular
Labral tear	Trochanteric bursitis
Loose bodies	Snapping hip (internal and external)
FAI: cam and/or pincer lesions	Iliopsoas bursitis
Osteochondral defects	Capsular laxity/instability
Crystalline arthropathies	
Infection	
Ligamentum injuries	

Abbreviation: FAI, femoral-acetabular. impingement.

explored, and treated appropriately to best eradicate the patients' pain.[1]

OSTEOARTHRITIS

The presence of osteoarthritis in any joint has been associated with poor long-term survivorship. Long-term studies on the knee have demonstrated that previously performed lavage of osteoarthritic knees have had outcomes that were no better than placebo.[3] Likewise, a review of the hip arthroscopy literature in the setting of osteoarthritis has generally has yielded poor Harris Hip Scores and a higher rate of conversion to total hip arthroplasty (THA).

In the authors' prior retrospective study, they reviewed 324 patients (340 hips) who underwent arthroscopy for pain and/or catching. Of 111 hips (106 patients) that had a minimum follow-up of 10 years (mean, 13 years; range, 10–20 years), they found a survivorship of 63%. The survivorship end point was determined at the time of the THA. The average nonarthritic hip score for non-THA patients was 87.3 ($\pm$12.1). The survivorship was greater for acetabular and femoral Outerbridge grades normal through II. The age at arthroscopy and Outerbridge grades independently predicted eventual THA. Gender and the presence of a labral tear did not influence long-term survivorship. In conclusion, a 20 to 60 times higher incidence of need for THA was noted in patients with a higher-grade osteoarthritis.[4]

Philippon and colleagues have written on several survivorship studies after hip arthroscopy with varying rates of THA conversion.[5] In 2008, a prospective analysis of 112 hips that underwent arthroscopy for femoroacetabular impingement (FAI) treatment had a 9% conversion rate at a mean of 16 months

(range 8–26 months). They found that preoperative modified harris hip score (mHHS), absence of joint space narrowing less than 2 mm and repair of labral pathology instead of debridement were associated with better outcomes.[5] In 2012, Philippon and colleagues[6] again examined survivorship of hip arthroscopy in a consecutive series of 153 patients aged 50 years or older who underwent treatment of FAI. Again, the length of time between arthroscopy and the need for conversion to THA was examined. Their findings revealed that conversion to THA was required in 20% of their patients. However, analysis of their 3-year follow-up data revealed survivorship of 90% in patients who had greater than 2 mm of joints space on plain radiographs. A 57% survivor rate was found in those patients with 2 mm or less. In patients who did not require THA, the mHHS and hip outcome score (HOS) scores significantly improved from 58 to 84 and 66 to 87 respectively.

Haviv and O'Donnell retrospectively reviewed 564 osteoarthritic patients that have had hip arthroscopy. Over a 7-year period, (mean follow-up of 3.2 years), they noted a 16% conversion to THA. Their findings noted that patients aged less than 55 years and with less arthritic changes had longer survivorship. Of note, the surgeon performed microfracture to any acetabular lesion that met the criteria. Importantly, patients who underwent femoral osteoplasty also had a lower conversion rate (16%) than those who did not (31%).[7]

Byrd and Jones, in their prospective 10-year follow-up, reported a 27% (14 of 52 hips) conversion rate to THA. They identified arthritis (defined as radiographic features of subchondral sclerosis or erosions, joint space narrowing, and osteophyte formation) as an indicator of poor long-term outcomes. The investigators, however, appropriately pointed out that neither the bony treatment of FAI nor labral repairs were performed on any of the patients because these current treatment options were not routinely being practiced arthroscopically at the time of surgery.[8]

Further preoperative radiologic predictors of survivorship were presented by Franco and colleagues.[9] In their analysis of 263 hips, they found the presence of subcortical acetabular cysts on preoperative magnetic resonance imaging (MRI) were 4 times more likely to require conversion to THA at 2 years. Finally, Larson and colleagues[10] noted no improvement in postoperative score measures in patients who had preoperative joint space narrowing greater than 50% or less than 2 mm of joint space remaining on plain radiographs. At a minimum 12-month follow-up on 210 patients (227 hips) treated for FAI, an overall failure rate of 52% was reported for the arthritic group, whereas the nonarthritic group was (12%). Based on their finding, the investigators noted decreased remaining joint space, advanced MRI chondral grade, and a longer duration of preoperative symptoms predicted lower scores and led to negative survivorship after hip arthroscopy.

A review of the literature for outcomes after hip arthroscopy for osteoarthritis yields scant long-term studies. Prior published studies fail to support arthroscopic intervention as beneficial for osteoarthritis, noting conversion to THA rates ranging from 9% to 37% (**Table 2**).[3–10] It should be pointed out that femoral osteoplasties and/or acetabuloplasties were not being routinely performed during many of the long-term studies because arthroscopic treatment of FAI had not grown in popularity until the midportion of the last decade. Likewise, labral repair was often not performed in these studies because many of the tears were managed with debridement. Future follow-up studies addressing both FAI treatment and survivorship after arthroscopy with higher levels of arthritis are warranted because THA conversion rates have been reported to be lower in those patients treated for FAI.[5,7,10]

OSTEOCHONDRAL DEFECTS

Osteochondral damage within the hip is often a silent lesion. Conventional radiographs often cannot identify these lesions, leaving them to be discovered during arthroscopy.[11,12] MRI arthrography has improved the identification of chondral injuries; however, lesions are still often underdiagnosed. Nevertheless, the severity of osteochondral defects can negatively impact long-term outcomes after hip arthroscopy.

In 2010, McCarthy and colleagues[4] performed a 10-year retrospective analysis of patients who underwent hip arthroscopy. It was found that patients who had Outerbridge scores of III or IV demonstrated a 20 to 58 times higher incidence of requiring a THA. Those with Outerbridge scores of O to II had zero conversions to THA and demonstrated a Modified Harris Hip Score (mHHS) of 87.3 ($\pm$12.1). It should be noted, however, that the treatment rendered to these patients did not address the pathology associated with FAI.

Byrd and Jones[8] likewise retrospectively reviewed 52 hips in 50 patients over 10 years. The spectrum of pathology treated included labral tears, osteoarthritis, chondral defects, and loose bodies. They noted a 25-point increase in the mHSS across all patients; however, they noted osteoarthritis to be a negative prognostic indicator for positive outcomes. Fourteen patients, all with noted osteoarthritis at the time of arthroscopy, were converted to THA. Underscoring the differentiation between chondral defects and arthritis was a 19-point improvement in the mHSS when patients with hallmark signs of arthritis were excluded. The investigators concluded that arthroscopic management of traumatic chondral lesions in the absence of arthritis can be quite favorable.

Philippon and colleagues[13] have reported on the successful management of full-thickness chondral lesions of the hip via microfracture. In their report on athletes, they found high success rates and high rates of returning to competitive sports. Karthikeyan and colleagues[14] were able to report the successful management of an isolate full-thickness chondral defect through microfracture. In their report, 20 hips met criteria for microfracture. At an average 17-month follow-up,

Table 2
Conversion rates to total hip arthroplasty after hip arthroscopy for osteoarthritis

	Conversion (%)	Mean Time to Conversion	Bony Procedure	Labral Procedure
McCarthy et al,[4] 2011	37	N/A	None	Debridement
Philippon et al,[19] 2008	9	16 mo	Femoral and/or acetabular	Debridement and/or repair
Philippon et al,[6] 2012	20	1.6 y	Femoral and/or acetabular	Debridement and/or repair
Haviv & O'Donnell,[7] 2010	16	1.5 y	16% of THA group 31% non-THA	7% Each of THA and non-THA groups
Byrd/Jones,[8] 2010	27	5 Patients (12–14 mo) 7 Patients (7 y or greater)	None	Debridement
Larson,[10] 2011	9	N/A	Femoral and/or acetabular	Repair

they were able to evaluate the cartilage via second-look arthroscopy, noting a 95% fill rate. Pain scores and function were also noted to have improved in the patients with successful fibrocartilage growth.

Recently, Philippon and colleagues[15] presented their findings on 5- to 7-year survivorship following hip arthroscopy for the treatment of labral pathology and FAI. They found that across 247 hips (average age of 41.7 years) the 5- and 7-year survivorship rate was 72% and 70%, respectively. However, most significant among their findings was that patients with diffuse changes in their cartilage at arthroscopy were 4.3 times more likely to undergo conversion to THA, with a survivorship at 5 years of 43%. Those patients without diffuse changes had a survivorship of 79%.

In 2004, McCarthy[16] noted that the severity of the chondral lesion has a highly correlative effect with the outcome of hip arthroscopy. Patients with an Outerbridge score of grade III or IV were 20 to 58 times more likely to require eventual THA. Osteochondral lesions are often missed during preoperative evaluation. Nevertheless, their presence has a negative effect on survivorship. Higher THA conversion rates have been found in patients identified with Outerbridge lesions of III or higher, with some conversions occurring as early as 1.4 years.[17] A lack of correlation between intraoperative Outerbridge scores and preoperative Tonnis scores has been cited repeatedly and may further necessitate the need to other preoperative predictors of long-term survivorship.[18] Horsiberger and colleagues found that preoperative radiographs and Tonnis grading were poor indicators of the intra-articular lesions actually found at the time of arthroscopy.[17] This finding again echoes the thought that early to midterm chondral damage that has yet to manifest itself into fulminant arthritis can be a setup for failed survivorship.[17] In an effort to further preoperative identifying indicators, Franco and colleagues[9] found that the presence of a subchondral acetabular cyst on presurgical MRI was noted to have higher sensitivity for predicting eventual THA conversion than other reported indicators, such as minimum joint space. Furthermore, they noted that these cysts led to similar conversion odds ratios as those reported by McCarthy and colleagues earlier.[4]

AGE

The ideal age of a hip arthroscopy candidate has been varied across the literature and from surgeon to surgeon. Hip arthroscopy has been reported on patients varying in age from as young as 11 years and as old as 82 years.[19,20] Narrow parameters may oftentimes lead to higher success rates; however, as the popularity of the procedure increases, so does the recognition and identification of patients with pathologic symptoms of FAI who may have been missed at a younger age. Although age does play a role in overall hip arthroscopy survivorship, it may also be a secondary criterion to factors such as arthritis, avascular necrosis, and FAI.

Philippon and colleagues[19] published a report on 16 patients aged 16 years or younger (mean age of 15 years) who underwent hip arthroscopy for FAI. All patients had labral pathology and cam, pincer, or mixed lesions. Seven patients were treated with suture anchor repair of the labrum and 9 with partial labral debridement. At a mean follow-up of 1.36 years, they noted excellent results, as quantified by an increase in scores of the following: mHHS (55–90), the HOS activities of daily living (ADL) (58–94), and the HOS sport (33–89). Building on that study, Fabricant and colleagues[21] retrospectively reviewed 27 hips in 21 patients 19 years of age or younger who underwent arthroscopic treatment for FAI. 24 of the 27 hips underwent cam decompression and labral pathology was addressed with either repair or debridement. At an average follow-up of 1.5 years, the mHHS demonstrated improvement by an average of 21 points, the ADL of the HOS improved by an average of 16 points, and the sports outcome subset of the HOS improved by an average of 32 points. Likewise, all patients' self-reported ability to engage in their preoperative level of athletic competition increased. Based on their short-term findings, the investigators concluded that early intervention for FAI and labral pathology in adolescents can lead to significantly improved outcomes. However, because of the relative short length of follow-up at the time of reporting, longer-term studies should be warranted to track the longevity of survivorship.

On the other end of the spectrum, Javed and O'Donnell[20] reported on 40 patients older than 60 years (mean 65, range 60–82) who underwent treatment of FAI. All patients underwent femoral osteoplasty, as well as any other indicated treatment for mechanical symptoms. Their results denoted a significant success distribution based on the level of arthritis. At a mean follow-up of 30 months (12–54 months), the mHHS improved by 19.2 points, whereas the mean non–arthritic hip score improved by 15.0 points. Conversion to THA was performed in 7 patients at a mean of 12 months (6–24 months). Of those patients converted to THA, the mean age was 63 years and higher levels of arthritis were noted to be present at time of arthroscopy. Despite this, the overall level of satisfaction was high via self-reporting.[20]

Similarly, Philippon and colleagues[6] examined survivorship of hip arthroscopy in a consecutive series of 153 patients aged 50 years or older who underwent treatment of FAI. Their findings revealed conversion to THA was required in 20% of their patients. The analysis of their 3-year follow-up data revealed survivorship of 90% in patients who had greater than 2 mm of joints space on plain radiographs; conversely, a 57% survivorship rate was found in those patients with 2 mm or less. In patients who did not require THA, the mHHS and HOS scores significantly improved from 58 to 84 and 66 to 87, respectively. Based on these findings, the investigators concluded that, arthritis, regardless of age, was found to most affect survivorship.

Cooper and colleagues[22] analyzed 88 patients who underwent hip arthroscopy (range 11–57, mean 24.3) and divided them into 2 groups: those older than 25 years and those younger. All patients were treated for symptomatic intra-articular hip pathology. Their findings noted increased mHHS across both age groups without significant statistical difference. Based on this, the investigators concluded that again age was not a significant factor in post–hip arthroscopy survivorship.

Finally, McCormick and colleagues[23] examined 176 consecutive patients who underwent hip arthroscopy for FAI and/or labral pathology with a minimum 2-year follow-up. The investigators identified those patients who were older than 40 years and/or had grade IV Outerbridge score changes as those most likely to have lower positive outcomes after arthroscopy. Likewise, they noted that patients younger than 40 years were predictive of good to excellent results.

Age as an independent predictor of survivorship does not seem to have a statistical significance after hip arthroscopy. However, age does have a relevance because osteoarthritis, which tends to progress with age, was found to have a corollary effect with age on outcomes. Considerations of age not fully identified include labral blood flow and healing potential, iatrogenic injury to the femoral head blood supply during joint distraction caused by decreased arterial elasticity, and potentially decreased ability to produce fibrocartilage after microfracture. As the age of the active population increases, so too does the potential for intra-articular hip joint pathology. Addressing these injuries seems relatively safe provided appropriate patient selection is performed. What has yet to be proven is the potential effect on decreasing possible chondral lesions or eventual arthritis by addressing femoral acetabular lesions in the young population. It can be extrapolated that removal of these inciting factors will be both protective and preventative; however, future studies need to be performed to further evaluate this hypothesis.

LABRAL PATHOLOGY

Over the past decade, the importance of the function of the acetabular labrum has grown. The role of the labrum is to create a fluid seal effect on the hip socket and to provide stability, pressure distribution, lubrication, and shock absorption. During the early stages of arthroscopic intervention for the hip, labral tears were routinely debrided or excised. However, more recent literature has advocated the benefit of labral repair and preservation to positively affect survivorship. These studies suggest that the labrum minimizes the risk of premature arthritis by maintaining proper biomechanical stability of the hip with the purpose of a labral repair to restore this function.[24–27]

Robertson and colleagues[28] performed a 25-year retrospective literature analysis on patients who underwent selective labral debridement without associated intra-articular pathology. Their finding, reported at an average of 3.5 years follow-up, demonstrated an overall 67% patient satisfaction level, improved mHSS, and nearly 50% resolution of mechanical symptoms after labral debridement. Byrd and Jones[29] also reviewed 31 hips up that underwent labral debridement with a minimum 10 years follow-up that underwent labral debridement. In 18 hips found to be without arthritis, 83% continued to show substantial improvement on their mHHS. Among the 8 patients with associated arthritis, 7 (88%) were converted to THA at a mean of 63 months. Two patients underwent repeat arthroscopy, which did not preclude a successful outcome at the 10-year follow-up. None of the patients underwent concomitant treatment of FAI. Based on this, they concluded that selective debridement of symptomatic tears can result in favorable long-term results, although the presence of arthritis remained a poor prognostic indicator of survivorship.

In a series reviewed by Larson and Giveans[30] for patients undergoing arthroscopy for pincer or combined pincer-cam lesions, higher mHHS were noted in the group treated with labral refixation as opposed to labral debridement at the 1-year follow-up. It was also noted that patients who underwent labral refixation subjectively reported good or excellent outcomes in 90% of cases, compared with 67% of labral debridement cases.[30] Espinosa and colleagues[31] found similar results in their retrospective review of 60 cases of arthroscopy for femoroacetabular impingement. In their consecutive series, 25 patients underwent labral debridement and the next 35 underwent labral refixation. At the 1- and 2-year follow-ups, clinical scores were significantly better in the refixation group. Likewise 76% of patients in the resection group and 94% in the refixation group reported good or excellent results.

The authors' retrospective study found an approximate 90% 10-year survivor rate after labral debridement provided there was little to no chondral damage. This finding again emphasizes the need for early detection and intervention of labral pathology before the onset of chondral injury.[4] Underscoring the importance of labral function has been the increased interest in labral reconstruction for those tears deemed nonsalvageable. Philippon and colleagues[32] reported on the follow-up of 47 patients who had undergone arthroscopic labral reconstructions using an illiotibial band (ITB) autograft in patients for advanced labral degeneration or deficiency (mean patient age 37years). At a mean follow-up of 18 months (12- to 32-month range), they noted the mean mHHS improved from 62 preoperatively to 85 postoperatively. Additionally, the median patient satisfaction was 8 out of 10 (range, 1–10). Improved outcomes and function were found in patients who were treated within 1 year of injury, had preserved joint space, and were of a younger age. Conversion to THA was performed in 4 patients (9%).[31] Similar results have been separately reported by both Walker and Madsuka on labral reconstruction. Unfortunately, because of the relative infancy of this procedure, long-term survivorship is unknown at this time and its benefits can only be extrapolated in the theory of recreating a suction-seal environment within the hip.[33,34]

Although effective results have been reported in the 10-year retrospective data with simple labral debridement, there has been a growing push toward labral repair.[35] The importance of the function of the labrum in the more recent literature has been emphasized, with some even advocating labral base fixation as an anatomic repair alternative to conventional repairs.[36] Despite this, only short-term and cadaveric laboratory studies exist at this time.[36,37] Nevertheless, the management of labral pathology can provide significant relief of symptoms; survivorship should be affected further if underlying FAI pathology is appropriately addressed at the time of the index procedure. Philippon and others[5,38] have noted that the longer the preoperative symptoms have existed has a negative impact on outcomes. This finding has to be caused by the increased chondral injuries caused by the abnormal joint forces created by an incompetent labrum or it may simply be caused by the increased damage to the symptomatic labrum resulting in decreasing amounts of healthy labrum after surgery.

FAI

FAI describes the phenomenon of abnormal congruency between the femoral head and the acetabulum. The results of this abnormal fit can lead to labral injury, chondral damage, and eventually arthritis. As has been increasingly reported, FAI can present in 3 patterns. Cam lesions are described as excess bone about the femoral head and neck, which can lead to abnormal contact against the labrum and chondral labral junction, particularly with flexion, adduction, and internal rotation of the hip. Pincer lesions are the result of acetabular overcoverage that leads to bony blockage of the femoral head during range of motion. The end result of this lesion is a crushed labrum and chondral damage to the femoral head-neck junction. The most common situation is a mixed cam and pincer pathology occurring along the anterior femoral neck and the anterior–superior acetabular rim.[13]

Addressing underlying FAI has been demonstrated in some reports to decrease the rate of conversion to THA in patients with osteoarthritis.[5,7,10] Similarly, failure to appropriately recognize and address FAI pathology has been shown to lead to high rates of failure or need for revision arthroscopy.[39] Heyworth and colleagues,[39] found in their review of 24 revision hip arthroscopies, that 79% of the revisions were caused by unaddressed bony pathology. Additionally, 25% of the patients who had undergone either cam or pincer treatment during the initial procedure required revision to address the corresponding lesion. Philippon and colleagues[40] echoed these findings in their 2007 review of hip arthroscopy failures. Thirty-two of their 27 revisions (95%) were noted to have unaddressed osseous lesions of the femoral head, acetabulum, or both. Incomplete decompression was found to still be a source of poor outcomes after hip arthroscopy, resulting in lower postsurgical mHHS and the need for potential revision. Furthermore, through retrospective review, they found all but 1 of these cases had preoperative FAI radiographic findings. In their early follow-up, survivorship and success was noted to be significantly improved over the index procedure with adequate addressing of the underlying bony abnormalities.[40]

Wenger and colleagues[41] reviewed 31 patients who had labral tears and found 87% had radiographic evidence of bony abnormalities about the femoral head or the acetabulum. Their findings were one of the first articles to suggest that isolated treatment of soft tissue pathologies may not be adequate without concomitantly addressing underlying structural abnormalities. As the recognition for the appropriate arthroscopic treatment of FAI has come to light, survivorships, at least at early and midterm reports, have improved. As noted earlier, Byrd and Jones[8] had a 27% conversion THA rate in their 10-year study in which most of the FAI lesions were not addressed arthroscopically. In a separate study in 2008, Byrd and Jones[42] this time reported on 207 hips that all underwent osseous deformity correction (163 cam lesions, 44 pincer lesions). At a mean of 16 months of follow-up (12–24 month range), they reported an average increase in the Harris hip score was 20 points and 0.5% converted to THA. Of note, the average age of these patients was lower in this population (33 years vs 38 years). Despite this, Byrd and Jones noted that most patients in the 2008 report had Outerbridge grade IV (107) or grade III (83) articular damage on at least one side of the joint, particularly the acetabular side. This finding may suggest further importance of the need for earlier detection and treatment of FAI in younger patients to prevent early chondral wear and ultimately improve survivorship.

Despite Byrd and Jones' findings on the treatment of FAI with advanced chondral damage, FAI in the face of advancement to osteoarthritis seems to still lead to poorer survivorship. Larson and Giveans[30] noted FAI correction with milder degrees of preoperative radiographic joint space narrowing resulted in improvements in pain and function at the short-term follow-up. However, patients with advanced radiographic joint space narrowing do not improve, and the authors think they should not be considered for arthroscopic FAI correction. Meftah and colleagues[43] also noted that coexisting pathology, especially arthritis and untreated FAI, can result in inferior outcomes.

FAI, as described by Ganz,[44] has grown in recognition and treatment over the past 10 to 15 years. Recent literature has identified good short- to midterm reports on outcomes after arthroscopic intervention for FAI; however, long-term survivorship studies are not available to date. Based off the work of Ganz and colleagues on the treatment of FAI via open surgical correction, there is the thought that arthroscopic intervention can offer a less invasive way to reduce pain and prevent osteoarthritis progression.[18,45] Ng and colleagues[35] performed a systematic review of the literature of 23 case study reports encompassing 970 cases. Based on patient outcome scores and effect size, all studies demonstrated improvement of patient symptoms. Across their search, they found that up to 30% of patients will eventually require THA. Within the subset of patients with poor outcomes, those patients with Outerbridge grade III or IV cartilage damage seen intraoperatively or with preoperative radiographs showing greater than Tonnis grade I osteoarthritis were identified as being predisposed for worse outcomes with treatment of FAI.

DEVELOPMENTAL DYSPLASIA OF THE HIP

Developmental dysplasia of the hip (DDH) (defined as abnormal bone morphology with a center edge angle of 25° or less) has typically been associated with poor long-term outcomes.[46,47] In patients with DDH, the acetabular labrum is often noted to be hypertrophic as a means of compensation for joint instability. Many times there are subsequent tears of these labrum or associated cartilage lesions caused by abnormal joint stresses. Typically, labral injuries are a result of a trauma or underlying FAI; however, in patients with DDH, there are often tears that originate more commonly because of the dysplastic head or acetabulum. It has been reported that patients with DDH can expect poor short- and long-term outcomes with arthroscopic intervention for labral tears unless the concomitant underlying cause of the DDH is addressed.[39,40,47] Matsuda and Khatod[48] additionally noted a rapid progression of osteoarthritis after labral repair in patients with DDH.

SUMMARY

Hip arthroscopy is a rapidly expanding field, attracting attention from patients and physicians alike. Although FAI and labral tears have presumably been around for hundreds of years, only in the past 2 decades or so have we come to understand the cause and pathology of the hip. Through trial and error and scholarly efforts, the arthroscopic community is rapidly gaining ground in handling and treating pathologies of the hip arthroscopically.

In assembling this article, it was interesting to note the shift in treatment algorithms. The removal of loose bodies has universally been known to be a successful procedure of hip arthroscopy. However, in the past 10 to 15 years, we have also come to recognize FAI and the function of the labrum. These realizations have led to successful treatment of cam and pincer lesions arthroscopically in the young and old alike.[35] It has been emphasized within the literature that early identification and treatment of these lesions be undertaken to minimize chondral and labral injury from repetitive insult. Having stated such, what will the next 10 to 15 years hold? Will arthroscopic surgeons become more aggressive with their indications in patients with asymptomatic or silent FAI?

The standard of care for labral tears has swung to repair or refixation as opposed to debridement. An increased understanding of the chondral protective effect of an intact labrum has changed the focus on the treatment of labral pathology, even despite the very successful outcomes with labral debridement.[49] Espinoza and colleagues[31] found a higher rate of progression of osteoarthritic changes in their subset of patients who underwent labral resection versus repair at a 1- to 2-year follow-up. Despite this, the results of the labral debridement noted in the few 10-year or longer studies has likewise demonstrated good results.[4,29] What is unknown still is the long-term survivorship in patients treated with either repair or debridement and concomitant FAI contouring. Retrospective analysis in the future will allow for adequate judgments to be made as to whether labral repair and refixation will truly increase survivorship after hip arthroscopy in the face of FAI.

Despite the many changes in philosophy across the literature, one axiom that has not wavered is that the presence of arthritis at the time of arthroscopy is a negative predictor of success. The identification of hips with Outerbridge grades III and IV have been proven throughout the review to lead to significant risk of THA conversion as soon as 1 year after arthroscopy.[4,16,17] As has been proven in the knee, lavage of an arthritic joint, even if concomitant pathology is addressed, can still lead to poor survivorship, even in the face of initial improved mHSS. Further diagnostic tools and improvements are still warranted, however. Repeatedly it was noted in the literature that there was a disconnect between Tonnis grades and the level of chondral injury found during arthroscopic evaluation.[9,11–13,15–18] Peters and Erickson,[12] among others, reported a high progression rate of osteoarthritis in patients found to have grade IV cartilage damage at the time of arthroscopy.[12] While using the Tonnis grades III and greater as a negative predictor of positive outcome, there is still a middle ground of those patients with Outerbridge scores of greater than III that has yet to convert these lesions to radiographic findings. Improvements in MRI arthrography quality has helped to stem some of these hidden lesions; however, further imaging indicators need to be explored to continue to identify patients who may best benefit from surgical intervention.

In closing, hip arthroscopy has evolved at an enormous rate, and the identification of our past mistakes has allowed us to advance the field.

The appropriate identification of risk factors for successful hip arthroscopy survivorship will guide the future outcomes and research in this ever-changing field. Future research should focus on the effect of body mass index on survivorship as well as the evaluation of labral allografts reconstructions and their outcomes. With the growth of surgical candidate parameters occurring daily, it will remain imperative to not blur the line between calculated expansion of criteria and negligence of understanding the aforementioned literature outlining factors that can negatively influence hip arthroscopy outcomes. The need for level I and level II midterm and long-term studies on factors affecting survivorship after hip arthroscopy continues. Diligence and dedication on the part of hip arthroscopists in this regard will allow for improved efficacy, further growth, and successful long-term outcomes in the art of hip arthroscopy.

REFERENCES

1. Kelly BT, Williams RJ III, Philippon MJ. Hip arthroscopy: current indications, treatment options, and management issues. Am J Sports Med 2003;31(6): 1020–37.
2. McCarthy JC, Lee JA. Arthroscopic intervention in early hip disease. Clin Orthop Relat Res 2004;(429): 157–62.
3. Moseley JB, O'Malley K, Petersen NJ, et al. A controlled trial of arthroscopic surgery for osteoarthritis of the knee. N Engl J Med 2002;347(2):81–8.
4. McCarthy JC, Jarrett BT, Ojeifo O, et al. What factors influence long-term survivorship after hip arthroscopy? Clin Orthop Relat Res 2011;469(2):362–71.
5. Philippon MJ, Briggs KK, Yen YM, et al. Outcomes following hip arthroscopy for femoroacetabular impingement with associated chondrolabral dysfunction: minimum two-year follow-up. J Bone Joint Surg Br 2009;91(1):16–23.
6. Philippon MJ, Schroder E, Souza BG, et al. Hip arthroscopy for femoroacetabular impingement in patients aged 50 years or older. Arthroscopy 2012; 28(1):59–65.
7. Haviv B, O'Donnell J. The incidence of total hip arthroplasty after hip arthroscopy in osteoarthritic patients. Sports Med Arthrosc Rehabil Ther Technol 2010;2:18.
8. Byrd JW, Jones KS. Prospective analysis of hip arthroscopy with 10-year followup. Clin Orthop Relat Res 2010;468(3):741–6.
9. Franco J, Maul R, Martin T. Preoperative predictors or early failures following hip arthroscopy. Arthroscopy 2011;27(10):e109.
10. Larson CM, Giveans MR, Taylor M. Does arthroscopic FAI correction improve function with

radiographic arthritis? Clin Orthop Relat Res 2011; 469(6):1667–76.

11. Beck M, Leunig M, Parvizi J, et al. Anterior femoroacetabular impingement: part II. Midterm results of surgical treatment. Clin Orthop Relat Res 2004; 418:67–73.

12. Peters CL, Erickson JA. Treatment of femoroacetabular impingement with surgical dislocation and debridement in young adults. J Bone Joint Surg Am 2006;88(8):1735–41.

13. Philippon M, Schenker M, Briggs K, et al. Femoroacetabular impingement in 45 professional athletes: associated pathologies and return to sport following arthroscopic decompression. Knee Surg Sports Traumatol Arthrosc 2007;15(7):908–14.

14. Karthikeyan S, Roberts S, Griffin D. Microfracture for acetabular chondral defects in patients with femoroacetabular impingement results at second-look arthroscopic surgery. Am J Sports Med 2012; 40(12):2725–30.

15. Philipon MJ, Herzog MM, Briggs KK. Five to seven year survivorship after hip arthroscopy. Chicago: Poster Presentation AAOS; March 19, 2013.

16. McCarthy JC. The diagnosis and treatment of labral and chondral injuries. Instr Course Lect 2004;53: 573–7.

17. Horisberger M, Brunner A, Herzog RF. Arthroscopic treatment of femoral acetabular impingement in patients with preoperative generalized degenerative changes. Arthroscopy 2010;26(5):623–9.

18. Larson CM, Giveans MR. Arthroscopic management of femoroacetabular impingement: early outcomes measures. Arthroscopy 2008;24(5):540–6.

19. Philippon MJ, Yen YM, Briggs KK, et al. Early outcomes after hip arthroscopy for femoroacetabular impingement in the athletic adolescent patient: a preliminary report. J Pediatr Orthop 2008;28(7): 705–10.

20. Javed A, O'Donnell JM. Arthroscopic femoral osteochondroplasty for cam femoroacetabular impingement in patients over 60 years of age. J Bone Joint Surg Br 2011;93(3):326–31.

21. Fabricant PD, Heyworth BE, Kelly BT. Hip arthroscopy improves symptoms associated with FAI in selected adolescent athletes. Clin Orthop Relat Res 2012;470(1):261–9.

22. Cooper AP, Basheer SZ, Maheshwari R, et al. Outcomes of hip arthroscopy. A prospective analysis and comparison between patients under 25 and over 25 years of age. Br J Sports Med 2013;47(4): 234–8.

23. McCormick F, Nwachukwu BU, Alpaugh K, et al. Predictors of hip arthroscopy outcomes for labral tears at minimum 2-year follow-up: the influence of age and arthritis. Arthroscopy 2012;28(10):1359–64.

24. Crawford MJ, Dy CJ, Alexander JW, et al. The 2007 Frank Stinchfield Award. The biomechanics of the hip labrum and the stability of the hip. Clin Orthop Relat Res 2007;465:16–22.

25. Groh MM, Herrera J. A comprehensive review of hip labral tears. Curr Rev Musculoskelet Med 2009;2: 105–17.

26. Kelly BT, Weiland DE, Schenker ML, et al. Arthroscopic labral repair in the hip: surgical technique and review of the literature. Arthroscopy 2005;21: 1496–504.

27. McCarthy JC, Noble PC, Schuck MR, et al. The Otto E. Aufranc Award: the role of labral lesions to development of early degenerative hip disease. Clin Orthop Relat Res 2001;393:25–37.

28. Robertson WJ, Kadrmas WR, Kelly BT. Arthroscopic management of labral tears in the hip: a systematic review of the literature. Clin Orthop Relat Res 2007; 455:88–92.

29. Byrd JW, Jones KS. Hip arthroscopy for labral pathology: prospective analysis with 10-year follow-up. Arthroscopy 2009;25(4):365–8.

30. Larson CM, Giveans MR. Arthroscopic debridement versus refixation of the acetabular labrum associated with femoroacetabular impingement. Arthroscopy 2009;25(4):369–76.

31. Espinosa N, Rothenfluh DA, Beck M, et al. Treatment of femoro-acetabular impingement: preliminary results of labral refixation. J Bone Joint Surg Am 2006;88(5):925–35.

32. Philippon MJ, Briggs KK, Hay CJ, et al. Arthroscopic labral reconstruction in the hip using iliotibial band autograft: technique and early outcomes. Arthroscopy 2010;26(6):750–6.

33. Walker JA, Pagnotto M, Trousdale RT, et al. Preliminary pain and function after labral reconstruction during femoroacetabular impingement surgery. Clin Orthop Relat Res 2012;470(12): 3414–20.

34. Matsuda DK, Burchette R. Arthroscopic hip labral reconstruction with gracilis autograft: surgical technique and preliminary outcomes. Paper 55; ISAKOS annual meeting. Rio de Janerio, May 15, 2011.

35. Ng VY, Arora N, Best TM, et al. Efficacy of surgery for femoralacetabular impingement: a systematic review. Am J Sports Med 2010;38(11):2337–45.

36. Fry R, Domb B. Labral base refixation in the hip: rationale and technique for an anatomic approach to labral repair. Arthroscopy 2010;26(No 9 Suppl 1): S81–9.

37. Cadet ER, Chan AK, Vorys GC, et al. Investigation of the preservation of the fluid seal effect in the repaired, partially resected, and reconstructed acetabular labrum in a cadaveric hip model. Am J Sports Med 2012;40(10):2218–23.

38. Philippon MJ. New frontiers in hip arthroscopy: the role of arthroscopic hip labral repair and capsulorrhaphy in the treatment of hip disorders. Instr Course Lect 2006;55:309–16.

39. Heyworth BE, Shindle MK, Voos JE, et al. Radiologic and intraoperative findings in revision hip arthroscopy. Arthroscopy 2007;23(12):1295–302.

40. Philippon MJ, Schenker ML, Briggs KK, et al. Revision hip arthroscopy. Am J Sports Med 2007; 35(11):1918–21.

41. Wenger DE, Kendell KR, Miner MR, et al. Acetabular labral tears rarely occur in the absence of bony abnormalities. Clin Orthop Relat Res 2004; 426:145–50.

42. Byrd TJ, Jones KS. Arthroscopic femoroplasty in the management of cam-type femoroacetabular impingement. Clin Orthop Relat Res 2009;467(3): 739–46.

43. Meftah M, Rodriguez JA, Panagopoulos G, et al. Long-term results of arthroscopic labral debridement: predictors of outcomes. Orthopedics 2011; 34(10):e588–92. http://dx.doi.org/10.3928/01477447-20110826-04.

44. Ganz R, Parvizi J, Beck M, et al. Femoroacetabular impingement: a cause for osteoarthritis of the hip. Clin Orthop Relat Res 2003;417:112–20.

45. Lavigne M, Parvizi J, Beck M, et al. Anterior femoroacetabular impingement: part I. Techniques of joint preserving surgery. Clin Orthop Relat Res 2004;418:61–6.

46. Byrd JW, Jones KS. Hip arthroscopy in the presence of dysplasia. Arthroscopy 2003;19(10):1055–60.

47. Parvizi J, Bican O, Bender B, et al. Arthroscopy for labral tears in patients with developmental dysplasia of the hip: a cautionary note. J Arthroplasty 2009; 24(Suppl 6):110–3.

48. Matsuda DK, Khatod M. Rapidly progressive osteoarthritis after arthroscopic labral repair in patients with hip dysplasia. Arthroscopy 2012;28(11): 1738–43.

49. Zaltz I. The biomechanical case for labral débridement. Clin Orthop Relat Res 2012;470(12):3398–405.

TRAUMA

Preface
Trauma Section

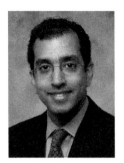

Saqib Rehman, MD
Editor

We have four interesting orthopedic trauma topics for the current issue of the *Orthopedic Clinics of North America*. Damage control orthopedics has gained popularity, although is a term that is often misused. Furthermore, identifying who needs to be treated with initial external fixation of the femur can be confusing, and most centers cannot check biomarkers such as IL-6 levels readily. Drs D'Alleyrand and O'Toole review the current evidence and practical applications of damage control theory. I am particularly in favor of the term they have named this, "Early Appropriate Care."

Many surgeons tend to be conservative with allowing weight-bearing after treatment of periarticular fractures, but with very little evidence to support their practice. Dr Kubiak and colleagues have reviewed this topic and present the available evidence on when we can allow our patients to weight-bear safely.

Talus fractures continue to be challenging injuries from a technical standpoint. Unfamiliar surgical approaches are often utilized and surgical strategies for achieving satisfactory outcomes are also not widely understood. Drs Shakked and Tejwani give an in-depth review of the surgical treatment of talus fractures in this volume.

Fractures from gun-related violence continue to be a regular phenomenon in our urban trauma centers. Many orthopedic surgeons often ask me what the basic principles are of management of these injuries, and what the evidence is behind our practice. Dr Tosti has done a fine job reviewing this topic, which rounds out this volume.

I hope you enjoy this particular issue!

Saqib Rehman, MD
Department of Orthopaedic Surgery
Temple University Hospital
3401 North Broad Street
Philadelphia, PA 19140, USA

E-mail address:
Saqib.Rehman@tuhs.temple.edu

Orthop Clin N Am 44 (2013) xv
http://dx.doi.org/10.1016/j.ocl.2013.07.007
0030-5898/13/$ – see front matter © 2013 Published by Elsevier Inc.

The Evolution of Damage Control Orthopedics
Current Evidence and Practical Applications of Early Appropriate Care

Jean-Claude G. D'Alleyrand, MD[a,b], Robert V. O'Toole, MD[b],*

KEYWORDS

- Damage control orthopedics • Early total care • Early appropriate care • Polytrauma

KEY POINTS

- The timing and fixation of extremity injury in polytrauma patients has evolved considerably over the past 40 years.
- Most polytrauma patients with femoral fractures can be treated safely with intramedullary nails in the first 24 hours; these are the "stable" patients.
- Polytrauma patients with femoral fractures who are unstable or in extremis should be treated initially with an external fixator and damage control orthopedics (DCO).
- Controversy continues regarding which "borderline" patients benefit from DCO and the ideal timing of fracture fixation surgery.
- Borderline patients with certain closed head injuries, poor response to resuscitation as measured by parameters such as lactate failing to normalize, and poor ventilator parameters are good candidates for DCO.

INTRODUCTION

The approach to treating major fractures in patients who have sustained severe trauma has evolved steadily over the past 40 years. Initially, patients who had sustained substantial trauma were viewed as too sick to undergo fracture surgery, but as increasing evidence was published linking prolonged recumbency with morbidity, these same patients became viewed as too sick *not* to undergo surgery. However, as the enthusiasm for early fracture fixation in these patients increased, it became clear that some patients paid a different physiologic price for too aggressive of a surgical approach after major trauma: multiorgan failure, particularly adult respiratory distress syndrome (ARDS). This paradoxic situation illuminated the need for a way to stabilize fractures early while minimizing

Commercial relationships: Dr O'Toole has no commercial relationships to report in direct relation to the topic of this article. Dr O'Toole is a consultant for Smith & Nephew (manufacturer of fracture care implants). Dr O'Toole was a former consultant for Synthes (maker of fracture care implants; ended 10/2010) and is an unpaid consultant for IMDS (biomedical device company), and his institution receives research support from Synthes and Stryker (maker of fracture care implants). Dr D'Alleyrand has no commercial relationships to report.
^a Department of Orthopaedics, Walter Reed National Military Medical Center, 8901 Wisconsin Avenue, Bethesda, MD 20889, USA; ^b Department of Orthopaedics, R Adams Cowley Shock Trauma Center, University of Maryland School of Medicine, 22 South Greene Street, Baltimore, MD 21201, USA
* Corresponding author.
E-mail address: rvo3@yahoo.com

Orthop Clin N Am 44 (2013) 499–507
http://dx.doi.org/10.1016/j.ocl.2013.06.004

orthopedic.theclinics.com

physiologic insult. From this need was born the concept of damage control orthopedics (DCO).

CHANGING THE NATURE OF STABILIZATION

Before the 1980s, patients who sustained severe multiple traumatic injuries were viewed as being too ill to tolerate the physiologic stressors associated with internal fixation of major fractures. Classically, these patients were treated in a staged fashion, as described by Wolff and colleagues.[1] Generally, patients were first resuscitated and emergency surgery performed for immediately life-threatening conditions. Patients then went through a stabilization phase for several days or weeks[2] in preparation for definitive surgery. Accordingly, patients were placed in traction for a period, until they seemed well enough to undergo fracture fixation. Unfortunately, a patient in prolonged traction is compelled to stay relatively immobilized in a recumbent position, which makes pulmonary toilet challenging, and the lack of fixation is thought to increase the likelihood of pulmonary complications, including thrombotic[3] and fat[4] embolism. With this method of treatment, the final rehabilitative phase is delayed until the fractures have been surgically stabilized or healed in traction, thus leaving patients bedridden and hospital-bound for long periods.

In the early 1970s, some groups began to take a more proactive approach to fracture stabilization. Seibel and colleagues[3] began performing immediate fracture fixation in patients who sustained blunt multitrauma during this period. Anecdotally, the investigators observed a surprising reduction in intensive care unit (ICU) days, pulmonary emboli, and fracture-related complications. Emboldened by these observations, they began to prospectively study the effects of timing of fixation on the clinical course of these patients.[3] Patients with femoral or acetabular fractures and a minimum injury severity score (ISS) of 22 were treated with fixation either within the first 24 hours or after 10 or more days of traction. Patients who underwent delayed fixation had more ICU and ventilator days, had a higher number of positive blood cultures, and required a greater number of antibiotics. The authors concluded that delaying fracture stabilization increased the risk of pulmonary complications from prolonged recumbency and nutritional depletion, narcotic use, and extrapulmonary sources of infection, such as open wounds and necrotic debris within fracture hematomas.

Additional studies were published in the mid to late 1980s, espousing the virtues of early fixation in polytrauma patients[5,6] in conjunction with early aggressive ventilatory support.[2] However, these studies were frequently heterogeneous with regard to the involved fractures or the associated injury patterns, and the single prospective series during this period had too small of a cohort ($N = 18$) for definitive conclusions to be drawn.[7]

THE ERA OF EARLY TOTAL CARE

To better evaluate the effects of the timing of fixation on the complications, clinical course, and cost associated with treating femoral fractures, Bone and colleagues[8] conducted a seminal prospective randomized study with 178 patients. Patients were randomized to femoral fracture internal fixation in less than 24 hours or greater than 48 hours. The authors found that in patients with isolated femoral fractures and an ISS less than 18, the timing of fixation had no appreciable effect on outcomes. However, with polytrauma patients (ISS>18), the timing of femoral fracture fixation did seem to play a major role in patients' clinical courses. Late fixation was associated with a higher incidence of ARDS, fat embolism syndrome, pulmonary emboli, and pneumonia. These patients also had a mean ICU stay and total length of stay that were 5 and 10 days longer, respectively, and an average cost of hospitalization that was 50% higher than that of the early fixation cohort. The study has been criticized for having unequal numbers of lung injuries in the 2 groups, no details of resuscitation, and limited statistical comparisons, but it clearly remains one of the most influential studies on this topic.

Following this paper, additional authors published studies supporting early fixation of all fractures (known as early total care [ETC]) in polytrauma patients.[9,10] However, some authors reported no benefit with early fixation.[11,12] In addition, some evidence suggested that although early fixation might be beneficial, fixation in the first 24 hours might be too early and might actually be detrimental to patients.[13–15] It began to become apparent that in certain patients,[1,16] particularly those with pulmonary[2,17] or traumatic brain injuries,[1,18,19] a less-aggressive approach to fracture fixation might be needed.

EMERGENCE OF THE 2-HIT MODEL

Over time, the concept of a 2-hit model of posttraumatic physiologic response began to emerge.[2,20] In the 1-hit model, the initial trauma is believed to generate a major inflammatory cascade with the potential for subsequent ARDS, independent of the timing of fracture fixation. The development of multiple organ failure is dependent on the extent of initial injury and the timing and quality of resuscitation.[3,21] In contrast, the 2-hit model suggests that the initial trauma generates a less-severe systemic inflammatory state. The immune system then becomes primed for an exaggerated inflammatory response after a second physiologic insult.[4,22] This second hit was initially thought to be from an infectious process,[3,23] such as pneumonia[5,6,24] or other sources of infection,[2,21] but some consideration was given to a noninfectious source of this second hit.

Anderson and Harken[22] described a mechanism of lung injury that begins with the priming of neutrophils and macrophages through inflammatory mediators generated by multisystem trauma. Once these cells are primed, a noninjurious or mildly injurious second stimulus causes an excessive inflammatory reaction that leads to cell-mediated lung injury.[7] The authors suggested that inhibiting this cellular priming could be an effective prophylaxis against secondary lung injury via this 2-hit phenomenon.

The work of Bone and colleagues[8] and of Waydhas and colleagues[25] supports this notion that inflammatory mediators play an important role in the response to polytrauma. In their series of patients, they prospectively followed 3 markers for inflammation: C-reactive protein, neutrophil elastase, and platelet count. They found that with 2 abnormal parameters, the probability of postoperative major organ failure was 73%, and if only 1 or no parameters were abnormal, that probability decreased to 17%. On further review of their data, the investigators found that nearly 80% of patients with postoperative organ failure despite low inflammatory markers had undergone extensive surgeries, such as fixation of pelvic or femoral fractures. Conversely, most patients (71%) who had a benign clinical course in the face of elevated inflammatory indicators had undergone mild procedures, such as fixation of facial fractures. Although no difference was seen in the timing of fixation between patients with and without organ failure, the authors concluded that surgeries more than 72 hours after trauma may induce a second-hit phenomenon and organ failure.

Eventually, it became apparent that the 2-hit model was not an all-or-none phenomenon, and that some patients could undergo early extensive fracture fixation without developing postoperative organ failure.[9,10,17] Pape and colleagues[17] reported on a retrospective series of 106 patients with an ISS greater than 18 who underwent reamed nailing of femoral shaft fractures. Patients who had an Abbreviated Injury Scale (AIS) thorax score of 2 or greater and underwent nailing in the first 24 hours after trauma had a significantly higher incidence of ARDS, had significantly longer

ventilator and ICU times, and trended toward a higher incidence of pneumonia compared with a cohort that had an AIS-thorax score of 1 or less. The authors posited that in the setting of a severe pulmonary contusion, the normal compensatory mechanisms of the lung may become taxed to their limits. The authors termed this a *borderline situation*, wherein the patient can no longer accommodate the added physiologic insult of prolonged surgery and intramedullary instrumentation. The authors then stated that the extent of pulmonary injury can be difficult to gauge in the early postinjury period. Accordingly, they recommended using external fixation or perhaps unreamed nailing in severely injured patients with associated thoracic trauma, despite having no unreamed nails in their series.

Reamed femoral nailing has been shown to increase lung capillary permeability in animal models[11,12,26] and to increase pulmonary arterial pressures in humans[13–15,27] when compared with unreamed femoral nailing. Unreamed femoral nailing has been shown to be safe when performed in the first 24 hours after trauma, despite severe thoracic injury (AIS$\geq$3).[16,28] However, early (<24 hours) reamed femoral nailing has not been shown to increase the incidence of ARDS in vivo,[17,29,30] even when performed in patients with an AIS-thorax score of 4 or greater.[31] With that in mind, reamed nailing has been shown to increase certain inflammatory markers to nearly significant levels (s-ICAM-1, $P = .052$; CD11b, $P = .08$),[32] which implies that the mode of initial fixation in borderline patients, not only the timing thereof, warrants some consideration.

DAMAGE CONTROL ORTHOPEDICS

It became increasingly evident that early fracture fixation needed to be performed while minimizing the secondary physiologic insult to the patient. After Townsend and colleagues[19] reported on hypotension observed in patients with brain injuries who underwent early femoral nailing, a question to the authors referenced the concept of "resuscitative orthopedics," specifically "minimal stabilization rather than definitive fixation." Two years later, Scalea and colleagues[33] reported on a 3-year series of patients who underwent a similar limited initial approach to femoral shaft fractures in polytrauma patients, terming it *damage control orthopedics* (DCO). The authors credited Rotondo and colleagues[34] with applying the naval war term *damage control* to the limited initial treatment of penetrating abdominal trauma.[35–37]

Scalea and colleagues[33] described damage control in 43 patients with femoral fractures and a median ISS of 27. These patients underwent early temporary external fixation for a median of 4 days before staged nailing. This cohort was compared with 281 patients who underwent primary femoral nailing with a median ISS of 17 (P = .001). The median operative time for external fixation was 35 minutes, compared with 135 minutes for primary intramedullary nailing. Despite a significantly higher incidence of laparotomy, AIS-head score of 3 or greater, shock on presentation, and days in the ICU, the damage control cohort had only 4 deaths (9% vs <1%; P = .001). The authors believed that femoral fractures should be fixed as early as possible but that some patients were not physiologically replete enough to withstand early nailing. Paradoxically, this subset of patients would be poor candidates for prolonged traction, and thus external fixation was a bridge to definitive treatment, affording the advantages of fixation with minimal operative time and physiologic insult. Before this era, external fixation of adult femoral fractures was uncommon and typically used only for definitive cases.[38,39] Temporary external fixation of femoral fractures had been described, but mainly for soft tissue management, not for resuscitative reasons.[40]

Clearly, minimizing the interval between provisional and definitive fixation has a direct effect on the length of hospitalization.[41] However, to mitigate the effects of a hyperstimulated immune response, delaying major fracture surgery in the first few days after injury seems to be advantageous in avoiding the second-hit phenomenon in certain polytrauma patients. Specifically, delaying secondary major fracture fixation until the fifth day after injury seems to have a significantly protective effect in terms of the inflammatory response and pulmonary and hepatic dysfunction.[42,43] The clinical ramifications of this are debated, but some clinicians delay definitive fixation after DCO until the fifth day based on this finding.

After its initial description in the literature, several papers on DCO were published, extolling its virtues in the multitrauma patient.[44–49] Before the published description of DCO, the Department of Orthopaedics and Trauma Surgery at Hannover Medical School had been performing staged fixation of femoral shaft fractures in polytrauma patients at risk for pulmonary complications for almost 10 years.[45] In 2002, Pape and colleagues[45] published a retrospective comparison of complication rates in this patient population before and after the implementation of this protocol. They found that the incidence of ARDS with primary nailing decreased from 55% to 27% after they began practicing DCO in selected patients. Moreover, the ARDS rate associated with primary

external fixation decreased from 97% to 22%, reflecting the use of this technique in borderline patients, as opposed to solely in patients in extremis.

The following year, Pape and colleagues[46] published a prospective, randomized, multicenter study comparing DCO with primary nailing of femoral shaft fractures in polytrauma patients. They found a significant increase in serum proinflammatory markers when primary nailing was performed, although they were unable to demonstrate an association with postoperative complications. External fixation was not associated with an increase in these markers and, interestingly, neither was the secondary nailing, performed a mean of 3 days later. This lack of a significant inflammatory response may have been because of a relatively quiescent inflammatory milieu or a type II error from a small sample size.

EARLY APPROPRIATE CARE

Nahm and colleagues[50] recently coined the term early appropriate care (EAC) to describe the preferential fixation of femoral fractures in the first 24 hours in contrast to other extremity fractures that could be splinted and fixed at a later date. This procedure would provide the benefits of early treatment while minimizing the length of the original surgery—a compromise between the staged treatment of DCO and the fixation of all fractures in ETC—and could be used in most patients, provided an aggressive approach to resuscitation was used.

The staged method of DCO has some potential negative aspects, mainly the possibility of infection after external fixation[51] and the need for additional surgery. The risk of secondary infection with staged nailing of femoral fractures has been estimated to be less than 3%,[33,52,53] even with many weeks of delay between external fixation and definitive fixation.[52] The infection risk for the tibia initially treated in external fixation is believed to be higher, at approximately 9%,[53] but this is less of an issue because closed tibias can be more easily splinted in borderline patients, and little of the current association with pulmonary dysfunction of nailing of femoral fractures is thought to apply to tibial fractures. As for the need for additional surgery, a staged nailing can be expected to increase the cost of hospitalization as a result of the cost of the external fixator and the potential increase in hospital length of stay (LOS). Although some evidence shows that DCO may not increase the LOS despite the additional surgical procedure,[49] evidence also exists to the contrary.[33,54]

Although use of DCO has been reported in up to 35% of femoral fractures in polytrauma patients

(ISS≥18),[45] DCO has been sparingly used in other series describing similar patient cohorts.[33,50,51,55] Despite using DCO in only 12% of femoral fractures with an ISS of 18 or greater, O'Toole and colleagues[55] reported rates of postnailing ARDS and mortality of only 1.5% and 2.0%, respectively. When comparing their findings with the ARDS rate of 26% described by Pape and colleagues,[45] the authors noted that their patients underwent primary nailing or DCO an average of 13 hours after admission, whereas virtually all of the patients in the series by Pape and colleagues underwent operative treatment in less than 8 hours.

Similarly, Nahm and colleagues[50] observed an ARDS rate of 1.7% in 492 patients with an ISS of 18 or greater who underwent femoral nailing in the first 24 hours. Patients with an AIS-thorax of 3 or greater who underwent early nailing experienced a 5.7% incidence of ARDS. The authors emphasized an aggressive resuscitation protocol, including the serial monitoring of blood pH and base deficit or lactate, throughout the preoperative period and during surgery.

The reason for the lower rate of ARDS observed after femoral nailing in polytrauma patients in multiple North American series compared with the German series is unknown. One possibility is that the German patients had worse lung injuries. O'Toole and colleagues[55] posited several other potential differences, such as genetic predisposition for ARDS, smoking rates, and differences in resuscitation or ICU care.

Patients with severe head injuries and concomitant extremity fractures constitute a particular subset of polytrauma patients, in that the possible hypotension or hypoxia associated with prolonged surgery may be especially deleterious.[56] The principles of EAC nonetheless seem to also apply to them. Jaicks and colleagues[18] found that early fixation of orthopedic injuries with an AIS-head of 2 or greater was associated with increased fluid requirements intraoperatively and in the immediate postoperative period, but they found no difference in neurologic complications during the initial hospitalization. Townsend and colleagues[19] observed a 2- to 8-fold increase in the incidence of intraoperative hypotension when femoral internal fixation was performed in the first 24 hours, although the Glasgow Coma Score (GCS) on discharge seemed to be related to the primary injury rather than the timing of fixation. Additional authors also found no effect of femoral internal fixation timing on neurologic outcomes in patients with severe head injuries, although resuscitation must be tailored to maximize cerebral perfusion pressures and oxygenation.[12,56–59]

PRACTICAL APPLICATIONS IN CURRENT PRACTICE

Particular attention has been paid to the timing of femoral fracture fixation in the trauma literature, perhaps because these fractures are typically sustained via a high-energy mechanism, associated with death, and frequently associated with multiple other injuries, including thoracic injury.[33] The femur is not amenable to splinting, thus requiring recumbency in traction before fixation, and the standard method of treatment involves some amount of medullary instrumentation, which contributes to augmenting the systemic inflammatory response and the creation of fat emboli. Therefore, it is fitting that the debate of ETC (or EAC) versus DCO be focused primarily on femoral fixation, but these principles can also be applied to the care of fractures of other major long bones or the pelvic ring.[6,47] Care of all of these injuries, particularly when more than one is present, involves a balance between the benefits of early mobilization and the physiologic tax of major surgery on a primed immunologic pathway and a traumatized pulmonary system.

Polytrauma patients can be grouped into 3 categories, and widespread agreement currently exists on the management of 2 of these: stable and unstable patients. Stable patients can be treated safely with EAC and intramedullary nails, with a low rate of postoperative ARDS and death, even those with associated lung injuries.[31,55,60] On the other hand, agreement exists that physiologically unstable patients and those in extremis, particularly those with significant respiratory compromise, should be treated initially with DCO to limit the second hit to the patient and additional pulmonary insult associated with intravasation of marrow in femoral nail placement. External fixators are placed on femoral and unstable pelvic fractures, amputations are completed, fasciotomies are performed if needed, and remaining fractures are splinted.

Controversy continues regarding the ideal treatment of so-called borderline patients and how to identify them. Borderline patients are those who fall between the categories of physiologically stable and unstable.[17,61,62] The second hit of fracture surgery may push them over the edge, but these patients are more difficult to identify than those at each end of the physiologic spectrum of stability.

Various authors have proposed criteria for identifying borderline polytrauma patients who may benefit from DCO of a femoral shaft fracture.[61,62] At the authors' institutions, 3 common indicators exist for DCO in borderline patients: (1) closed head injury, (2) poor response to resuscitation in the first 12 hours, and (3) poor respiratory status at the time of fracture treatment.

DCO for Closed Head Injuries

Closed head injuries are common in these patients. No firm guideline seems to exist regarding which closed head injuries are safe to receive nail fixation. At many centers this is typically left to the judgment of the neurosurgery team. Concern for additional brain injury from blood pressure fluctuations during extensive fracture surgery makes neurosurgery hesitant to clear patients for the operating room.[12,18,19,56–59] However, the potential benefit of DCO and the minimal physiologic insult of placing an external fixator allows for almost all patients with closed head injuries to be appropriate for external fixation of a femoral shaft fracture initially. Frequently this requires a discussion with the neurosurgery attending to explain that the goals of DCO are to help the respiratory status and overall physiology of the patient, not merely to better align the limb.

DCO for Poor Response to Resuscitation

The authors' center (R Adams Cowley Shock Trauma Center) typically prefers to observe that the markers for resuscitation are normalizing before nail fixation. The rationale for this is that underresuscitation is thought to place the lungs at additional risk for damage from the insult that happens whenever a nail is placed in a femur.[63] The center uses a lactate approaching 2.5 mmol/L as a rough clinical measure of the patient's resuscitation status,[55] but other measures such as base deficit are also very reasonable, and clinical judgment is needed in this determination.

DCO for Respiratory Issues

The presence of a lung injury unto itself is no longer an indication for DCO in polytrauma patients with femoral shaft fractures.[31,60,61,64,65] However, before undertaking femoral nailing, the authors routinely evaluate how well the patient's lungs are performing based on several ventilator parameters, including fraction of inspired oxygen and peak airway pressure. The ventilator mode affects this, and therefore this factor requires significant communication with the team managing the lungs to determine how well the patient is doing. The patient's oxygen saturation is not a helpful marker, because the ventilator parameters will be adjusted to keep this measure high at all costs. A reasonable test question is, "If the decision were based only on the lung performance now, might the patient be extubated?" The answer often gives useful data to clinicians who are not familiar with how to interpret ventilator parameters.

The ideal timing for a patient to receive either DCO or ETC is still unknown. A recent large study suggests that femoral fixation within 12 hours of injury may be too early, particularly in patients with concomitant abdominal injury, and might place the patient at increased risk of mortality.[66] One possible explanation for this effect is that patients benefit from additional time for resuscitation before femoral nailing, but the mechanism is not certain. At the authors' center, the decision for ETC versus DCO typically results in fixation with a mean time to the operating room of approximately 13 hours,[55] and they attempt to have external fixation performed within the first 24 hours if possible. This practice is not possible for all patients and is based on limited guidelines,[8,61,64,66] and further work is therefore needed to determine the ideal timing for fixation of femoral shaft fractures.

It is important to remember, particularly in patients with multiple fractures, that physiologic stability is dynamic and requires continuous evaluation before early fracture fixation is performed. If patients begin to manifest physiologic signs of hypoperfusion, then the surgical tactic must change to one of damage control. Orthopedic surgeons must stay abreast of the patient's resuscitation status throughout the procedure. No guarantee exists that the anesthesia provider will recognize the significance of a slowly increasing lactate or base deficit while the surgeon is contemplating fixing successive fractures. Furthermore, the orthopedic surgeon must communicate to the anesthesia provider the possible link between penetrating the femoral canal and acute deterioration of pulmonary status so that femoral nailing can be aborted in patients who show acute signs of not tolerating the procedure. Thus, the surgeon must remain more aware of the overall physiology of the polytrauma patient.

Even with a set of guidelines delineating which borderline patients should get DCO, the decision is often not clear-cut and a gray zone exists for clinical interpretation. Despite publication of low rates of ARDS with infrequent use of DCO,[55] the authors believe that clinicians should err toward overuse of DCO in these cases. DCO for a patient who did not need it results in delay in definitive fixation and might delay discharge. ETC for a patient who needed DCO may result in ARDS and death, which is obviously a much more serious consequence.

SUMMARY

The literature over the past 3 decades has reflected conflicting views regarding the best treatment for polytrauma patients with major pelvic and extremity fractures. Over the years, the pendulum has swung between delayed and immediate treatment, and modifications thereof, until the current conceptual balance was reached: that of EAC.

Although surgeons must tailor their approach to their own practice setting, evidence is emerging that resuscitation and timing of treatment are important parameters for any treatment strategy. A generalized algorithm is often useful to help manage these complex patients. Once adequate tissue oxygenation seems to be meeting metabolic demand, definitive fracture fixation seems prudent and beneficial. In patients who have sustained severe trauma, this typically involves a prolonged period of resuscitation with the early use of blood products.[55] A risk-adapted evaluation of patient's suitability for early fixation is then performed, based on the constellation of injuries and the response to resuscitation attempts.[67] Provided the patient is responding appropriately, the resuscitation is continued in the operating room while major fracture fixation is performed. Although the safety of treating most polytrauma femoral fractures with femoral nailing has been established, when in doubt, treating the patient with DCO is probably safest. Significant progress has been made in this domain, but more work is needed to better define the ideal treatment algorithm in clinical practice.

REFERENCES

1. Wolff G, Dittmann M, Rüedi T, et al. Koordination von Chirurgie und Intensivmedizin zur Vermeidung der posttraumatischen respiratorischen Insuffizienz. Unfallheilkunde 1978;81(6):425–42.
2. Goris RJ, Gimbrère JS, van Niekerk JL, et al. Early osteosynthesis and prophylactic mechanical ventilation in the multitrauma patient. J Trauma 1982; 22(11):895–903.
3. Seibel R, LaDuca J, Hassett JM, et al. Blunt multiple trauma (ISS 36), femur traction, and the pulmonary failure-septic state. Ann Surg 1985;202(3): 283–93 [discussion: 293].
4. Riska EB, Bonsdorff von H, Hakkinen S, et al. Prevention of fat embolism by early internal fixation of fractures in patients with multiple injuries. Injury 1976;8(2):110–6.
5. Johnson KD, Cadambi A, Seibert GB. Incidence of adult respiratory distress syndrome in patients with multiple musculoskeletal injuries: effect of early operative stabilization of fractures. J Trauma 1985;25(5):375–84.
6. Goldstein A, Phillips T, Sclafani SJ, et al. Early open reduction and internal fixation of the disrupted pelvic ring. J Trauma 1986;26(4):325–32 [discussion: 332–3].
7. Lozman J, Deno DC, Feustel PJ, et al. Pulmonary and cardiovascular consequences of immediate fixation or conservative management of long-bone fractures. Arch Surg 1986;121(9):992–9.
8. Bone LB, Johnson KD, Weigelt J, et al. Early versus delayed stabilization of femoral fractures. A prospective randomized study. J Bone Joint Surg Am 1989;71(3):336–40.
9. Behrman SW, Fabian TC, Kudsk KA, et al. Improved outcome with femur fractures: early vs. delayed fixation. J Trauma 1990;30(7):792–7 [discussion: 797–8].
10. Charash WE, Fabian TC, Croce MA. Delayed surgical fixation of femur fractures is a risk factor for pulmonary failure independent of thoracic trauma. J Trauma 1994;37(4):667–72.
11. Pelias ME, Townsend MC, Flancbaum L. Long bone fractures predispose to pulmonary dysfunction in blunt chest trauma despite early operative fixation. Surgery 1992;111(5):576–9.
12. Poole GV, Miller JD, Agnew SG, et al. Lower extremity fracture fixation in head-injured patients. J Trauma 1992;32(5):654–9.
13. Fakhry SM, Rutledge R, Dahners LE, et al. Incidence, management, and outcome of femoral shaft fracture: a statewide population-based analysis of 2805 adult patients in a rural state. J Trauma 1994;37(2):255–60 [discussion: 260–1].
14. Rogers FB, Shackford SR, Vane DW, et al. Prompt fixation of isolated femur fractures in a rural trauma center: a study examining the timing of fixation and resource allocation. J Trauma 1994;36(6):774–7.
15. Reynolds MA, Richardson JD, Spain DA, et al. Is the timing of fracture fixation important for the patient with multiple trauma? Ann Surg 1995;222(4): 470–81.
16. Pape HC, Schmidt RE, Rice J, et al. Biochemical changes after trauma and skeletal surgery of the lower extremity: quantification of the operative burden. Crit Care Med 2000;28(10):3441–8.
17. Pape HC, Auf'm'Kolk M, Paffrath T, et al. Primary intramedullary femur fixation in multiple trauma patients with associated lung contusion—a cause of posttraumatic ARDS? J Trauma 1993;34(4):540–7 [discussion: 547–8].
18. Jaicks RR, Cohn SM, Moller BA. Early fracture fixation may be deleterious after head injury. J Trauma 1997;42(1):1–5 [discussion: 5–6].
19. Townsend RN, Lheureau T, Protetch J, et al. Timing fracture repair in patients with severe brain injury (Glasgow Coma Scale score). J Trauma Acute Care Surg 1998;44(6):977–83.
20. Faist E, Baue AE, Dittmer H, et al. Multiple organ failure in polytrauma patients. J Trauma 1983; 23(9):775–87.

21. Meakins JL. Etiology of multiple organ failure. J Trauma 1990;30(Suppl 12):S165–8.

22. Anderson BO, Harken AH. Multiple organ failure: inflammatory priming and activation sequences promote autologous tissue injury. J Trauma 1990; 30(Suppl 12):S44–9.

23. Barton R, Cerra FB. The hypermetabolism. Multiple organ failure syndrome. Chest 2006;96(5):1153–60.

24. Sauaia A, Moore FA, Moore EE, et al. Pneumonia: cause or symptom of postinjury multiple organ failure? Am J Surg 1993;166(6):606–11.

25. Waydhas C, Nast-Kolb D, Trupka A, et al. Posttraumatic inflammatory response, secondary operations, and late multiple organ failure. J Trauma 1996;40(4):624–30 [discussion: 630–1].

26. Pape HC, Dwenger A, Regel G, et al. Pulmonary damage after intramedullary femoral nailing in traumatized sheep–is there an effect from different nailing methods? J Trauma 1992;33(4):574–81.

27. Pape HC, Regel G, Dwenger A, et al. Influences of different methods of intramedullary femoral nailing on lung function in patients with multiple trauma. J Trauma 1993;35(5):709–16.

28. Weninger P, Figl M, Spitaler R, et al. Early unreamed intramedullary nailing of femoral fractures is safe in patients with severe thoracic trauma. J Trauma 2007;62(3):692–6.

29. Norris BL, Patton WC, Rudd JN, et al. Pulmonary dysfunction in patients with femoral shaft fracture treated with intramedullary nailing. J Bone Joint Surg Am 2001;83-A(8):1162–8.

30. Carlson DW, Rodman GH, Kaehr D, et al. Femur fractures in chest-injured patients: is reaming contraindicated? J Orthop Trauma 1998;12(3):164–8.

31. Bosse MJ, MacKenzie EJ, Riemer BL, et al. Adult respiratory distress syndrome, pneumonia, and mortality following thoracic injury and a femoral fracture treated either with intramedullary nailing with reaming or with a plate. A comparative study. J Bone Joint Surg Am 1997;79(6):799–809.

32. Giannoudis PV, Smith RM, Bellamy MC, et al. Stimulation of the inflammatory system by reamed and unreamed nailing of femoral fractures. An analysis of the second hit. J Bone Joint Surg Br 1999; 81(2):356–61.

33. Scalea TM, Boswell SA, Scott JD, et al. External fixation as a bridge to intramedullary nailing for patients with multiple injuries and with femur fractures: damage control orthopedics. J Trauma 2000;48(4):613–21 [discussion: 621–3].

34. Rotondo MF, Schwab CW, McGonigal MD, et al. "Damage control": an approach for improved survival in exsanguinating penetrating abdominal injury. J Trauma 1993;35(3):375–82.

35. Wall MJ, Soltero E. Damage control for thoracic injuries. Surg Clin North Am 1997;77(4):863–78.

36. Reilly PM, Rotondo MF, Carpenter JP, et al. Temporary vascular continuity during damage control: intraluminal shunting for proximal superior mesenteric artery injury. J Trauma 1995;39(4):757–60.

37. Scalea TM, Mann R, Austin R, et al. Staged procedures for exsanguinating lower extremity trauma: an extension of a technique—case report. J Trauma 1994;36(2):291–3.

38. Mohr VD, Eickhoff U, Haaker R, et al. External fixation of open femoral shaft fractures. J Trauma Acute Care Surg 1995;38(4):648–52.

39. Murphy CP, D'Ambrosia RD, Dabezies EJ, et al. Complex femur fractures: treatment with the Wagner external fixation device or the Grosse-Kempf interlocking nail. J Trauma 1988;28(11):1553–61.

40. Alonso J, Geissler W, Hughes JL. External fixation of femoral fractures. Indications and limitations. Clin Orthop Relat Res 1989;(241):83–8.

41. Maurer DJ, Merkow RL, Gustilo RB. Infection after intramedullary nailing of severe open tibial fractures initially treated with external fixation. J Bone Joint Surg Am 1989;71(6):835–8.

42. Pape H, Stalp M, Weinberg A, et al. Optimal timing for secondary surgery in polytrauma patients: an evaluation of 4,314 serious-injury cases. Chirurg 1999;70(11):1287–93 [in German].

43. Pape HC, van Griensven M, Rice J, et al. Major secondary surgery in blunt trauma patients and perioperative cytokine liberation: determination of the clinical relevance of biochemical markers. J Trauma 2001;50(6):989–1000.

44. Harwood PJ, Giannoudis PV, van Griensven M, et al. Alterations in the systemic inflammatory response after early total care and damage control procedures for femoral shaft fracture in severely injured patients. J Trauma 2005;58(3):446–54.

45. Pape HC, Hildebrand F, Pertschy S, et al. Changes in the management of femoral shaft fractures in polytrauma patients: from early total care to damage control orthopedic surgery. J Trauma 2002;53(3):452–61 [discussion: 461–2].

46. Pape HC, Grimme K, van Griensven M, et al. Impact of intramedullary instrumentation versus damage control for femoral fractures on immunoinflammatory parameters. J Trauma 2003; 55(1):7–13.

47. Giannoudis PV, Pape HC. Damage control orthopaedics in unstable pelvic ring injuries. Injury 2004;35(7):671–7.

48. Taeger G, Ruchholtz S, Waydhas C, et al. Damage control orthopedics in patients with multiple injuries is effective, time saving, and safe. J Trauma 2005; 59(2):409–16.

49. Tuttle MS, Smith WR, Williams AE, et al. Safety and efficacy of damage control external fixation versus early definitive stabilization for femoral shaft

fractures in the multiple-injured patient. J Trauma 2009;67(3):602–5.

50. Nahm NJ, Como JJ, Wilber JH, et al. Early appropriate care: definitive stabilization of femoral fractures within 24 hours of injury is safe in most patients with multiple injuries. J Trauma 2011; 71(1):175–85.

51. Scalea TM. Optimal timing of fracture fixation: have we learned anything in the past 20 years? J Trauma 2008;65(2):253–60.

52. Nowotarski PJ, Turen CH, Brumback RJ, et al. Conversion of external fixation to intramedullary nailing for fractures of the shaft of the femur in multiply injured patients. J Bone Joint Surg Am 2000; 82(6):781–8.

53. Bhandari M, Zlowodzki M, Tornetta P, et al. Intramedullary nailing following external fixation in femoral and tibial shaft fractures. J Orthop Trauma 2005; 19(2):140–4.

54. Scannell BP, Waldrop NE, Sasser HC, et al. Skeletal traction versus external fixation in the initial temporization of femoral shaft fractures in severely injured patients. J Trauma 2010;68(3):633–40.

55. O'Toole RV, O'Brien M, Scalea TM, et al. Resuscitation before stabilization of femoral fractures limits acute respiratory distress syndrome in patients with multiple traumatic injuries despite low use of damage control orthopedics. J Trauma 2009; 67(5):1013–21.

56. Nahm NJ, Vallier HA. Timing of definitive treatment of femoral shaft fractures in patients with multiple injuries. J Trauma Acute Care Surg 2012;73(5): 1046–63.

57. Scalea TM, Scott JD, Brumback RJ, et al. Early fracture fixation may be "just fine" after head injury: no difference in central nervous system outcomes. J Trauma 1999;46(5):839–46.

58. Brundage SI, McGhan R, Jurkovich GJ, et al. Timing of femur fracture fixation: effect on outcome in patients with thoracic and head injuries. J Trauma 2002;52(2):299–307.

59. Giannoudis PV, Veysi VT, Pape HC, et al. When should we operate on major fractures in patients with severe head injuries? Am J Surg 2002; 183(3):261–7.

60. Bone LB, Giannoudis P. Current concepts review femoral shaft fracture fixation and chest injury after polytrauma. J Bone Joint Surg Am 2011;93: 311–7.

61. Boulton CL. Damage control orthopaedics. Orthopaedic Knowledge Online. Available at: http://orthoportal.aaos.org/oko/article.aspx?article=OKO_TRA044#abstract. Accessed July 29, 2013.

62. Pape HC, Giannoudis P, Krettek C. The timing of fracture treatment in polytrauma patients: relevance of damage control orthopaedic surgery. Am J Surg 2002;183(6):622–9.

63. Tiansheng S, Xiaobin C, Zhi L, et al. Is damage control orthopaedics essential for the management of bilateral femoral fractures associated or complicated with shock? An animal study. J Trauma 2009; 67(6):1402–11.

64. Crist BD, Ferguson T, Murtha YV, et al. Surgical timing of treating injured extremities an evolving concept of urgency. J Bone Joint Surg Am 2012; 94:1515–24.

65. Pape HC, Rixen D, Morley J, et al. Impact of the method of initial stabilization for femoral shaft fractures in patients with multiple injuries at risk for complications (borderline patients). Ann Surg 2007;246(3):491–501.

66. Morshed A, Miclau T, Bembom O, et al. Delayed internal fixation of femoral shaft fracture reduces mortality among patients with multisystem trauma. J Bone Joint Surg Am 2009;91:3–13.

67. Rixen D, Grass G, Sauerland S, et al. Evaluation of criteria for temporary external fixation in risk-adapted damage control orthopedic surgery of femur shaft fractures in multiple trauma patients: evidence-based medicine versus reality in the trauma registry of the German Trauma Society. J Trauma 2005;59(6):1375–95.

Weight Bearing After a Periarticular Fracture
What is the Evidence?

Justin M. Haller, MD, Michael Q. Potter, MD,
Erik N. Kubiak, MD*

KEYWORDS

- Weight bearing • Periarticular fracture • Lower extremity • Tibial plateau fracture
- Acetabular fracture • Tibial plafond fracture • Calcaneus fracture • Ankle fracture

KEY POINTS

- There is some evidence that patients autoregulate weight bearing based on the amount of fracture healing.
- Current methods of evaluating weight-bearing status are unreliable.
- Patient compliance with existing weight-bearing restrictions is poor.
- Studies of early weight bearing for acetabular, tibial plateau, tibial plafond, ankle, and calcaneus fractures demonstrate no increased risk for loss of reduction or nonunion compared with restricted weight bearing.
- Early weight bearing may return patients to function earlier.

INTRODUCTION

Anatomic fracture reduction, stable fixation, preservation of the surrounding soft tissues, and early mobilization are essential to the successful treatment of lower extremity articular injuries. However, because of concerns about loss of reduction, orthopedic surgeons are often hesitant to permit early mobilization of the injured limb. Restricted weight bearing after a periarticular fracture is thought to decrease the forces at the fracture site and the implant and reduce the risk of malreduction. Less mechanical stress on the implant is thought to lead to fewer construct failures and revisions. In contrast, animal studies have shown greater callus volume and faster time to union in extremities that were axially loaded as compared with those that were not loaded.[1,2] Early weight bearing may also expedite the return to work and minimize the economic impact of lower extremity injury. The authors review the available clinical evidence on early weight bearing after periarticular lower extremity fractures.

EFFECTS OF RESTRICTED WEIGHT BEARING

Weight-bearing restrictions can impart a significant physiologic toll on patients. In healthy patients, restricted weight bearing

- Results in a 4-fold increase in the energy expended for ambulation, when compared with full weight bearing, as measured by the physiologic cost index[3]
- Alters gait mechanics[4]
- Shifts the weight distribution from the forefoot and hallux to the heel[4]

Despite concerns for the increased risk of venous thromboembolism following surgery and

Department of Orthopaedics, University of Utah, 590 Wakara Way, Salt Lake City, UT 84108, USA
* Corresponding author.
E-mail address: erik.kubiak@hsc.utah.edu

Orthop Clin N Am 44 (2013) 509–519
http://dx.doi.org/10.1016/j.ocl.2013.06.005
0030-5898/13/$ – see front matter Published by Elsevier Inc.

restricted weight bearing, available studies have demonstrated no change in the venous return in the lower extremities affected by restricted weight bearing.[5]

WEIGHT BEARING AFTER FRACTURE

Clinicians routinely prescribe partial weight bearing for a lower extremity fracture in an attempt to produce an optimal mechanical environment at various stages of fracture healing. Partial weight bearing involves a gradual increase in the amount of weight that is placed on the affected limb. The partial-weight-bearing recommendation for patients varies based on the type of fracture, the extent of the injury, and the discretion of the clinician. For periarticular fractures, the standard partial-weight-bearing protocol includes 10 to 12 weeks of non–weight bearing followed by 4 to 6 weeks of progressive weight bearing whereby in the first week patients bear weight at 25% of their body weight and increase the amount of weight bearing by 25% each week until they are able to bear their full weight.[6]

There are few studies in the laboratory setting that examine axial fracture loading in humans. In a study of 27 patients with a tibia fracture treated with external fixation and early weight bearing, the initial axial motion across the fracture site was shown to be small at 5 weeks after the fracture (mean 0.28 mm), peaked at 11 weeks (mean 0.43 mm), and then decreased at later time points as fracture healing progressed.[7] This same group identified a similar trend when this study was performed with a larger clinical series of 45 patients.[8]

Koval and colleagues[9] performed gait analysis testing on elderly patients with operatively treated intracapsular and extracapsular hip fractures. Patients were allowed to bear weight as tolerated immediately after surgery. Over time, these patients voluntarily increased the weight applied to the injured limb from 51% at 1 week to 87% at 12 weeks when compared with the uninjured, contralateral limb. None of these patients experienced loss of fixation or other complications associated with immediate weight bearing.

Similarly, patients instructed to bear weight as tolerated after operative fixation of tibia fractures progressively increased axial loading across their injured extremity to around 85% that of the uninjured, contralateral extremity at 6 weeks postoperatively. All fractures successfully went on to union. The 2 patients in this series that developed a delayed union were only able to place 40% of their body weight on the affected limb at 20 weeks postoperatively.[10]

Axial loading studies have shown that

- Initial axial motion across the fracture site is small after the fracture and decreases as the fracture healing progresses.[8]
- No loss of fixation or other complications are associated with immediate weight bearing.[9]
- Progressive increases in axial loading result in successful union.[10]

PATIENT COMPLIANCE

Available data suggests patient compliance with physician restrictions on weight bearing is poor.[11–15] Standard clinical techniques to monitor weight-bearing compliance include the use of bathroom scales and a therapist estimating the load with palpation or observation. The scale has been shown to be effective; however, this is only useful for standing but not ambulation.[16,17] Both palpation and observation by a therapist have proven to be unreliable, regardless of the therapist's experience.[11,13,17–19] Multiple investigations of compliance demonstrate that patients exceed the prescribed amount of partial weight bearing even when they thought themselves to have been compliant.[12–15]

In efforts to improve compliance, investigators have used devices that provide real-time feedback on weight bearing.[12–15,20,21] In 2 separate studies, investigators found audible feedback to be ineffective in preventing overloading of the limb because of a lag between auditory perception and motor response.[13,14] Furthermore, patients trained to partially bear weight with audio feedback during their hospital stay were unable to replicate the prescription when walking unsupervised at home 21 days later.[20]

Winstein and colleagues[21] demonstrated that delayed verbal feedback by a therapist improved patient compliance with partial weight bearing more than device-based real-time audio feedback. Based on the available evidence, it is difficult to know if patients are actually abiding by weight-bearing restrictions, particularly outside the hospital setting.

Patients routinely

- Exceed the prescribed amount of partial weight bearing[12–15]
- Are unable to make use of audible feedback for compliance[13,14,20,21]

ACETABULAR FRACTURE

Malreduction after an acetabular fracture has been shown to be associated with poor patient outcome and development of posttraumatic arthritis.[22,23]

Given the potential consequences of fixation failure with subsequent loss of reduction, few studies have been performed permitting early weight bearing after acetabular fracture.

Mouhsine and colleagues[24] allowed elderly patients (mean 81 years of age) with column, transverse, or T-type fractures fixed percutaneously to begin unrestricted weight bearing at 4 weeks. With a minimum 2-year follow-up, the investigators reported no failure of fixation; all fractures healed an average of 12 weeks postoperatively. Similarly, 22 patients (mean 49 years of age, range 18–83 years) treated with percutaneous fixation of either an anterior column or an anterior column posterior hemitransverse fracture were permitted immediate full weight bearing postoperatively. There was no loss of reduction, and patient outcomes were similar to other reported studies at a minimum of 12 months of follow-up.[25]

A study of mostly elderly patients who participated in early weight bearing after total hip arthroplasty for acetabular fracture reported no early loosening, hardware failure, or revision surgery for osteolysis at a mean of 8.1 years postoperatively.[26] Based on these available studies, early weight bearing does not seem to be an excessive risk for fracture displacement in select operatively treated acetabular fractures.

Classically, postoperative protocols for acetabular fractures allow for touchdown weight bearing to decrease the joint reactive forces on the acetabulum as compared with strict non–weight bearing. However, peak pressures on the acetabulum during sit-to-stand activities performed during restricted weight bearing are nearly 3 times the forces seen during walking.[27] Much of the force during sit-to-stand activities is directed posteriorly, whereas during ambulation more load is distributed to the superior lateral aspect of the roof.[27,28]

Although few studies have examined weight bearing in patients with acetabular fractures, it is known that

- Immediate postoperative full weight bearing has not been shown to result in loss of reduction.[25]
- Early weight bearing after total hip arthroplasty for an acetabular fracture does not result in early loosening, hardware failure, or revision surgery for osteolysis.[26]
- Early weight bearing may not place patient at excessive risk for fracture displacement.[25,26]

TIBIAL PLATEAU FRACTURE

The knee joint experiences forces between 220% and 350% of a person's body weight during normal daily activities.[29] A 3-mm step-off in the tibial plateau can increase the cartilage contact stresses by 75%, thus raising concerns that loss of reduction could lead to worse patient outcomes.[30] However, the tibial plateau has been shown to tolerate some malreduction without change in outcome.[31,32]

Segal and colleagues[33] reported on a consecutive series of 86 lateral tibial plateau fractures treated operatively or nonoperatively based on an initial fracture displacement cut-off of 5 mm. Both groups were permitted to bear weight immediately in a fracture brace. The investigators reported superior outcomes among the operatively treated group; no patient in either group showed radiographic fracture displacement greater than 2 mm (**Table 1**).

More recently, 32 patients with partial articular plateau fractures (AO 41-B) were treated operatively with locking plate fixation and prescribed immediate (n = 12) or delayed (n = 20) weight bearing postoperatively. There was no evidence of radiographic fracture displacement in either group, and both groups had a similar rate of complications.[34] Similarly, Solomon and colleagues[35] reported on 7 patients with Schatzker II tibial plateau fractures treated with plate fixation and immediate partial weight bearing of 20 kg. The investigators reported a mean fracture displacement of 0.34 mm at 1 year using radiostereometric analysis.

Higher-energy plateau fractures are associated with increased fracture comminution and greater soft tissue injury, both of which can distribute more load to the fixation construct and create concern for failure. Eggli and colleagues[36] performed dual plating on 14 patients with these high-energy patterns and permitted immediate 10 kg of weight bearing. All patients achieved union by 12 weeks, and none experienced loss of fixation or subsidence as judged on radiographs.

In a study of elderly patients with bicondylar plateau treated with external ring fixator and early full weight bearing, 10 of 11 patients achieved a good result without loss of fixation; one patient experienced subsidence of the lateral plateau and underwent corrective osteotomy.[37] In a prospective, randomized study of high-energy tibial plateau fractures, a group of 43 patients underwent fixation with ring external fixation and were permitted to bear full weight. At the minimum 2-year follow-up, there was no difference in reoperations, articular incongruity, or development of radiographic signs of osteoarthritis as compared with a cohort of 40 patients that underwent open reduction and internal fixation with restricted weight bearing.[38]

Table 1
Tibial plateau fracture

Authors, Year	Study Type	Fracture Type	Treatment	Outcomes Measured	Results
Segal et al,[33] 1993	Retrospective	Lateral tibial plateau	ORIF (n = 44) and nonop (n = 42); both with WB in cast	Pain, swelling, ROM, and XR at 6, 12, 24 mo	Superior clinical outcomes in operative group; no loss of reduction in either group
Haak et al,[34] 2012	Retrospective	Lateral tibial plateau	ORIF with immediate WB (n = 12) vs delayed WB (n = 20)	Pain, reoperation, ROM, and XR at 6–8 wk	No difference in reoperations; no loss of reduction in either group
Solomon et al,[35] 2011	Prospective cohort	Lateral tibial plateau	ORIF and PWB (20 kg) (n = 7)	Fracture displacement at 2, 6, 12, 18, 26, 52 wk	Mean fracture displacement of 0.34 mm at 52 wk
Eggli et al,[36] 2008	Prospective cohort	Bicondylar plateau	ORIF and PWB (10 kg) (n = 14)	Pain, Lysholm knee score, ROM, and XR at 8, 12, 24, 52 wk	Improved knee scores; no loss of reduction
Ali et al,[37] 2003	Prospective cohort	Bicondylar plateau	Ringed EF and WB (n = 11)	ROM, SF-36, Rasmussen scale, Iowa knee, XR	3 Pts with valgus malunion, 82% satisfactory results
COTS[38] 2006	Multicenter prospective RCT	Bicondylar plateau	Ringed EF and WB (n = 43) vs ORIF and NWB (n = 40)	HSS knee score, WOMAC, SF-36, XR, ROM	No difference in patient outcomes or loss of reduction Fewer secondary surgeries with EF and WB

Abbreviations: EF, external fixator; HSS, Hospital Special Surgery; nonop, nonoperative; NWB, non–weight bearing; ORIF, Open reduction internal fixation; Pts, patients; PWB, partial weight bearing; RCT, randomized controlled trial; ROM, range of motion; SF-36, 36-Item Short Form Health Survey; WB, weight bearing; WOMAC, Western Ontario and McMasters Universities Arthritis Index; XR, radiograph.

Based on limited evidence, early weight bearing after tibial plateau fracture has been shown to

- Result in limited fracture displacement[33–35]
- Result in limited loss of fixation and subsidence[36]
- Have similar outcomes as restricted weight bearing[33]

TIBIAL PLAFOND FRACTURE

Tibial plafond fractures are associated with high rates of posttraumatic arthritis.[39,40] A 2-mm malreduction of the tibial plafond can result in a nearly 200% elevation in surrounding contact pressures.[41] Given the concern of loss of reduction and the potential development of posttraumatic osteoarthritis, there is limited literature evaluating early weight bearing after tibial plafond fractures.[42]

In a series of 26 patients with AO type C plafond fractures treated with dynamic external fixator and allowed partial weight bearing at 3 weeks, the investigators reported one case requiring arthrodesis and 2 cases of collapse after the fixator was removed. The remainder of the patients achieved bony union at a mean of 14 weeks.[43]

A nonrandomized series comparing 28 patients with AO type C plafond fractures treated with locked plate fixation and non–weight bearing to 14 patients treated with the Ilizarov technique and allowed to bear weight immediately showed nonsignificant trends in the Ilizarov group toward a faster time to union (mean 24 weeks vs 39 weeks) with a trend toward higher associated rates of nonunion, malunion, and infection.[44] Similarly, a series of 27 patients treated with internal fixation and restricted weight bearing were compared with 18 patients treated with external fixation and early weight bearing. There was no difference in postoperative articular congruity, but there were significantly more malunions in the external fixation group.[45] In addition, several small case series of comminuted plafond fractures treated with ring external fixation and full weight bearing within 3 weeks of surgery have shown good results (**Table 2**).[46–48]

In a large study with 51 patients with comminuted plafond fractures treated with a variety of fixation techniques, almost half were treated with internal fixation and early partial weight bearing without a cast. When compared with the other patients treated with external fixation and restricted weight bearing, there was no difference in the rates of reoperation, development of post traumatic osteoarthritis (PTOA), or pain. Patients with early weight bearing returned to previous employment significantly more frequently than those who underwent restricted weight bearing.[49]

With the limited data available for early weight bearing after tibial plafond fracture, it is difficult to make recommendations on this fracture pattern.

ANKLE FRACTURE

The best available evidence for weight bearing after periarticular lower extremity fractures is found in the literature on ankle fractures. A Cochrane meta-analysis of early versus late weight bearing after ankle fractures showed no difference between the groups in range of motion, functional scores, or radiographic outcomes at 1 year after the injury.[50] This analysis was based on 3 studies that directly compared early and late weight bearing after ankle fractures without other confounding variables; all 3 were published before 1990 and did not evaluate modern implants or fixation techniques (**Table 3**).[51–53]

Finsen and colleagues[52] randomized 56 patients to one of 3 groups: early range of motion and delayed weight bearing with no immobilization, late range of motion and immediate weight bearing as tolerated in a cast, or late range of motion and delayed weight bearing in a cast. At up to 2 years of follow-up, there were no consistent differences in the functional outcomes between the 3 groups at 9, 18, 36, 52, or 104 weeks.

Similarly, in a 2-part trial performed by Ahl and colleagues,[51,53] 93 patients were randomized to one of 4 groups: early range of motion (orthosis) and delayed weight bearing, early range of motion and early weight bearing, late range of motion (cast) and delayed weight bearing, or late range of motion and early weight bearing. They found a trend toward improved functional outcomes in the early weight bearing, early motion group that reached statistical significance at 3 and 6 months but not at 1 year or 18 months.

Gul and colleagues[54] reported 25 patients with ankle fractures treated through surgical stabilization followed by immediate weight bearing without protective immobilization. Their outcomes compared favorably with a historical control group treated with postoperative plaster cast immobilization and non–weight bearing. They found no difference in hospital stays, pain intensities, or functional outcomes; however, patients in the early weight-bearing group had a significant decrease in the time to return to work (91.3 ± 20.2 vs 54.6 ± 15.5 days).

In a study of 81 patients treated with operative fixation of an ankle fracture and randomized to immediate weight bearing in a plaster cast or non–weight bearing for 4 weeks without a cast, the investigators found significant improvement

Table 2
Tibial plafond fracture

Authors, Year	Study Type	Fracture Type	Treatment	Outcomes Measured	Results
Bacon et al,[43] 2008	Retrospective	OTA 43-C	Dynamic EF with PWB at 3 wk (n = 26)	Pain, swelling, ROM, and XR at 6, 12, 24 mo	3 Cases failure; 67% & 71% good-excellent results in subjective and objective criteria
Bacon et al,[44] 2007	Prospective Cohort	OTA 43-C	ORIF with NWB (n = 28) vs Ilizarov with WB (n = 14)	Time to union, malunion, nonunion, complications	No difference in outcome measures
Zarek et al,[46] 2002	Retrospective	OTA 43-C	Ilizarov and WB (n = 8)	ROM, pain, XR	1 case of malunion
McDonald et al,[47] 1996	Retrospective	OTA 43-C	Ilizarov and WB (n = 13)	Pain, ROM, and XR	2 cases of delayed/nonunion
Kapukaya et al,[48] 2005	Retrospective	OTA 43-C	Ilizarov and WB (n = 14)	ROM, pain, XR	1 case malunion
Blauth et al,[49] 2001	Retrospective	OTA 43-C	ORIF with PWB (n = 15) vs EF then ORIF with PWB (n = 8) vs EF with NWB (n = 28)	ROM, pain, XR	Patients with EWB returned to employment more frequently; no difference in other outcomes

Abbreviations: EF, external fixator; EWB, early weight bearing; NWB, non-weight bearing; ORIF, Open reduction internal fixation; OTA, Orthopaedic Trauma Association; ROM, range of motion; WB, weight bearing; XR, radiograph.

Table 3
Ankle fracture

Authors, Year	Study Type	Control Group	Treatment Group	Outcomes Measured	Results
Ahl et al,[53] 1986	Prospective RCT	ORIF and immediate WB in plaster cast (n = 22)	ORIF and WB in plaster cast at 4 wk (n = 24)	Pain, swelling, ROM, and XR at 3, 6, 18 mo	No difference; no loss of reduction in either group
Ahl et al,[51] 1987	Prospective RCT	ORIF and immediate WB in plaster cast (n = 25)	ORIF and WB in plaster cast at 4 wk (n = 28)	Pain, swelling, ROM, and XR at 3, 6, 18 mo	No difference; no loss of reduction in either group
Ahl et al,[51] 1993	Prospective RCT	ORIF and WB in removable orthosis at 1 wk (n = 26)	ORIF and WB in orthosis at 8 wk (n = 25)	Pain, swelling, ROM, and XR at 3, 6, 18 mo	Better DF in tx group at 3 mo; no loss of reduction
Ahl et al, 1993	Prospective RCT	ORIF and WB in removable orthosis at 1 wk (n = 26)	ORIF and WB in orthosis at 8 wk (n = 25)	Pain, swelling, ROM, and XR at 3, 6, 18 mo	No difference; no loss of reduction in either group
Finsen et al,[52] 1989	Prospective RCT	ORIF and immediate WB in plaster cast (n = 19)	ORIF and WB in plaster cast at 6 wk (n = 19)	ROM, activity questionnaire, RTW, XR	No difference; mortise widening in 3 of 19 each group
Gul et al,[54] 2007	Prospective cohort	ORIF and immediate WB w/o orthosis (n = 25)	ORIF and NWB in plaster cast for 6 wk (n = 25)	Pain, functional score, LOS, RTW, XR	Faster RTW (~45 d), one loss of reduction at 1 wk in early WB group
van Laarhoven et al,[55] 1996	Prospective RCT	ORIF and WB in plaster cast at 1 wk (n = 41)	ORIF and NWB in plaster cast for 6 wk (n = 40)	Pain, patient satisfaction, RTW, XR	Greater patient satisfaction at 10 d and 6 wk in early WB group

Abbreviations: DF, dorsiflexion; LOS, length of stay; NWB, non–weight bearing; ORIF, open reduction internal fixation; RCT, randomized controlled trial; ROM, range of motion; RTW, return to work; WB, weight bearing; w/o, without; XR, radiograph.

in subjective ankle scores at 6 weeks in the immediate weight-bearing group with no difference at later time points up to 1 year from the injury. There was no difference in wound complications, reoperation, or loss of reduction between the two groups. The patients in the early weight-bearing group returned to part-time work an average of 20 days sooner than those with weight-bearing restrictions. However, the return to full-time work was no different between the groups.[55]

Several level I and II studies investigating the effects of early ankle motion in postoperative care, with or without immediate weight bearing, have reported no long-lasting improvement in outcomes.[56–62] In a meta-analysis of early versus late mobilization of the ankle joint after operative fixation of ankle fractures, Thomas and colleagues[63] found that early ankle range of motion, with or without early weight bearing, improved range of motion and functional scores at 9 to 12 weeks after treatment. At 1 year, there was no difference between the groups. Despite similar long-term functional outcomes, early motion has been associated with a higher rate of superficial and deep wound complications.[54,57,62]

No long-term significant functional improvements have been shown with early weight bearing and early motion protocols, but they may offer short-term functional and socioeconomic benefits. Several investigators have reported a decrease in the time before the return to work with early motion protocols, but this finding has not been universal.[52,54,55,57–59,62]

Early weight bearing after ankle fracture has been shown to result in

- No difference between groups in range of motion, functional scores, or radiographic outcomes at 1 year after injury[50]
- No consistent differences in short-term functional outcomes[52]
- No difference in hospital stays, pain intensities, or functional outcomes[54]
- No difference in wound complications, reoperation, or loss of reduction[55]

CALCANEUS FRACTURE

In patients with a calcaneal fracture with significant soft tissue compromise, external fixation offers the ability to minimize further damage to the surrounding soft tissue envelope. Ali and colleagues[64] used an Ilizarov external fixator on displaced calcaneal fractures in 25 patients (10 Sanders type II, 9 type III, and 6 type IV). Partial weight bearing was encouraged 3 weeks postoperatively. There were no reported revision surgeries, and 68%

excellent or good outcomes according to the American Orthopaedic Foot and Ankle Society's (AOFAS) scale. Eleven of the patients developed subtalar arthritis, primarily in the type III and IV injuries. McGarvey and colleagues[65] reported similar results in a study of 18 patients treated with an Ilizarov external fixator and immediate full weight bearing.

Several small series of patients with intraarticular calcaneus fractures treated with open reduction and ring external fixation followed by immediate full weight bearing yielded acceptable results. Paley and Fischgrund[66] reported maintenance of reduction in 6 of 7 patients (86%) treated in this fashion. None of the patients had heel pain at 2 years, which the investigators attributed to desensitization from early weight bearing. Talarico and colleagues[67] described 25 patients (17 Sanders type II, 6 type III, and 2 type IV) treated similarly with no loss of reduction and 92% good or excellent results at 2 years using the Maryland Foot Score.

In a study of 39 patients with a displaced calcaneal fracture treated with minimal internal fixation (2–3 3.5-mm cancellous screws) and an external fixator, Fu and colleagues[68] reported no loss of reduction or collapse of the subtalar joint with patients that began partial weight bearing at 4 weeks.

A retrospective comparison of patients with intraarticular calcaneal fractures treated with open reduction and locking plate fixation showed no difference in pain or the AOFAS scores between patients restricted to 10 kg of weight bearing for 12 weeks (n = 58) or those allowed earlier progressive weight bearing beginning at 6 weeks (n = 78).[69] Additionally, Hyer and colleagues[70] reported on 17 calcaneus fractures whereby progressive weight bearing in a walking boot was allowed at an average of 4.8 weeks after open reduction and locked plate fixation. The average Bohler angle was 30.1° at the first postoperative visit and 28.5° at the final follow-up, with no patients showing significant loss of calcaneal height, loss of reduction, or hardware failure.

In a study that combined calcaneal perimeter plate with calcium phosphate bone cement in 10 patients, Thordarson and Latteier[71] reported that none experienced failure of fixation with early weight bearing. In contrast, a study of 40 patients treated with 3 AO mini-fragment plates placed laterally and early weight bearing of 15 kg reported significant decreases in the Gissane and Bohler angles at a minimum of 24 months of follow-up.[72]

Results of early weight bearing after calcaneus fracture have shown

- No reported revision surgeries and 68% excellent or good outcomes according to the AOFAS scale[64]
- No heel pain at 2 years postoperative[66]
- No loss of reduction and 92% good or excellent results at 2 years, using the Maryland Foot Score[67]
- No significant loss of calcaneal height, loss of reduction, or hardware failure[70]

SUMMARY

Despite their willingness to comply, patients often do not follow weight-bearing restrictions. Based on the few laboratory-based studies available, patients seem to advance their weight bearing as fracture healing progresses. The evidence available for early weight bearing following fixation of acetabular, tibial plateau, tibial plafond, ankle, and calcaneus fractures suggests that patients are not at a higher risk of loss of fixation as compared with patients with restricted weight bearing. Prospective, randomized studies comparing weight-bearing protocols are needed to help guide treatment recommendations.

REFERENCES

1. Bailon-Plaza A, van der Meulen MC. Beneficial effects of moderate, early loading and adverse effects of delayed or excessive loading on bone healing. J Biomech 2003;36:1069–77.
2. Gardner MJ, van der Meulen MC, Demetrakopoulos D, et al. In vivo cyclic axial compression affects bone healing in the mouse tibia. J Orthop Res 2006;24:1679–86.
3. Westerman RW, Hull P, Hendry RG, et al. The physiological cost of restricted weight bearing. Injury 2008;39:725–7.
4. North K, Potter MQ, Kubiak EN, et al. The effect of partial weight bearing in a walking boot on plantar pressure distribution and center of pressure. Gait Posture 2012;36(3):646–9.
5. Eisele R, Weickert E, Eren A, et al. The effect of partial and full weight-bearing on venous return in the lower limb. J Bone Joint Surg Br 2001;83(7):1037–40.
6. Ruedi TP, Buckely RE, Moran CG. AO principles of fracture management. 2nd edition. New York: Thieme; 2008.
7. Cunningham JL, Evans M, Kenwright J. Measurement of fracture movement in patients treated with unilateral external skeletal fixation. J Biomed Eng 1989;11:118–22.
8. Kershaw CJ, Cunningham JL, Kenwright J. Tibial external fixation, weight bearing, and fracture movement. Clin Orthop Relat Res 1993;28–36.
9. Koval KJ, Sala DA, Kummer FJ, et al. Postoperative weight-bearing after a fracture of the femoral neck or an intertrochanteric fracture. J Bone Joint Surg Am 1998;80:352–6.
10. Joslin CC, Eastaugh-Waring SJ, Hardy JR, et al. Weight bearing after tibial fracture as a guide to healing. Clin Biomech 2008;23:329–33.
11. Hurkmans HL, Bussmann JB, Selles RW, et al. The difference between actual and prescribed weight bearing of total hip patients with a trochanteric osteotomy: long-term vertical force measurements inside and outside the hospital. Arch Phys Med Rehabil 2007;88:200–6.
12. Hustedt JW, Blizzard DJ, Baumgaertner MR, et al. Is it possible to train patients to limit weight bearing on a lower extremity? Orthopedics 2012;35:e31–7.
13. Warren CG, Lehmann JF. Training procedures and biofeedback methods to achieve controlled partial weight bearing: an assessment. Arch Phys Med Rehabil 1975;56:449–55.
14. Chow DH, Cheng CT. Quantitative analysis of the effects of audio biofeedback on weight-bearing characteristics of persons with transtibial amputation during early prosthetic ambulation. J Rehabil Res Dev 2000;37:255–60.
15. Crews RT, Armstrong DG, Boulton AJ. A method for assessing off-loading compliance. J Am Podiatr Med Assoc 2009;99:100–3.
16. Gray FB, Gray C, McClanahan JW. Assessing the accuracy of partial weight-bearing instruction. Am J Orthop 1998;27:558–60.
17. Youdas JW, Kotajarvi BJ, Padgett DJ, et al. Partial weight-bearing gait using conventional assistive devices. Arch Phys Med Rehabil 2005;86(3):394–8.
18. Bohannon RW, Tinti-Wald D. Accuracy of weight bearing estimation by stroke versus healthy subjects. Percept Mot Skills 1991;72:935–41.
19. Hurkmans HL, Bussmann JB, Benda E. Validity and interobserver reliability of visual observation to assess partial weight-bearing. Arch Phys Med Rehabil 2009;90(2):309–13.
20. Hurkmans HL, Bussmann JB, Benda E, et al. Effectiveness of audio feedback for partial weight-bearing in and outside the hospital: a randomized controlled trial. Arch Phys Med Rehabil 2012;93:565–70.
21. Winstein CJ, Pohl PS, Cardinale C, et al. Learning a partial-weight-bearing skill: effectiveness of two forms of feedback. Phys Ther 1996;76:985–93.
22. Matta JM. Fractures of the acetabulum; accuracy of reduction and clinical results in patients managed operatively within three weeks after the injury. J Bone Joint Surg Am 1996;78:1632–45.
23. Tannast M, Najibi S, Matta JM. Two to twenty-year survivorship of the hip in 810 patients with operatively treated acetabular fractures. J Bone Joint Surg Am 2012;94(17):1559–67.

24. Mouhsine E, Garofalo R, Borens O, et al. Percutaneous retrograde screwing for stabilisation of
acetabular fractures. Injury 2005;36:1330–6.

25. Kazemi N, Archdeacon MT. Immediate full weight
bearing after percutaneous fixation of anterior
column acetabulum fractures. J Orthop Trauma
2012;26:73–9.

26. Mears DC, Velyvis JH. Acute total hip arthroplasty
for selected displaced acetabular fractures: two to
twelve-year results. J Bone Joint Surg Am 2002;84:
1–9.

27. Yoshida H, Faust A, Wilckens J, et al. Three-dimensional dynamic hip contact area and pressure distribution during activities of daily living. J Biomech
2006;39:1996–2004.

28. Bergmann G, Deuretzbacher G, Heller M, et al. Hip
contact forces and gait patterns from routine activities. J Biomech 2001;34:859–71.

29. Kutzner I, Heinlein B, Graichen F, et al. Loading of
the knee joint during activities of daily living
measured in vivo in five subjects. J Biomech
2010;43(11):2164–73.

30. Brown TD, Anderson DD, Nepola JV, et al. Contact
stress aberrations following imprecise reduction of
simple tibial plateau fractures. J Orthop Res 1988;
6:851–62.

31. Lansinger O, Bergman B, Korner L, et al. Tibial
condylar fractures. A twenty-year follow-up. J Bone
Joint Surg Am 1986;68:13–9.

32. Stevens DG, Beharry R, McKee MD, et al. The
long-term functional outcome of operatively treated
tibial plateau fractures. J Orthop Trauma 2001;15:
312–20.

33. Segal D, Mallik AR, Wetzler MJ, et al. Early weight
bearing of lateral tibial plateau fractures. Clin
Orthop Relat Res 1993;232–7.

34. Haak KT, Palm H, Holck K, et al. Immediate
weight-bearing after osteosynthesis of proximal
tibial fractures may be allowed. Dan Med J 2012;
59:A4515.

35. Solomon LB, Callary SA, Stevenson AW, et al.
Weight-bearing-induced displacement and migration over time of fracture fragments following split
depression fractures of the lateral tibial plateau: a
case series with radiostereometric analysis.
J Bone Joint Surg Br 2011;93:817–23.

36. Eggli S, Hartel MJ, Kohl S, et al. Unstable bicondylar tibial plateau fractures: a clinical investigation.
J Orthop Trauma 2008;22(10):673–9.

37. Ali AM, Burton M, Hashmi M, et al. Treatment of
displace bicondylar tibial plateau fractures (OTA-
41C2&3) in patients older than 60 years of age.
J Orthop Trauma 2003;17(5):346–52.

38. Canadian Orthopaedic Trauma Society. Open
reduction and internal fixation compared with circular fixator application for bicondylar tibial plateau
fractures. Results of a multicenter, prospective,

randomized clinical trial. J Bone Joint Surg Am
2006;88(12):2613–23.

39. Marsh JL, Weigel DP, Dirschl DR. Tibial plafond
fractures. How do these ankles function over
time? J Bone Joint Surg Am 2003;85A(2):287–95.

40. Harris AM, Patterson BM, Sontich JK, et al. Results
and outcomes after operative treatment of high energy tibial plafond fractures. Foot Ankle Int 2006;
27(4):256–65.

41. McKinley TO, McKinley T, Rudert MJ, et al. Stance-
phase aggregate contact stress gradient changes
resulting from articular surface stepoffs in human
cadaveric ankles. Osteoarthr Cartil 2006;14(2):
131–8.

42. Anderson DD, Van Hofwegen C, Marsh JL, et al. Is
elevated contact stress predictive of post-traumatic
osteoarthritis for imprecisely reduced tibial plafond
fractures? J Orthop Res 2010;29(1):33–9.

43. Mitkovic MB, Bumbasirevic MZ, Lesic A, et al. Dynamic external fixation of comminuted intra-
articular fractures of the distal tibia (type C pilon
fractures). Acta Orthop Belg 2002;68(5):508–14.

44. Bacon S, Smith WR, Morgan SJ, et al.
A retrospective analysis of comminuted intra-
articular fractures of the tibial plafond: open reduction and internal fixation versus external Ilizarov
fixation. Injury 2008;39:196–202.

45. Richards JE, Magill M, Tressler MA, et al. External
fixation versus ORIF for distal intra-articular tibia
fractures. Orthopedics 2012;35(6):862–7.

46. Zarek S, Othman M, Macias J. The Ilizarov method
in the treatment of pilon fractures. Ortop Traumatol
Rehabil 2002;4:427–33.

47. McDonald MG, Burgess RC, Bolano LE, et al. Ilizarov treatment of pilon fractures. Clin Orthop Relat
Res 1996;325:232–8.

48. Kapukaya A, Subasi M, Arslan H. Management of
comminuted closed tibial plafond fractures using
circular external fixators. Acta Orthop Belg 2005;
71(5):582–9.

49. Blauth M, Bastian L, Krettek C, et al. Surgical options for the treatment of severe tibial pilon fractures: a study of three techniques. J Orthop
Trauma 2001;15(3):153–60.

50. Lin CW, Donkers NA, Refshauge KM, et al. Rehabilitation for ankle fractures in adults. Cochrane Database Syst Rev 2012;(11):CD005595.

51. Ahl T, Dalen N, Holmberg S, et al. Early weight
bearing of displaced ankle fractures. Acta Orthop
Scand 1987;58:535–8.

52. Finsen V, Saetermo R, Kibsgaard L, et al. Early
postoperative weight-bearing and muscle activity
in patients who have a fracture of the ankle.
J Bone Joint Surg Am 1989;71:23–7.

53. Ahl T, Dalen N, Holmberg S, et al. Early weight
bearing of malleolar fractures. Acta Orthop Scand
1986;57:526–9.

54. Gul A, Batra S, Mehmood S, et al. Immediate un-protected weight-bearing of operatively treated ankle fractures. Acta Orthop Belg 2007;73:360–5.

55. Van Laarhoven CJ, Meeuwis JD, van der Werken C. Postoperative treatment of internally fixed ankle fractures: a prospective randomised study. J Bone Joint Surg Br 1996;78:395–9.

56. Cimino W, Ichtertz D, Slabaugh P. Early mobilization of ankle fractures after open reduction and internal fixation. Clin Orthop Relat Res 1991;152–6.

57. Vioreanu M, Dudeney S, Hurson B, et al. Early mobilization in a removable cast compared with immobilization in a cast after operative treatment of ankle fractures: a prospective randomized study. Foot Ankle Int 2007;28:13–9.

58. DiStasio AJ, Jaggears FR, DePasquale LV, et al. Protected early motion versus cast immobilization in postoperative management of ankle fractures. Contemp Orthop 1994;29:273–7.

59. Egol KA, Dolan R, Koval KJ. Functional outcome of surgery for fractures of the ankle. A prospective, randomised comparison of management in a cast or a functional brace. J Bone Joint Surg Br 2000; 82:246–9.

60. Tropp H, Norlin R. Ankle performance after ankle fracture: a randomized study of early mobilization. Foot Ankle Int 1995;16:79–83.

61. Hedstrom M, Ahl T, Dalen N. Early postoperative ankle exercise. A study of postoperative lateral mal-leolar fractures. Clin Orthop Relat Res 1994;(300): 193–6.

62. Lehtonen H, Jarvinen TL, Honkonen S, et al. Use of a cast compared with a functional ankle brace after operative treatment of an ankle fracture. A pro-spective, randomized study. J Bone Joint Surg Am 2003;85:205–11.

63. Thomas G, Whalley H, Modi C. Early mobilization of operatively fixed ankle fractures: a systematic re-view. Foot Ankle Int 2009;30(7):666–74.

64. Ali AM, Elsaied MA, Elmoghazy N. Management of calcaneal fractures using the Ilizarov external fixa-tor. Acta Orthop Belg 2009;75(1):51–6.

65. McGarvey WC, Burris MW, Clanton TO, et al. Calcaneal fractures: indirect reduction and external fixation. Foot Ankle Int 2006;27(7):494–9.

66. Paley D, Fischgrund J. Open reduction and circular external fixation of intraarticular calcaneal frac-tures. Clin Orthop Relat Res 1993;(290):125–31.

67. Talarico LM, Vito GR, Zyryanov SY. Management of displaced intraarticular calcaneal fractures by us-ing external ring fixation, minimally invasive open reduction, and early weight bearing. J Foot Ankle Surg 2004;43:43–50.

68. Fu TH, Liu HC, Su YS, et al. Treatment of displaced intra-articular calcaneal fractures with combined transarticular external fixation and minimal internal fixation. Foot Ankle Int 2013;34(1):91–8.

69. Kienast B, Gille J, Queitsch C, et al. Early weight bearing of calcaneal fractures treated by intraoper-ative 3D-fluoroscopy and locked-screw plate fixa-tion. Open Orthop J 2009;3:69–74.

70. Hyer CF, Atway S, Berlet GC, et al. Early weight bearing of calcaneal fractures fixated with locked plates: a radiographic review. Foot Ankle Spec 2010;3:320–3.

71. Thordarson DB, Latteier M. Open reduction and in-ternal fixation of calcaneal fractures with a low pro-file titanium calcaneal perimeter plate. Foot Ankle Int 2003;24(3):217–21.

72. Brunner A, Muller J, Regazzoni P, et al. Open reduction and internal fixation of OTA type C2-C4 fractures of the calcaneus with a triple-plate tech-nique. J Foot Ankle Surg 2012;51(3):299–307.

Surgical Treatment of Talus Fractures

Rachel J. Shakked, MD[a], Nirmal C. Tejwani, MD[b],*

KEYWORDS

- Talus fracture • Hawkins classification • Hawkins sign • Post-traumatic arthritis
- Snowboarder's fracture

KEY POINTS

- Talus fractures result from high-energy mechanisms and may be associated with other injuries to the foot and ankle.
- Talar neck fractures are most common and are classified using Hawkins classification. Functional outcome scores have been shown to vary inversely with increasing Hawkins grade.
- Prompt reduction of dislocation and surgical treatment of open fractures help decrease complications.
- Open anatomic reduction and internal fixation using dual incisions should be performed as soon as the patient is stable for the operating room.
- Hawkins sign as seen on radiographs at 6 weeks indicates intact blood supply and is a good prognostic indicator.
- Long-term complications after talus fractures include osteonecrosis, malunion, and arthritis of ankle and subtalar joints.

Management of talus fractures is a challenge because of the historically poor outcomes and high incidence of complications. Talus fractures account for 2% of all lower extremity injuries and are typically associated with a high-energy mechanism.[1]

ANATOMY

Sixty percent of the talar surface is articular cartilage, and no muscles insert on or originate from the talus.[2] The limited nonarticular surface of the talus available for vascular supply potentially contributes to the high risk of osteonecrosis following fractures of the talus.

Osteology

The superior surface of the talar body articulates with the tibial plafond, and the articular surface extends medially and laterally to articulate with the malleoli. The inferior aspect of the body articulates with the posterior facet of the calcaneus, and the talar head articulates with the navicular. The lateral process of the talus is also involved in the articulation with the posterior facet of the calcaneus. The posterior process of the talus is composed of the medial and lateral tubercles between which the flexor hallucis longus traverses. Ligamentous and capsular expansions attach to the talar neck, which is relatively devoid of articular cartilage and is an important location of vascular supply.[1]

Blood Supply

The posterior tibial artery supplies the anastomotic sling of vessels in the tarsal sinus and the tarsal canal that make up the primary arterial blood

Disclosures: Royalties: Biomet; Consultant/Speaker's Bureau: Stryker; Zimmer; No conflicts with the subject of this article (N.C. Tejwani). None (R.J. Shakked).
a Department of Orthopaedic Surgery, NYU Hospital for Joint Diseases, 301 East 17th Street, New York, NY 10003, USA; b Department of Orthopaedics, New York University Medical Center, 550 First Avenue, CD4-102, New York, NY 10016, USA
* Corresponding author.
E-mail address: Nirmal.Tejwani@NYUMC.org

supply to the talus.[2,3] These branches enter the talus via the inferior aspect of the neck and course posterolaterally to supply the talar body in a retrograde fashion.[2] A branch of the anterior tibial artery enters the talus at the dorsal aspect of the neck and supplies the talar head, and a branch of the peroneal artery contributes to the artery of the sinus tarsi. The blood supply to the talus is summarized in **Fig. 1**.

TALAR NECK FRACTURES

Approximately 45% of talus fractures occur at the neck.[4] The mechanism of injury has been described as hyperdorsiflexion of the ankle and fracture through the talar neck due to impingement of the anterior tibia.[5] There is a rotational component implied by the presence of medial comminution and concurrent medial malleolar fracture in 11% to 28% of cases.[4,6–8] The mechanism is typically high energy, as suggested by high rates of associated fractures in 54% to 64% of cases and open fractures in approximately 20% of cases.[4,7]

Classification

The most commonly used classification system was described by Hawkins and modified by Canale and Kelly (**Fig. 2**).[6,9] This classification system has been shown to correlate with prognosis as shown in **Table 1**.[6] Use of a computed tomography (CT) scan improves the interobserver correlation of the modified Hawkins classification as compared with radiographs alone.[10]

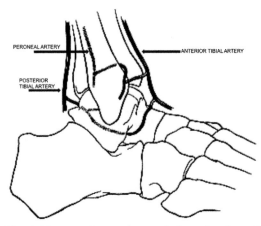

Fig. 1. The vascular anatomy of the talus from 3 major vessels: anterior tibial, peroneal, and posterior tibial. (*Adapted from* Adelaar RS, Madrian JR. Avascular necrosis of the talus. Orthop Clin North Am 2004;35(3):384; with permission.)

Clinical Evaluation

Patients with talar neck fractures typically present after a high-energy mechanism with foot swelling. There may be gross deformity and skin tenting with associated dislocations. Dislocations of the talus should be reduced urgently to reduce the risk of osteonecrosis and skin compromise. Type 2 fracture dislocation is the most common, and the reduction maneuver is plantar flexion and inversion or eversion. Up to 38% of Hawkins type 3 fractures are open, and in these cases, the talus may be partially or completely extruded.[8] Neurovascular status of the foot should be assessed. The patient should also be evaluated for other injuries given the high-energy mechanism.

Radiographic Evaluation

Radiographic evaluation of the injured extremity should include anteroposterior, oblique, and lateral views of the foot and the ankle. To better visualize the talar neck, an additional view can be obtained as described by Canale and Kelly and shown in **Fig. 3** (Canale view).[6] CT scans are useful to assess for comminution, intra-articular fragments, and congruent reduction of subtalar, tibiotalar, and talonavicular joints.

Treatment: Nonoperative

Type 1 fractures are usually amenable to nonoperative treatment if CT scan truly demonstrates no displacement of the talar neck. As little as 2 mm of displacement has been shown to alter contact pressures of the subtalar joint, which can lead to arthritis.[11] The patient is placed in a short-leg cast for 6 weeks with no weight bearing permitted. Weekly radiographic confirmation with a Canale view that no displacement of the talar neck has developed is recommended.[6] After 6 weeks of cast immobilization, the patient can be converted to a fracture boot for an additional 6 weeks with restricted weight bearing.

Treatment: Operative

Anteromedial
The anteromedial approach to the talus is performed using an incision medial to the anterior tibial tendon to visualize the talar neck. An osteotomy of the medial malleolus can be performed using this approach for better visualization of the talar body. Care should be taken to avoid stripping the dorsal aspect of the neck and deltoid ligament attachment to preserve what remains of the blood supply. This approach by itself may be insufficient if there is medial comminution or impaction, because judgment of the reduction

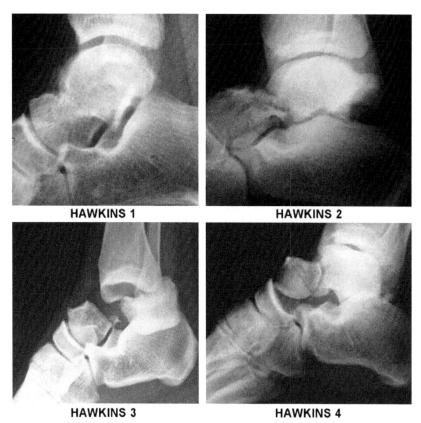

Fig. 2. Hawkins classification. (*From* Williams T, Barba N, Noailles T, et al. Total talar fracture—inter- and intra-observer reproducibility of two classification systems (Hawkins and AO) for central talar fractures. Orthop Traumatol Surg Res 2012;98:S60; with permission.)

may be inadequate without visualizing the lateral aspect of the neck.

Anterolateral

To approach the talar neck using the anterolateral approach, an incision is made lateral to the extensor digitorum longus. If this incision is used

in conjunction with the anteromedial approach, an adequate skin bridge should be left to avoid skin necrosis. It is especially important to avoid injury to the vessels in the tarsal sinus when utilizing this approach. Provisional fixation with Kirschner wires is performed, and then medial and/or lateral screws and plates are placed from

Table 1
Hawkins classification system for talar neck fractures and rates of osteonecrosis

Talar Neck Fracture	Associated Joint Subluxation or Dislocation	Rate of Osteonecrosis (%)
1 Nondisplaced	None	13[6]
2 Displaced	Subtalar	50[6]
3 Displaced	Subtalar Tibiotalar	80[6,9]
4 Displaced	Subtalar Tibiotalar Talonavicular	50[6]

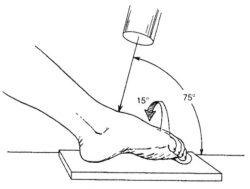

Fig. 3. Positioning for a Canale view to demonstrate the talar neck. (*From* Juliano PJ, Dabbah M, Harris TG. Talar neck fractures. Foot Ankle Clin 2004;9(4):725; with permission.)

a point just off the articular surface of the head and directed posteriorly into the body. Cannulated screws are useful to better control the position of the screw.

Posterolateral

Screws can also be placed from posterior to anterior, allowing for a configuration that is perpendicular to the fracture line. The approach is lateral to the Achilles tendon between the flexor hallucis longus and peroneal tendons, revealing the posterior process of the talus. The ideal location of the screws is starting at the lateral tubercle and angled anteromedially.[12] Risks of this approach include screw penetration of the subtalar joint, involvement of the talonavicular joint, and injury to the peroneal artery and saphenous nerve.

Percutaneous fixation

Displaced talar neck fractures should be fixed in anatomic position. Closed reduction is sometimes achieved with the foot in equinus, but this can lead to contracture. If closed reduction is possible, and there is no significant comminution, percutaneous screw fixation is an option. Low rates of osteonecrosis and malunion have been described when closed reduction is performed using Schanz screws, and percutaneous screw fixation is performed in Hawkins grades 2, 3, and 4.[13] Percutaneous screw fixation can also be performed in nondisplaced talar neck fractures to begin early range of motion. Screws (usually 4.5 mm diameter) can be placed from a posterolateral or anterior approach. In general, when using screws to fix talar neck fractures, the surgeon should consider using titanium screws so that magnetic resonance imaging (MRI) can be used postoperatively to assess for bony healing and/or avascular necrosis.

Open reduction and internal fixation

Anterior-to-posterior screws versus posterior-to-anterior screws If the decision is made to use screw fixation, Swanson and colleagues[14] showed superior mechanical strength using the posterior-to-anterior technique. A trend toward increased strength of posterior-to-anterior compared with anterior-to-posterior screws was also found by Attiah and colleagues[15] in a biomechanical study.

Screws alone versus plate and screws Plate fixation is performed in a bridging fashion if there is significant comminution as shown in **Fig. 4**.[16] The plate may be placed medially or laterally depending on the location of comminution.[16] Plate fixation has been shown to effect a more precise reduction and avoids malalignment due to compression through areas of comminution that can occur when using only compression screws.[17] Combined plate and screw fixation is not as strong as using screws alone as measured by Charlson and colleagues[17] in a biomechanical cadaver study, but this difference is not clinically significant. Another cadaveric study found no significant difference in strength when comparing various screw combinations to screw with medial plate fixation.[15]

Small fragment screws versus headless screws When using screws to fix the talar neck, countersinking or headless screws will prevent impingement of the screw head and restricted range of motion. No biomechanical difference between variable-pitch cannulated headless screws was identified in a biomechanical study compared with standard cannulated screws.[18]

Timing of surgery

Talar neck fractures were traditionally considered orthopedic emergencies requiring surgical treatment within 6 hours. Lindvall and colleagues[19] compared early operative intervention within 6 hours to delayed treatment (6–504 hours) after presentation, and no differences in union rates, osteonecrosis, arthritis, and functional outcome scores were identified. Vallier and colleagues[20] also showed no correlation between osteonecrosis and surgical delay as long as any associated dislocation was urgently reduced. Rather than the timing of surgery, osteonecrosis was associated with degree of comminution of the talar neck and the presence of open fractures in 1 study.[20] Time between injury and operative treatment did not increase patients' risk of developing complications and requiring additional surgery in the future.[21] However, although definitive fixation can be done in a delayed fashion, dislocations must be reduced urgently, and open fractures must be addressed as soon as the patient is stable to go to the operating room.

Postoperative management

If stable fixation is attained and there is no significant comminution or joint instability, early range of motion can be initiated. If there is any concern for the integrity of the fixation, casting for 6 weeks is recommended. Radiographs at 6 weeks may show a radiolucent line, indicating the presence of intact blood supply (Hawkins sign). However, the absence of one does not necessarily mean that the patient will develop osteonecrosis. Regardless, patients should remain nonweight-bearing until there is evidence of healing, usually for around 3 months.

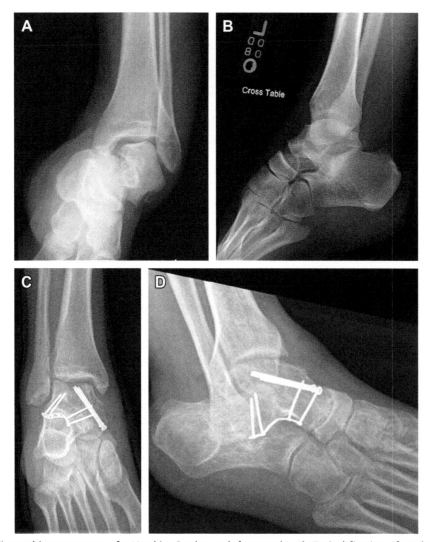

Fig. 4. Radiographic appearance of a Hawkins 3 talar neck fracture (*A, B*). Typical fixation of a talar neck fracture using a lateral plate and medial screws (*C, D*). (*Courtesy of* Nirmal C. Tejwani, MD, New York, NY; with permission.)

TALAR BODY FRACTURES

Fractures of the talar body involve the tibiotalar and subtalar joints and therefore necessitate anatomic reduction. These fractures have the highest incidence of tibiotalar and subtalar joint arthrosis among talus fractures.[4] Axial load is the typical mechanism of injury, and up to 50% of patients have associated talar neck fractures.[20] Radiologic evaluation should include CT of the talus, because articular injury is underestimated on standard radiographs.

Treatment: Nonoperative

Closed treatment of talar body fractures generally has poor outcomes, and surgical management is preferred to ensure anatomic reconstruction of involved articular surfaces.[22]

Treatment: Open Reduction and Internal Fixation

Standard approaches as described for fixation of talar neck fractures can be used for open reduction and internal fixation of talar body fractures using minifragment screws and plates (**Fig. 5**). Countersunk or headless screws can be used to avoid prominent hardware. To expose the talar dome, medial malleolar osteotomy may be performed. This is preferable to violating the deltoid ligament, which contains an important source of blood supply to the talus. If the size of the fracture fragments preclude fixation, excision can be

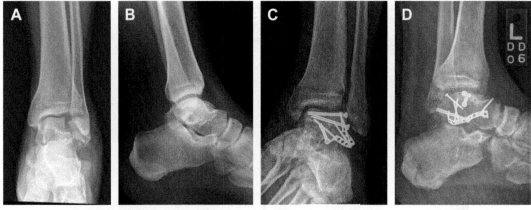

Fig. 5. Injury (*A, B*) and postoperative radiographs (*C, D*) of a talar body fracture. (*Courtesy of* Nirmal C. Tejwani, MD, New York, NY; with permission.)

performed; this should be limited to small fragments not affecting ankle stability. In cases of significant subchondral impaction, bone grafting should be considered.

TALAR HEAD FRACTURES

The incidence of talar head fractures is lower than talar body and neck fractures. The mechanism of injury is axial compression of the talar head into the navicular, and the talonavicular joint surface is therefore usually involved. Standard radiographs should be supplemented with a CT scan to assess articular displacement.

Treatment: Nonoperative

In a nondisplaced talar head fracture, nonoperative treatment with a short-leg cast and nonweight-bearing can be performed.

Treatment: Open Reduction and Internal Fixation

An anteromedial approach is used to fix the fracture with screws. Bone grafting is recommended for significant impaction in order to restore articular reduction.

Postoperatively, early range of motion can be initiated if the talonavicular joint is felt to be stable at the time of operation. If unstable, 6 weeks of immobilization and nonweight-bearing should ensue prior to range of motion and weight bearing. Compared with other portions of the talus, the talar head has sufficient blood supply to allow rapid healing, and the rates of osteonecrosis are low.[2]

LATERAL PROCESS FRACTURES (SNOWBOARDER'S FRACTURE)

Lateral process fractures are commonly missed and are often seen with snowboarding accidents.[23] The lateral process of the talus is part of the subtalar and talofibular articulations. Fracture patterns may be small avulsion fragments or larger articular fragments. The mechanism of injury is thought to be axial load, forced dorsiflexion, and external rotation.[23,24] Standard ankle radiographs do not demonstrate lateral process fractures well, and a CT scan is usually required to visualize the fracture and determine whether operative intervention is necessary.

Treatment: Nonoperative

Small lateral process fractures or nondisplaced fractures can be treated nonoperatively with ankle immobilization and progressive weight bearing.

Treatment: Open Reduction and Internal Fixation

Larger and displaced lateral process fractures require fixation using lag screws or a minifragment plate using the posterolateral approach. Primary surgical treatment has been shown to have better outcomes, reduced risk of subtalar arthritis, and return to same level of preinjury activity.[24]

OUTCOMES

Patient outcomes after talus fracture are highly variable, but in general, lateral and posterior process fractures have the best outcomes, followed by neck fractures and then body fractures.[4] Eighty percent of patients with a lateral process fracture return to preinjury sport level.[24] Functional outcome scores have been shown to vary inversely with increasing Hawkins grade.[7] On average, 56% of patients have good-to-excellent functional outcomes after talar neck fracture, and 44% have poor-to-fair outcomes.[25] If the patient with a talus fracture has a concomitant calcaneal fracture, the outcome is known to be worse. Sixty-two percent of patients with an open injury required below-knee amputation (BKA) in a retrospective study by Aminian and colleagues.[26] In addition, 80% of patients who did not undergo BKA developed subtalar arthritis.

COMPLICATIONS
Osteonecrosis

The incidence of osteonecrosis after talar neck fracture varies with Hawkins stages.[27] Approximately 80% of Hawkins stage 3 or 4 fractures will result in osteonecrosis.[27] More recent studies have reported a lower incidence of osteonecrosis, which may be attributable to early and anatomic fixation. Osteonecrosis is also seen more commonly in open talus fractures. Lindvall and colleagues[19] reported osteonecrosis in 13 of 26 talus fractures and in 6 out of 7 open fractures. Twenty-five percent of Hawkins 2 talar neck fractures and 42% of Hawkins 3 talar neck fractures developed osteonecrosis in a series published by Elgafy and colleagues.[4] This complication can be identified on radiographs between 4 weeks and 6 months after injury. It is demonstrated by relative opacity of the talus compared with the surrounding bones. The presence of subchondral osteopenia, classically known as the Hawkins sign, at 6 to 8 weeks after injury predicts that development of osteonecrosis is unlikely, with 91% to 100% sensitivity.[7,28] However, the absence of the Hawkins sign is not useful for predicting osteonecrosis. In addition to radiographic evaluation, MRI can be used to detect early osteonecrosis.

Treatment

Only 41% of cases of osteonecrosis after talus fracture have been reported to be symptomatic.[7] There is no obvious relationship between prolonged nonweight-bearing and eventual bony collapse or development of arthritis in patients with osteonecrosis. Revascularization of the talus can take as long as 2 years, if at all.[29] An offloading orthosis can be used if patients have pain. If conservative treatment fails and arthrosis develops, arthrodesis of the involved joints can be performed, and all osteonecrotic bone should be excised to allow for successful fusion. Recently, early reports of total ankle replacement have shown somewhat encouraging results.[20,30]

Post-traumatic Arthrosis

Post-traumatic arthrosis develops at the ankle and subtalar joints secondary to articular damage at time of injury or abnormal joint mechanics following healing. The incidence of post-traumatic arthritis has been reported to be as high as 74% and varies directly with increasing Hawkins grade.[7]

Treatment

Post-traumatic arthritis can be treated conservatively with bracing and pain medication, or with fusion of the involved joints. Twenty-five percent of patients with talar body and neck fractures eventually required subtalar, talocrural, talonavicular, or combined arthrodesis for arthritis.[7]

Malunion

The rate of malalignment after talar neck repair is approximately 30%.[7,21] Talar neck fractures tend to result in varus malunion because of the medial comminution. Medially placed screws can compress through this area of comminution and lead to varus malunion. Because of this tendency to overcompress, a plate should be used to ensure anatomic reduction in combination with screws. Reduction can also be difficult to assess, especially when a single incision is used. Parameters of an acceptable reduction as described by Canale and colleagues[6] are less than 5 mm of displacement and 5° of angulation or varus, although greater than 2 mm of displacement affects the biomechanics of the subtalar joint.[11] CT is the best modality to assess malunion, although both radiograph and CT scan have been shown to underestimate the actual amount of displacement.[31] Varus malunion causes the patient's foot to be in a supinated, internally rotated position with medial column shortening that requires reconstructive osteotomy. Dorsal malunion also can occur, which results in restricted dorsiflexion because of impingement on the anterior tibia. This is treated with resection of the dorsal prominence.

Treatment

If malunion is associated with arthritis, fusion of the affected joints can be performed. However, if there is no evidence of arthritis, talar osteotomy can be performed to correct the malunion.

Skin Complications and Infections

The skin around the ankle is relatively devoid of subcutaneous soft tissue and is more fragile than other areas of the body. Skin tenting after talus fractures caused by associated dislocations can place the soft tissues at risk and should be promptly reduced. Displaced fractures need to be reduced in order to reduce tension on dorsal skin. Open fractures are associated with a high rate of infection, especially with partial or total extrusion of the talus.[4,20,32]

REFERENCES

1. Sanders DW. Talus fractures. In: Bucholz RW, Court-Brown CM, Heckman JD, et al, editors. Rockwood and green's fractures in adults. 7th edition. Philadelphia: Lippincott Williams and Wilkins; 2010. p. 2022–63.
2. Kelly PJ, Sullivan CR. Blood supply of the talus. Clin Orthop Relat Res 1963;30:37–44.
3. Haliburton RA, Sullivan CR, Kelly PJ, et al. The extra-osseous and intra-osseous blood supply of the talus. J Bone Joint Surg Am 1958;40:1115–20.
4. Elgafy H, Ebraheim NA, Tile M, et al. Fractures of the talus: experience of two level 1 trauma centers. Foot Ankle Int 2000;21(12):1023–9.
5. Anderson HG. The medical and surgical aspects of aviation. London: Oxford University Press; 1919.
6. Canale ST, Kelly FB Jr. Fractures of the neck of the talus. Long-term evaluation of seventy-one cases. J Bone Joint Surg Am 1978;60(2):143–56.
7. Fournier A, Barba N, Steiger V, et al. Total talar fracture—long-term results of internal fixation of talar fractures. A multicentric study of 114 cases. Orthop Traumatol Surg Res 2012;98:S48–55.
8. Lorentzen JE, Christensen SB, Krogsoe O, et al. Fractures of the neck of the talus. Acta Orthop Scand 1977;48(1):115–20.
9. Hawkins LG. Fractures of the neck of the talus. J Bone Joint Surg Am 1970;52(5):991–1002.
10. Williams T, Barba N, Noailles T, et al. Total talar fracture—inter- and intra-observer reproducibility of two classification systems (Hawkins and AO) for central talar fractures. Orthop Traumatol Surg Res 2012;98:S56–65.
11. Sangeorzan BJ, Wagner UA, Harrington RM, et al. Contact characteristics of the subtalar joint: the effect of talar neck misalignment. J Orthop Res 1992;10(4):544–51.
12. Ebraheim NA, Mekhail AO, Salpietro BJ, et al. Talar neck fractures: anatomic considerations for posterior screw application. Foot Ankle Int 1996;17(9):541–7.
13. Abdelgaid SM, Ezzat FF. Percutaneous reduction and screw fixation of fracture neck talus. Foot Ankle Surg 2012;18(4):219–28.
14. Swanson TV, Bray TJ, Holmes GB Jr. Fractures of the talar neck. A mechanical study of fixation. J Bone Joint Surg Am 1992;74(4):544–51.
15. Attiah M, Sanders DW, Valdivia G, et al. Comminuted talar neck fractures: a mechanical comparison of fixation techniques. J Orthop Trauma 2007;21(1):47–51.
16. Fleuriau Chateau PB, Brokaw DS, Jelen BA, et al. Plate fixation of talar neck fractures: preliminary review of a new technique in twenty-three patients. J Orthop Trauma 2002;16(4):213–9.
17. Charlson MD, Parks BG, Weber TG, et al. Comparison of plate and screw fixation and screw fixation alone in a comminuted talar neck fracture model. Foot Ankle Int 2006;27(5):340–3.
18. Capelle JH, Couch CG, Wells KM, et al. Fixation strength of anteriorly inserted headless screws for talar neck fractures. Foot Ankle Int 2013;34(7):1012–6.
19. Lindvall E, Haidukewych G, DiPasquale T, et al. Open reduction and stable fixation of isolated, displaced talar neck and body fractures. J Bone Joint Surg Am 2004;86(10):2229–34.
20. Vallier HA, Nork SE, Barei DP, et al. Talar neck fractures: results and outcomes. J Bone Joint Surg Am 2004;86(8):1616–24.
21. Sanders DW, Busam M, Hattwick E, et al. Functional outcomes following displaced talar neck fractures. J Orthop Trauma 2004;18(5):265–70.
22. Sneppen O, Christensen SB, Krogsoe O, et al. Fracture of the body of the talus. Acta Orthop Scand 1977;48(3):317–24.
23. Bladin C, McCrory P. Snowboarding injuries. An overview. Sports Med 1995;19(5):358–64.
24. Valderrabano V, Perren T, Ryf C, et al. Snowboarder's talus fracture: treatment outcome of 20 cases after 3.5 years. Am J Sports Med 2005;33(6):871–80.
25. Halvorson JJ, Winter SB, Teasdall RD, et al. Talar neck fractures: a systematic review of the literature. J Foot Ankle Surg 2013;52(1):56–61.
26. Aminian A, Howe CR, Sangeorzan BJ, et al. Ipsilateral talar and calcaneal fractures: a retrospective review of complications and sequelae. Injury 2009;40(2):139–45.
27. Metzger MJ, Levin JS, Clancy JT. Talar neck fractures and rates of avascular necrosis. J Foot Ankle Surg 1999;38(2):154–62.
28. Tezval M, Dumont D, Sturmer KM. Prognostic reliability of the Hawkins sign in fractures of the talus. J Orthop Trauma 2007;21(8):538–43.
29. Adelaar RS, Madrian JR. Avascular necrosis of the talus. Orthop Clin North Am 2004;35(3):383–95.
30. Lee KB, Cho SG, Jung ST, et al. Total ankle arthroplasty following revascularization of avascular necrosis of the talar body: two case reports and literature review. Foot Ankle Int 2008;29(8):852–8.
31. Chan G, Sanders DW, Yuan X, et al. Clinical accuracy of imaging techniques for talar neck malunion. J Orthop Trauma 2008;22(6):415–8.
32. Juliano PJ, Dabbah M, Harris TG. Talar neck fractures. Foot Ankle Clin 2004;9(4):723–36.

Surgical Management Principles of Gunshot-Related Fractures

Rick Tosti, MD*, Saqib Rehman, MD

KEYWORDS

• Ballistic • Bullet • Fracture • Gunshot • Wound

KEY POINTS

- Initial assessment should begin with Advanced Trauma Life Support principles, inspection of soft-tissue damage and contamination, a thorough neurovascular examination, local wound care, imaging, and fracture stabilization.
- High-risk wounds are those involving high-energy weapons, delayed presentation, large soft-tissue deficits, multiple projectiles, exposed bone, and those occurring on a battlefield or farm environment.
- Most low-risk gunshot fractures can be treated similarly to closed fractures. Stable injuries can be treated with cast immobilization, antibiotics, and daily wound care.
- Operative intervention is indicated for unstable fracture patterns, wounds with exposed bone, high-risk wounds, associated vascular injury, or associated compartment syndrome.
- Bullet tracts do not decompress compartments, and compartment syndrome should be managed with full-length fasciotomies.

INTRODUCTION

Nonfatal gunshot injuries are a common problem, estimated to occur approximately 60,000 to 80,000 times per year in the United States.[1,2] Several studies have reported that roughly half of all hospital admissions for gunshot wounds require fracture care, underscoring the importance of the orthopedic surgeon in the overall management of these patients.[1–4] Gunshot missiles most commonly penetrate the bones of the spine, femur, tibia and fibula, hand, and forearm, and may acutely result in life-threatening or limb-threatening injuries.[2] Furthermore, despite appropriate initial treatment, early and late sequelae such as compartment

syndrome, nerve palsy, bone and soft-tissue deficits, and lead toxicity may additionally incur a significant morbidity in this population. The purpose of this review is to discuss contemporary management strategies for gunshot-related fractures, with special attention paid to the initial evaluation, role of debridement, principles of fixation, need and duration of antibiotic therapy, and management of sequelae.

INITIAL EVALUATION

The Advanced Trauma Life Support (ATLS) protocol should be the initial priority in a gunshot-wound victim. After primary stabilization, a history and

Conflict of Interest Statement: Each author certifies that he or she has no commercial associations (eg, consultancies, stock ownership, equity interest, patent/licensing arrangements, and so forth) that might pose a conflict of interest in connection with the submitted article.
Location Statement: Research for this article was conducted at Temple University Hospital and its affiliates.
Department of Orthopaedic Surgery and Sports Medicine, School of Medicine, Temple University, 3401 N Broad St, Philadelphia, PA 19140, USA
* Corresponding author.
E-mail address: rtosti@temple.edu

Orthop Clin N Am 44 (2013) 529–540
http://dx.doi.org/10.1016/j.ocl.2013.06.006
0030-5898/13/$ – see front matter © 2013 Elsevier Inc. All rights reserved.

secondary survey should be performed by the orthopedic surgeon. The patient or law enforcement officers may provide clues relating to the weapon involved in the shooting. Shotguns are considered low-velocity weapons but with a high injury potential as a result of multiple, high-mass projectiles. More extensive tissue damage is associated with multiple shots, close range, higher-velocity weapons, and expanding missiles (eg, hollow-point ammunition) (**Figs. 1** and **2**). Although forensic science can help to determine entry versus exit wounds, ammunition type by examination of wounds, and the position of the patient at the time of missile entry, it is not the job, nor within the scope of expertise, of the treating physician to attempt to establish these facts. The forensic information is generally not helpful for treating the patient at hand. Furthermore, these conclusions can be erroneous, leading to legal confusion in later criminal proceedings.

The patient should be fully exposed and examined for wounds, and the anatomic structures in the trajectory of each bullet wound should be evaluated thoroughly. The appearance of the limb should be inspected for color, soft-tissue damage, gross contamination, compartment swelling, joint effusion, and the presence of exposed bone fragments. Wounds presenting with pulsatile bleeding and/or diminished distal pulses should raise suspicion for vascular injury, and may require emergent surgical exploration.[5] Even in the presence of normal pulses, one should consider checking an ankle-brachial index on all gunshot-related injuries of the extremities, and obtain angiography or ultrasonic vascular testing for ratios less than 0.9. A thorough neurologic examination, including testing with pinprick for sharp/dull sensation, should also be documented as a baseline. All wounds can be labeled with a metallic marker for easier identification on radiographs, and all missiles should then be accounted for either with a retained bullet fragment or an exit wound. Characterization of periarticular or perivascular injuries may be enhanced via computed tomography (CT). All wounds are then copiously irrigated and dressed; the authors generally pack small wounds daily with ¼-inch iodinated gauze strips, and dress larger wounds with iodinated vaseline gauze sheets. Tetanus prophylaxis is considered in all patients with an unknown immunization status. Fractures are reduced and stabilized with padded plaster splints. Fractures involving retained fragments in the hip joint or fractures of the femur that cannot be immediately treated are stabilized with skeletal traction via distal transosseous pins.

ROLE OF DEBRIDEMENT

The common myth that bullets fired from a gun are sterile has been disproved in several studies.[3,6,7] Bacteria and clothing debris are commonly translocated into the wound from the blast effect, and cause contamination. However, despite the fact that many surgeons consider the wound contamination to be similar to that of open fractures, current evidence has demonstrated that not all wounds require debridement as is done for open fractures. For example, Dickey and colleagues[7] presented a prospective randomized trial of 73 patients with stable, nonoperatively managed gunshot-related fractures, and noted similar infection rates between those with and without antibiotic prophylaxis. Knapp and colleagues[8] reported on 222 stable long-bone fractures treated nonoperatively, and similarly found no difference in infection rates between those treated with intravenous or oral antibiotics. The authors' preference for stable low-energy gunshot fractures without exposed bone is to allow the wounds to close by secondary intention via daily packing changes; additionally, a 5-day course of an oral first-generation cephalosporin as prophylaxis is prescribed, because of the unknown degree of initial contamination and the potential for poorer personal hygiene in the urban population. Stable

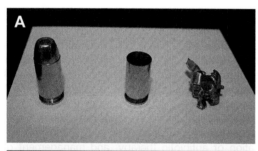
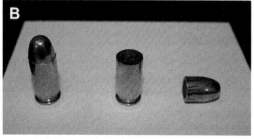

Fig. 1. Hollow-point (expanding) versus full-metal-jacket ammunition. (*A*) .45 Automatic Colt Pistol Federal 230 grain HydraShok (Hollow point). Shot at 850 feet per second (fps) from a SIG 220 gun. (*B*) .45 Automatic Colt Pistol Remington 230 grain, full metal jacket. Shot at 860 fps from a SIG 220 gun. Note that the hollow-point bullet collapses on itself and disperses its kinetic energy to the surrounding tissue in the body.

Type of weapon	Full metal-jacketed and solid bullets	Deforming and fragmentation bullets
	A	**B**
Rifle		
	C	**D**
Handgun		

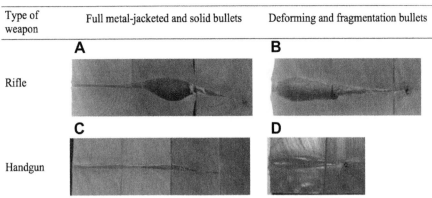

Fig. 2. Comparison of rifle and handgun ammunition as they penetrate soap blocks. (*A*) A jacketed rifle cartridge is fired into a soap block. The permanent cavity can be seen at both ends of the block whereas in the middle, the large temporary cavity is more prominent. It forms as a result of the pressure changes that take place as the bullet penetrates the block. (*B*) The entire trajectory of the jacketed bullet seems to show the permanent cavity. However, in low-velocity firearms such as handguns, the temporary cavity still forms but to such a small degree that it nearly matches the permanent cavity (narrow channel). On close examination, a small increase in the cavity volume in the center of the trajectory is observed. (*C, D*) The bullet is not jacketed, so during its flight it partially disintegrates, deforms, or breaks into fragments, causing the large temporary cavity to form early on in the trajectory, toward the point of entrance. (*D*) The penetration of the bullet is not as great because it was fired from a low-velocity handgun.

fractures of the tibia and humerus, for example, can be placed into an appropriately molded cast or splint with a window to allow for wound care. Unstable fractures are treated using operative principles similar to those for closed fractures (**Figs. 3** and **4**).

It is important to bear in mind that the aforementioned studies are reports of low-risk bullet wounds; that is, low-velocity handgun injuries resulting in mildly comminuted fractures in urban environments. On the other hand, surgical debridement of gunshot wounds still has a role in high-risk wounds, which need to be evaluated on an individual basis. Those wounds involving high-energy weapons (military rifles or shotguns), delayed presentation, large soft-tissue deficits, and multiple projectiles, and those occurring on a battlefield or farm environment carry an increased risk of infection, and such wounds should be managed operatively. From their experience the authors also argue that even low-velocity gunshot fractures over subcutaneous bones, such as the clavicle or tibia, would also benefit from surgical debridement and coverage of the exposed bone (**Fig. 5**).

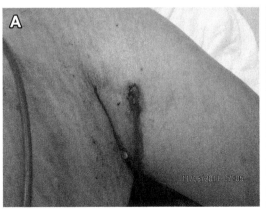
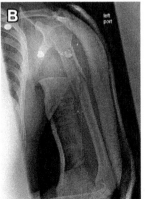
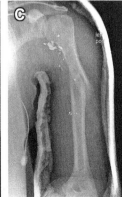

Fig. 3. Presumed low-velocity handgun injury causing humerus fracture. (*A*) Clinical photograph demonstrating a small entrance wound with no exposed bone. (*B, C*) Radiographs show a fragmented missile, although it is unclear whether this is a hollow-point, frangible, or simple lead bullet. This injury was treated with a short course of antibiotics, local wound care, and splinting. Soft-tissue swelling was not suggestive of significant injury. Nonoperative management generally suffices.

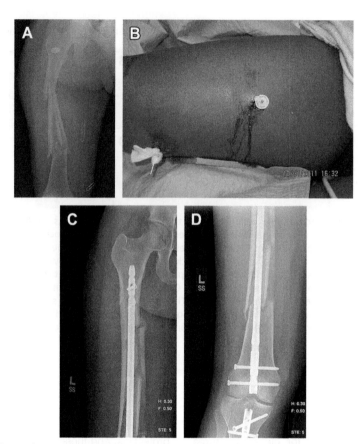

Fig. 4. Presumed low-velocity gunshot wounds to the thigh and leg resulting in femur and tibia fractures. (*A*) Preoperative radiograph demonstrating a segmental femur fracture with a bullet noted proximally. (*B*) Small entrance wounds and acceptable soft-tissue swelling were noted, without evidence of any vascular injury. (*C, D*) Other than antibiotics and simple local wound care, surgical treatment did not differ from that for closed fractures, which consisted of closed intramedullary nailing.

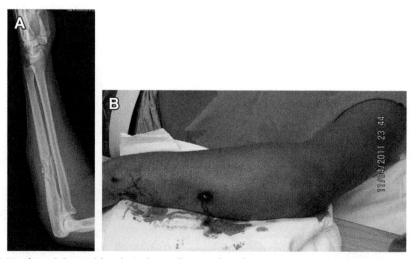

Fig. 5. (*A, B*) Handgun injury with relatively small wounds. After irrigation and inspection in the emergency department, exposed bone at the fracture site was clearly visible. This injury needs to be carefully evaluated for fractures in subcutaneous bones such as the ulna, tibia, and clavicle. In this case, formal debridement in the operating room should be considered.

The key principle of gunshot-wound debridement is removal of necrotic and contaminated tissue. High-energy wounds with extensive soft-tissue damage require debridement of devitalized tissue, and the "4 Cs" (color, capacity to bleed, consistency, contractility) have been recommended as a guide to determine muscle tissue viability. Shotgun injuries possess a dual infection risk in that large, soft-tissue damage may be accompanied by contaminated shotgun wadding or the plastic shell. An attempt should be made to remove these gross materials along with any obvious pellets, but an exhaustive search to remove each individual pellet is likely to cause unnecessary secondary injury. Debridement may also be performed during fixation of unstable fractures. If implanting hardware, the bullet tract can be excised with an elliptical incision and closed primarily after a thorough debridement and irrigation.

Transabdominal gunshot wounds that are associated with fractures of the spine, pelvis, and proximal femur represent a unique concern, as the presence of free intestinal contents increases the risk for infection. Although fractures to the spine with concurrent viscus perforation may lead to meningitis, vertebral osteomyelitis, or abscess formation, the current evidence suggests that bony debridement is not necessary if broad-spectrum antibiosis is continued for 7 to 14 days.[9–11] Furthermore, extraction of retained bullets has not been proved to decrease the risk of infection, and should only be reserved for deteriorating neurologic function, acute lead toxicity, or location in an intervertebral disk space causing mechanical symptoms.[9] Similar findings have been observed in the pelvis and hip joints. In a review at the authors' institution, 84 patients with gunshot-related pelvic fractures were studied. Perforated viscus injury was seen in 50 patients, hip joint involvement in 15 patients, and sacroiliac joint injury in 3 patients. Only 1 patient experienced an infection from a transcolonic missile that resulted in a retained fragment in the hip joint, and that patient was treated with an initial debridement. The investigators concluded that extra-articular fractures, even in the presence of intestinal injury, did not require orthopedic debridement.[12] Several other studies have corroborated a similar conclusion that debridement should be reserved only for intra-articular violation from a transabdominal bullet or for any trajectory injury with retained joint fragments.[12–14]

Intra-articular retained fragments represent an undisputed surgical indication (**Fig. 6**). Regardless of the joint, metallic fragments can lead to irreversible mechanical disruption of articular cartilage and/or lead toxicity.[15] Otherwise, bullet extraction is usually not indicated unless it is retained within a synovial joint, is associated with acute lead toxicity, or positioned in a painful anatomic region such as the subcutaneous tissue, the foot, or the hand. Bullets retained in the foot are especially not well tolerated during weight-bearing activities, and a similar argument can be made for bullets lodged within the hand that cause discomfort with dexterous activities.[16,17]

PRINCIPLES OF FIXATION

Gunshot projectiles cause fractures via 3 mechanisms: (1) direct crushing of tissue, (2) the sonic wave, and (3) the temporary cavity. The degree of energy transfer often causes significant comminution, which complicates operative planning and outcomes. In general, the operative fixation principles follow those of nonpenetrating trauma, but a brief review by anatomic region is given here.

Articular Injury

Chondral injuries can be managed by arthroscopic or open approaches. Arthroscopy allows for greater visualization of the joint surfaces, but an open arthrotomy may be necessary for more

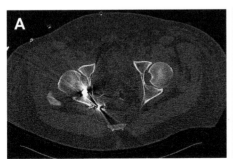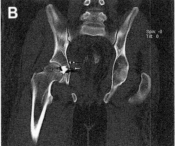

Fig. 6. (*A, B*) Low-velocity handgun injury to the hip joint with concomitant rectal injury, with retained intra-articular missile. Although most extra-articular pelvic gunshot fractures do not require urgent formal debridement, the risk of intra-articular sepsis in this case necessitates urgent debridement and missile removal.

complex reconstructions. If an arthroscopic method is chosen, care should be taken to monitor the adjacent compartments (including the retroperitoneal space and abdomen for hip arthroscopy), as fluid may extravasate from the spaces between fracture fragments, causing compartment syndrome and possibly death.[18] Regardless of the method, gross contaminants, bullet fragments, and/or small loose bodies may cause posttraumatic arthritis and should be removed from the joint. Acutely, large osteochondral fragments can be repaired with headless compression screws, and small defects can be treated with debridement and microfracture. Severely comminuted joints or those with advanced degenerative disease may benefit from delayed hemiarthroplasty or total joint arthroplasty.

Extra-Articular Injury

Upper extremity

Fractures of the proximal humerus and humeral shaft can often be managed nonoperatively, similarly to closed fractures. The usual indications for repair of the proximal humerus apply (ie, displacement of 1 cm or angulation of 45°), and may be repaired via plating, pinning, or nailing, depending on the surgeon's preference. Fractures of the humeral shaft can be treated with plating, nailing, or external fixation, although recent meta-analyses suggest that the rates of reoperation are lower for plating.[19] Fractures with significant comminution can be bridged with locked plates, and those with significant bone loss may require an additional procedure such as wave plating with cancellous bone graft, vascularized fibular graft, titanium mesh cage with bone graft, or bone transport with an Ilizarov frame.[20–23] Fractures of the distal humerus are more challenging to reconstruct, and posttraumatic stiffness often complicates these injuries. Typically the medial and lateral columns are fixed with 3.5-mm plates, which may need to be augmented with bone graft (tricortical iliac crest or cancellous with a bridge plate). External fixation may initially be required if irreparable comminution or excessive swelling is present. At the proximal ulna, surgery is often required to reestablish articular congruity and early motion. Open reduction and internal fixation is often the treatment of choice, but severe comminution may require external fixation or excision with triceps advancement. For late complications of stiffness or pain, arthrodesis or total elbow arthroplasty are salvage options, and whole-elbow allografting may reestablish bone stock if an insufficient amount precludes these procedures.[24] Nondisplaced fractures of the forearm can be managed expectantly with local wound care, but operative management of displaced forearm fractures has been shown to have superior outcomes.[25] Finally, the challenge with gunshot fractures to the hand lies in managing the multiple tissue injuries.[16] For example, a tendon injury would require early motion, but a nerve injury would ideally require immobilization. Another example of conflicting rehabilitation protocols is seen with a concomitant flexor and extensor tendon injury. The authors' preference is to allow motion of the tendons if a tensionless repair can be achieved on the nerves; in the case of concomitant flexor and extensor injury, the flexor tendon protocol takes precedence, as revision repair of the extensor tendon is less complicated. Unstable fractures of the metacarpals and phalanges require rigid fixation to allow early motion, which may be accomplished by plates or miniature external fixators. Large soft-tissue defects can be managed with limited debridement; questionable tissue should actually be initially left behind, as the hand possesses a unique regeneration potential. In a study by Pereira and colleagues,[26] 55 complex hand injuries from gunshots were reviewed; 44 required primary closure, 4 required local rotational flaps, 1 required a free flap, and 1 required a digital amputation. Although 61% had good subjective functional scores, 65% still reported being "disabled from work."

Lower extremity

Most civilian handgun injuries to the femur result in mild to moderately comminuted fractures with a low degree of soft-tissue loss. In such cases, standard reamed intramedullary nailing techniques are generally preferred, and have been shown to have outcomes comparable with those of closed fractures.[27] In higher-energy wounds with extensive loss of bone and soft tissue, external fixation may be used either as a temporary measure until adequate soft-tissue coverage can be achieved, or as a definitive treatment. External fixation may be necessary in a critically injured patient who requires a "damage control" approach. In study by Mack and colleagues,[28] provisional external fixation was required in 39 of 41 open proximal femur fractures in the combat setting. In their study, blast wounds and high-energy gunshot wounds were responsible for 71% and 20% of the fractures, respectively, and reoperation for complications was required in 56% of patients, with infection being the most common indication. In general, the external fixation is exchanged within 2 weeks of its application for a static locked intramedullary nail, but the fixator may be used definitively in cases with severe bone loss by converting it to a ring construct for bone transport. Distal femoral shaft and supra-condylar fractures can similarly be stabilized with intramedullary nailing, albeit in a retrograde direction. Distal femur periarticular plates are another option, and are more appropriate for fractures with intra-articular extension. Fractures of the tibia metaphysis and shaft are treated similarly to those of the femur, except that low-energy shaft fractures can effectively be treated with casting and wound care.[29] Often an intact fibula maintains length and the ability to perform straight leg raise, which can mislead initial responders. Fractures with inadequate alignment are preferably treated with static locked intramedullary nails, although no prospective or retrospective trials examining exclusively gunshot-related fractures exist. Periarticular fractures are best managed with anatomic reduction of the joint fragments and rigid fixation with plate-and-screw constructs. Bone graft or substitutes may be necessary to fill structural voids. In either the shaft or periarticular regions, excessive soft-tissue swelling or deficits can be managed with bridging external fixation devices, which may be used temporarily or definitively. Fractures of the foot are often treated nonoperatively with weight bearing as tolerated, as long as the bullet has been removed. These patients often experience stiffness, but the degree to which this occurs is usually not disabling.[30]

Spine and pelvis

Gunshot fractures to the spine are common but infrequently require surgical fixation. Unless the bullet has a transverse trajectory across both facets or unless the bullet is large in comparison with a small spine (such as in a child), the spine usually remains stable.[31,32] Although not originally designed for penetrating trauma, some spine surgeons use the 3-column model of Denis to guide treatment. In the cervical spine, if 1 column is disrupted then a C-collar is applied, but if 2 or more are disrupted then the patient is placed in halo traction. In the thoracic and lumbar spine, if 1 column is disrupted then observation is warranted, but if 2 or more columns are involved then a thoracolumbar spinal orthosis (TLSO) can be worn by the patient when out of bed. Alternatively, in unstable patterns such as disruption of 2 or more columns or bilateral facet destruction, short-segment posterior spinal fusion allows early rehabilitation and mobilization.[32] Unstable fractures of the pelvis are rare. External fixation or plate-and-screw constructs may be used to stabilize an anteriorly or posteriorly disrupted pelvic ring.

NEED AND DURATION OF ANTIBIOTIC THERAPY

No universal protocol exists for antibiotic prophylaxis in gunshot fractures. Several studies have shown that low-risk wounds can be managed with local wound care and either oral or no antibiotics.[3,7,8,33] Wounds defined as high risk (ie, high-energy ballistics, large soft-tissue deficit, delayed presentation, soil contamination, or joints with intestinal contamination) are often managed with debridement and 48 hours of intravenous antibiotics. Debridement is not necessarily required in intra-articular violation with low-velocity missiles without environmental or visceral contamination; however, these injuries should be managed with 48 hours of antibiotics.[33] Gunshot-related fractures of the foot also represent a higher infectious risk; Boucree and colleagues[34] studied 81 gunshot-related fractures and noted a 12% rate of infection evenly distributed among high-velocity and low-velocity injuries; they subsequently recommended 72 hours of intravenous antibiotics for these injuries. The choice of appropriate antibiotic therapy is variable in the current literature. The authors prefer to treat low-risk wounds with an oral cephalosporin, and high-risk wounds with intravenous cephalosporin and gentamycin. Penicillin can also be added to the latter regimen in the presence of soil contamination.

MANAGING SEQUELAE OF GUNSHOT INJURIES

Management of early and late sequelae can be time consuming and frustrating for both the surgeon and the patient, which often necessitates a multidisciplinary approach. This section briefly describes commonly encountered sequelae.

Vascular Injury

Vascular injuries may complicate up to 15% of penetrating injuries to the upper extremity, and represent an emergent multidisciplinary surgical approach.[2] In a study of long-bone fractures with vascular injuries by McHenry and colleagues,[35] complications and lengths of stay were less when the vascular defect was repaired first and the orthopedic was defect repaired second, rather than the converse. The surgical sequence of these injuries is still somewhat controversial, as proponents of the "fracture first" philosophy contend that an orthopedic repair may jeopardize the vascular repair. Supporters of the "vascular first" approach cite that immediate resolution of limb ischemia is the most critical factor in salvaging the extremity. Several investigations at the authors' institution have concluded that either approach is acceptable in the appropriate patient, and that an early discussion between the vascular and orthopedic teams facilitates the best outcome.[36,37] If the vascular team anticipates the need for stabilized length and the orthopedic procedure can be completed quickly, the orthopedic team may proceed. On the other hand, if limb ischemia appears to be threatening the limb, the vascular repair should take priority. The authors usually prefer to first reestablish perfusion with a temporary shunt followed by orthopedic fixation for bony length and then, finally, the definitive vascular repair.

Compartment Syndrome

Decompression of the anatomic compartments is not accomplished by a bullet tract. Signs of increasing edema, hematoma, or associated vascular injury should raise suspicion for compartment syndrome, and a full-length fasciotomy should be performed in such cases. Fracture pattern or degree of comminution is not necessarily related to the risk of developing a compartment syndrome. Compartment pressure monitoring can be used for equivocal cases or

cases for which a physical examination cannot be obtained (eg, an intubated patient). A difference less than 30 mm Hg between the compartment pressure and diastolic blood pressure is a commonly used criterion for diagnosing compartment syndrome (**Fig. 7**). Definitive internal fixation should be avoided until the wounds are closed, and external fixation is often the fixation method of choice in the acute period. Once the swelling subsides, wounds can be gradually closed or may require a skin graft.

Massive Loss of Soft Tissue and Bone

High-energy wounds resulting from gunshots can be challenging; soft-tissue contractures, flap failure, and infections commonly complicate soft-tissue coverage methods (**Fig. 8**). Initially the wounds can be covered with negative-pressure wound therapy (NPWT) or antibiotic bead pouches. The wounds should be debrided every 2 to 3 days until a clean wound bed allows for optimal definitive soft-tissue coverage. Frequently, gunshot injuries with massive soft-tissue loss also result in highly comminuted fractures, and are treated with standard open fracture debridement protocols. This procedure typically results in

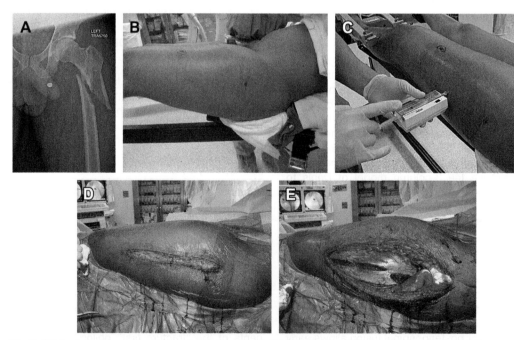

Fig. 7. (A) Presumed low-velocity gunshot injury to the thigh with simple femur fracture and a small, nonexpanding/nonfragmented projectile. (B) Clinical examination demonstrates a small entrance wound and signs and symptoms concerning for compartment syndrome. (C–E) Compartment pressure monitoring confirmed the diagnosis. This injury was treated with emergent fasciotomy and fracture fixation. The hematoma encountered was not particularly large for a femur fracture. No vascular injury was diagnosed. One could speculate that destructive wound ballistics caused a more severe soft-tissue injury, leading to compartment syndrome.

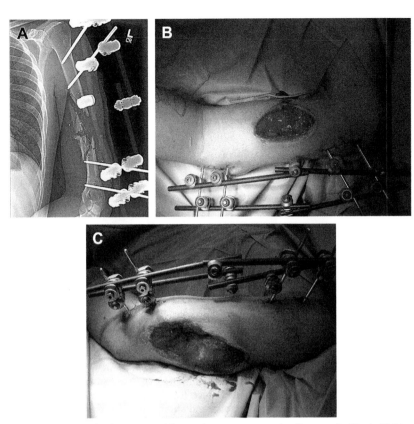

Fig. 8. (*A–C*) Shotgun injury to the humerus with massive entrance and exit wounds. The initial treating surgeon did not consider emergent debridement because "gunshot injuries aren't really open fractures." Clearly, this requires urgent debridement and application of open fracture treatment principles. This injury was also treated with external fixation as shown.

debridement of the multiple devitalized fragments, thereby leaving a bony defect that requires subsequent treatment. The authors have treated these injuries with antibiotic cement beads and spacers with delayed conversion (at 6 weeks) to autogenous bone grafting (ie, Masquelet technique) (**Fig. 9**). By contrast, gunshot-related fractures from presumed low-velocity missiles with small entry and exit wounds and no exposed bone frequently have the same degree of comminution but are not treated with formal debridement unless exposed bone is present. In wounds with extensive soft-tissue loss, skin grafts, rotational flaps, or free tissue transfer may be required. Kumar and colleagues[38] reported on 26 free tissue transfers for open fractures sustained in battle. The investigators performed serial debridements every 2 to 3 days until the wound beds were optimal for coverage. On average, wound beds were not appropriate for coverage until 31 days, but a 96% success rate of tissue transfers was reported, with 1 flap failure and an 8% infection rate. *Acinetobacter calcoaceticus baumannii* was the most commonly cultured wound contaminant.

Nerve Injury

A complete injury to the central nervous system is more common with penetrating trauma than with a closed injury.[39] Although the second National Acute Spinal Cord Injury Study (NASCIS 2) trial excluded penetrating injury, 2 retrospective studies have also concluded that high-dose steroids did not result in significantly different rates of neurologic recovery, but did result in increased rates of complications.[40–42] The prognosis of complete spinal cord injuries is not favorable, but incomplete injuries may improve over 6 months to a year. Improvement of penetrating trauma has been shown to be less than that of nonpenetrating trauma.[43]

Peripheral nerve injuries to the extremities are common. Most low-energy gunshot wounds induce a neuropraxia or axonotmesis, but higher-energy wounds are more likely to result in a complete rupture.[44,45] Fractures with an associated vascular injury are also more likely to have a structural defect of a peripheral nerve.[46] Nerve injury may be present in 30% to 40% of gunshot wounds

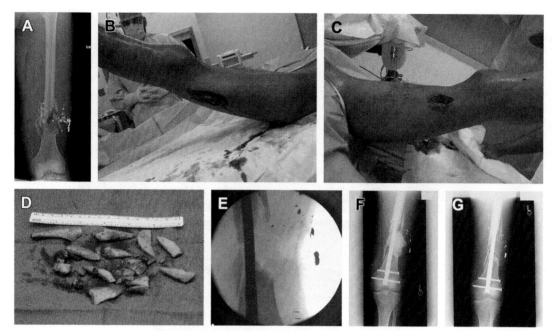

Fig. 9. Supposed handgun injury with a comminuted distal femur fracture. (*A*) Radiograph demonstrates significant comminution, and suggests the possibility of exposed bone and metallic fragments. (*B, C*) Massive lacerating entrance and exit wounds shown before initial debridement, which was done urgently. (*D*) After irrigation and debridement, several devitalized fragments were noted and excised. (*E, F*) Intramedullary nailing was performed, and an antibiotic cement spacer was placed into the defect. (*G*) After 6 weeks and no sign of infection, the patient returned to the operating room for spacer removal and autogenous iliac crest bone grafting. If this patient had typical small entrance and exit wounds without exposed bone or bullet fragments, formal debridement would not even have been done.

to the hand, but improvement may be expected 70% to 90% with conservative management.[47] The indications to explore a malfunctioning nerve are controversial. Most nerves are found to be intact during exploration, and thus have a potential for recovery. However, nerves that do not show signs of improvement by 3 months are more likely to have been ruptured or trapped within callus or scar tissue. The management of such lesions is variable among centers; the authors generally prefer to follow nerve function with electrodiagnostic studies and physical examination. Such a protocol requires a baseline electrodiagnostic study at 3 weeks and then again at 3 months. The 3-week study allows enough time for the signs of Wallerian degeneration to appear in the electrodiagnostics, and the 3-month study establishes a trend. Each clinical examination should also document a thorough sensory examination with pinprick testing and graded muscle-strength testing. An advancing Tinel sign may also herald nerve regeneration. Patients without evidence of improvement at 3 months are indicated to undergo exploration. Immediate exploration may be indicated for lesions associated with high-energy wounds, vascular injury, or an associated fracture that

requires exposure for fixation. Neurolysis is the most common intervention on exploration, as the nerve is most often found in continuity. Ruptured nerves or those with a neuroma can be directly repaired or nerve grafted. Sensory nerves of the hand with small gaps may additionally be repaired with synthetic nerve conduits, but at present no data exist on the efficacy of nerve conduits as a primary repair method of motor or mixed nerves. Outcomes following surgical repair vary depending on the location and severity of the lesion. Radial nerve injuries generally have better outcomes than those of brachial plexus, ulnar nerve, or peroneal nerve injuries. The results of the latter group are complicated by the nature of their mixed sensory and motor fibers, and long distances to the motor end plates. In such cases, nerve transfers or tendon transfers may be a more appropriate means of improving functional outcomes.

Lead Toxicity

Synovial fluid acts as a solvent on the lead core of the bullet, and may cause synovitis or systemic plumbism. Toxicity is confirmed with a blood lead level greater than 10 µg/dL, but symptoms such as fatigue, headache, anemia, abdominal pain, nausea, renal failure, encephalopathy, or peripheral neuropathy generally occur at levels higher than 24 μg/dL. A peripheral blood smear will show basophilic stippling. The time between injury and lead toxicity is variably reported as 2 days to 40 years, depending on the location of the bullet and the metabolic state of the patient.[2–4] In general, the risk of lead toxicity from gunshots is low, as avascular fibrous tissue rapidly envelops the missile. However, involved extraskeletal tissues may elute lead faster if within a cyst or within an intervertebral disk, or if a concurrent hypermetabolic condition accelerates lead elution from body storage sites.[2–4,48,49] Surprisingly, bullets retained in cerebrospinal fluid actually do not rapidly elute lead, and may remain in situ if not causing neurologic compromise or plumbism.[33] If lead toxicity is suspected the missile should be extracted, serial lead levels trended, and chelation therapy offered.

SUMMARY

Fractures caused by firearms in the civilian population are typically caused by handgun injuries. Although many of these fractures and their associated wounds can be treated similarly to closed fractures with the addition of minimal wound care and a short course of antibiotics, patients must be treated on a case-by-case basis, as there are several indications for formal open treatment. It cannot be assumed that low-velocity missiles are involved, and injuries with larger wounds and more significant soft-tissue injury can occur, requiring urgent debridement. Urgent operative treatment is also required in gunshot-related fractures with exposed bone, vascular disruption, and injuries with compartment syndrome.

REFERENCES

1. Centers for Disease Control, National Center for Injury Prevention and Control. WISQUARS fatal injuries: mortality reports. Available at: http://webappa.cdc.gov/sasweb/ncipc/mortrate.html. Accessed November 10, 2008.
2. Dougherty PJ, Vaidya R, Silverton CD, et al. Joint and long-bone gunshot injuries. J Bone Joint Surg Am 2009;91(4):980–97.
3. Bartlett CS, Helfet DL, Hausman MR, et al. Ballistics and gunshot wounds: effects on musculoskeletal tissues [Review]. J Am Acad Orthop Surg 2000;8(1): 21–36.
4. Bartlett CS. Clinical update: gunshot wound ballistics [Review]. Clin Orthop Relat Res 2003;(408): 28–57.
5. Cornwell EE 3rd. Current concepts of gunshot wound treatment: a trauma surgeon's perspective. Clin Orthop Relat Res 2003;(408):58–64.
6. Vennemann B, Grosse Perdekamp M, Kneubuehl BP, et al. Gunshot-related displacement of skin particles and bacteria from the exit region back into the bullet path. Int J Legal Med 2007; 121(2):105–11.
7. Dickey RL, Barnes BC, Kearns RJ, et al. Efficacy of antibiotics in low-velocity gunshot fractures. J Orthop Trauma 1989;3:6–10.
8. Knapp TP, Patzakis MJ, Lee J, et al. Comparison of intravenous and oral antibiotic therapy in the treatment of fractures caused by low-velocity gunshots. A prospective, randomized study of infection rates [Review]. J Bone Joint Surg Am 1996;78(8):1167–71.
9. Bono CM, Heary RF. Gunshot wounds to the spine [Review]. Spine J 2004;4(2):230–40.
10. Kumar A, Wood G, Whittle A. Low-velocity gunshot injuries of the spine with abdominal viscus trauma. J Orthop Trauma 1998;12:514–7.
11. Roffi R, Waters R, Adkins R. Gunshot wounds to the spine associated with a perforated viscus. Spine 1989;14:808–11.
12. Rehman S, Slemenda C, Kestner C, et al. Management of gunshot pelvic fractures with bowel injury: is fracture debridement necessary? J Trauma 2011;71(3):577–81.
13. Becker VV Jr, Brien WW, Patzakis M, et al. Gunshot injuries to the hip and abdomen: the association of joint and intra-abdominal visceral injuries. J Trauma 1990;30:1324–9.
14. Long WT, Brien EW, Boucree JB Jr, et al. Management of civilian gunshot injuries to the hip. Orthop Clin North Am 1995;26:123–31.
15. Rehman MA, Umer M, Sepah YJ, et al. Bullet-induced synovitis as a cause of secondary osteoarthritis of the hip joint: a case report and review of literature. J Med Case Rep 2007;1:171.
16. Wilson RH. Gunshots to the hand and upper extremity [Review]. Clin Orthop Relat Res 2003;(408): 133–44.
17. Holmes GB Jr. Gunshot wounds of the foot [Review]. Clin Orthop Relat Res 2003;(408):86–91.
18. Bartlett CS, DiFelice GS, Buly RL, et al. Cardiac arrest as a result of intraabdominal extravasation of fluid during arthroscopic removal of a loose body from the hip joint of a patient with an acetabular fracture. J Orthop Trauma 1998;12(4):294–9.
19. Kurup H, Hossain M, Andrew JG. Dynamic compression plating versus locked intramedullary nailing for humeral shaft fractures in adults. Cochrane Database Syst Rev 2011;(6):CD005959.
20. Attias N, Lehman RE, Bodell LS, et al. Surgical management of a long segmental defect of the humerus using a cylindrical titanium mesh cage and plates: a case report. J Orthop Trauma 2005;19:211–6.

21. Heitmann C, Erdmann D, Levin LS. Treatment of segmental defects of the humerus with an osteoseptocutaneous fibular transplant. J Bone Joint Surg Am 2002;84:2216–23.

22. Mandrella B, Abebaw TH, Hersi ON. Defect fractures of the upper arm and their treatment in difficult circumstances: three case reports from Ethiopian and Somalian provincial hospitals. Unfallchirurg 1997;100:154–8 [in German].

23. Ring D, Allende C, Jafarnia K, et al. Ununited diaphyseal forearm fractures with segmental defects: plate fixation and autogenous cancellous bone-grafting. J Bone Joint Surg Am 2004;86:2440–5.

24. Dean GS, Holliger EH IV, Urbaniak JR. Elbow allograft for reconstruction of the elbow with massive bone loss: long-term results. Clin Orthop Relat Res 1997;341:12–22.

25. Lenihan MR, Brien WW, Gellman H, et al. Fractures of the forearm resulting from low-velocity gunshot wounds. J Orthop Trauma 1992;6:32.

26. Pereira C, Boyd JB, Olsavsky A, et al. Outcomes of complex gunshot wounds to the hand and wrist: a 10-year level I urban trauma center experience. Ann Plast Surg 2012;68(4):374–7.

27. Nowotarski P, Brumback RJ. Immediate interlocking nailing of fractures of the femur caused by low- to mid-velocity gunshots. J Orthop Trauma 1994;8: 134–41.

28. Mack AW, Freedman BA, Groth AT, et al. Treatment of open proximal femoral fractures sustained in combat. J Bone Joint Surg Am 2013;95(3):e13(1-8).

29. Leffers D, Chandler RW. Tibial fractures associated with civilian gunshot injuries. J Trauma 1985;25: 1059–64.

30. Durkin RC, Coughlin RR. Management of gunshot wounds to the foot. Injury 1997;28:6–10.

31. Kitchel SH. Current treatment of gunshot wounds to the spine. Clin Orthop Relat Res 2003;(408): 115–9.

32. Waters RL, Sie IH. Spinal cord injuries from gunshot wounds to the spine. Clin Orthop Relat Res 2003;(408):120–5.

33. Simpson BM, Wilson RH, Grant RE. Antibiotic therapy in gunshot wound injuries [Review]. Clin Orthop Relat Res 2003;(408):82–5.

34. Boucree JB Jr, Gabriel RA, Lezine-Hanna JT. Gunshot wounds to the foot. Orthop Clin North Am 1995;26:191–7.

35. McHenry TP, Holcomb JB, Aoki N, et al. Fractures with major vascular injuries from gunshot wounds: implications of surgical sequence. J Trauma 2002; 53(4):717–21.

36. Fowler J, Macintyre N, Rehman S, et al. The importance of surgical sequence in the treatment of lower extremity injuries with concomitant vascular injury: a meta-analysis. Injury 2009;40(1):72–6.

37. Rehman S, Salari N, Codjoe P, et al. Gunshot femoral fractures with vascular injury: a retrospective analysis. Orthop Surg 2012;4(3):166–71.

38. Kumar AR, Grewal NS, Chung TL, et al. Lessons from the modern battlefield: successful upper extremity injury reconstruction in the subacute period. J Trauma 2009;67(4):752–7.

39. Young JA, Burns PE, McCutchen R, editors. Spinal cord injury statistics: experience of the regional spinal cord injury systems. Phoenix (AZ): Good Samaritan Medical Center; 1982. p. 1–152.

40. Bracken MB, Shoemaker WC, Avakian S, et al. A randomized, controlled trial of methylprednisolone or naloxone in the treatment of acute spinal-cord injury. Results of the Second National Acute Spinal Cord Injury Study. N Engl J Med 1990;322:1405–11.

41. Heary RF, Vaccaro AR, Mesa JJ, et al. Steroids and gunshot wounds to the spine. Neurosurgery 1997; 41:576–83 [discussion: 583–4].

42. Levy ML, Gans W, Wijesinghe HS, et al. Use of methylprednisolone as an adjunct in the management of patients with penetrating spinal cord injury: outcome analysis. Neurosurgery 1996;39:1141–8 [discussion: 1148–9].

43. Green BA, Eismont FJ, Close KJ, et al. A comparison of open versus closed spinal cord injuries during the first year post injury. Annual Meeting of the American Spinal Injury Association. New Orleans, April, 1981.

44. Secer HI, Daneyemez M, Tehli O, et al. The clinical, electrophysiologic, and surgical characteristics of peripheral nerve injuries caused by gunshot wounds in adults: a 40-year experience. Surg Neurol 2008; 69(2):143–52.

45. Beidas OE, Rehman S. Civilian gunshot extremity fractures with neurologic injury. Orthop Surg 2011; 3(2):102–5.

46. Bercik MJ, Kingsbery J, Ilyas AM. Peripheral nerve injuries following gunshot fracture of the humerus. Orthopedics 2012;35(3):e349–52.

47. Omer GE. Injuries to the nerves of the upper extremity. J Bone Joint Surg Am 1974;56:1615.

48. Dougherty PJ, van Holsbeeck M, Mayer TG, et al. Lead toxicity associated with a gunshot-induced femoral fracture. A case report. J Bone Joint Surg Am 2009;91(8):2002–8.

49. Beazley WC, Rosenthal RE. Lead intoxication 18 months after a gunshot wound. Clin Orthop 1984; 190:199–203.

PEDIATRICS

Preface

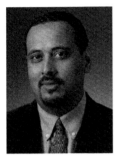

Shital N. Parikh, MD, FACS
Editor

A 9-year-old wrestler with a SLAP IV tear in his shoulder (**Fig. 1**). A 12-year-old pitcher with partial articular-side rotator cuff tear. Injuries that were once thought to be nonexistent in the pediatric population are now being diagnosed and treated. Then there are injuries exclusive to children, such as the Little League Shoulder and physeal fractures of the proximal humerus. Last, but not the least, management of an unstable shoulder poses challenging issues in skeletally immature patients. Dashe, Roocroft, Bastrom, and Edmonds provide a comprehensive review, and an epidemiologic study, related to the spectrum of shoulder injuries in skeletally immature patients. This review helps in the evaluation and management of a child with shoulder symptoms.

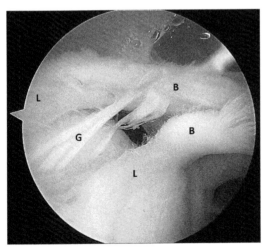

Fig. 1. A 9-year-old boy with right shoulder pain after a wrestling injury. Patient is in a beach-chair position with the arthroscope in the posterior portal. At arthroscopy, the SLAP IV tear was identified and treated. B, split biceps tendon; G, glenoid; L, labrum.

With year-round sports participation and increased competitiveness, there is an increase in overuse sports injuries in children. In 2007, The American Orthopaedic Society for Sports Medicine initiated a public outreach program, known as the STOP (Sports Trauma and Overuse Prevention) campaign, to promote safe play in children.[1] Paterno, Taylor-Hass, Myer, and Hewett provide an exclusive review of injury prevention efforts, focusing on lower extremities. Overuse injuries sustained during running, like medial tibial stress syndrome, patellofemoral pain syndrome, and iliotibial band syndrome, are discussed. Similarly, prevention of injuries during cutting and pivoting maneuvers, such as anterior cruciate ligament tears, and the latest research supporting such prevention programs are reviewed.

Gray described the earliest case of osteogenesis imperfecta in a mummy dating back to circa 1000 BC.[2] At the time of excavation, the strange appearance of the bones were mistaken for a mummified monkey. Scientific knowledge has come a long way since then. Laron and Pandya provide us with historical aspects, genetic basis, and diagnostic advances related to osteogenesis imperfecta. The role of bisphosphonates in the management of these patients has been reviewed. In the end, the authors discuss the evolution of surgical treatment, including latest generation of telescoping rods. These rods have provided promising results for the prevention and treatment of fracture and deformity.

Although the term "femoroacetabular impingement" was coined in 1999, the condition has long been recognized in studies on patterns of osteoarthritis of the hip.[3–5] There are controversies as to what constitutes the disease, since the radiographic findings of the "Cam" and "Pincer" lesions have been identified in asymptomatic individuals.

Orthop Clin N Am 44 (2013) xvii–xviii
http://dx.doi.org/10.1016/j.ocl.2013.07.006
0030-5898/13/$ – see front matter © 2013 Published by Elsevier Inc.

orthopedic.theclinics.com

Also, it is unknown if impingement is a cause or the result of osteoarthritis. Sankar, Matheney, and Zaltz review the best available evidence and summarize the key issues, including imaging and the range of surgical treatment options from arthroscopy to surgical hip dislocation.

Shital N. Parikh, MD, FACS
Cincinnati Children's Hospital Medical Center
University of Cincinnati School of Medicine
3333, Burnet Av., Cincinnati, OH 45229, USA

E-mail address:
Shital.Parikh@cchmc.org

REFERENCES

1. Available at: www.stopsportsinjuries.org. Accessed July 24, 2013.
2. Gray PH. A case of osteogenesis imperfecta, associated with dentinogenesis imperfecta, dating from antiquity. Clin Radiol 1970;21(1):106–8.
3. Myers SR, Eijer H, Ganz R. Anterior femoroacetabular impingement after periacetabular osteotomy. Clin Orthop Relat Res 1999;363:93–9.
4. Murray RO. The aetiology of primary osteoarthritis of the hip. Br J Radiol 1965;38(455):810–24.
5. Solomon L. Patterns of osteoarthritis of the hip. J Bone Joint Surg Br 1976;58(2):176–83.

Spectrum of Shoulder Injuries in Skeletally Immature Patients

Jesse Dashe, MD[a], Joanna H. Roocroft, MA[b],
Tracey P. Bastrom, MA[b], Eric W. Edmonds, MD[c],*

KEYWORDS

• Childhood • Shoulder • Sports-related injuries • Fractures

KEY POINTS

- Pediatric shoulder injuries behave and heal different than adult shoulder injuries because of the biomechanics of the open physis.
- Fractures are more common in younger patients, whereas instability is common in older and more skeletally mature patients.
- Proximal humerus fractures are more likely to require surgery than clavicle fractures in children, although younger children can tolerate more displacement than older children.
- The increased participation in single year-round sports leads to a specific overuse injuries such as Little League shoulder.
- Treatment of overhead shoulder injuries, such as internal impingement, includes rest, strengthening exercises, and proper throwing mechanics education; however, surgery may be necessary for intra-articular disorders that fail to improve.
- Dislocation and instability can be treated with physical therapy, but the recurrence rate is high in this young population.

INTRODUCTION

With about 45 million children and adolescents in organized youth athletics, injuries are common and there are approximately 2 million high school athletic injuries annually.[1] Shoulder injuries are a common component of that number (**Fig. 1**), accounting for nearly 1 million outpatient visits per year in the general population.[2] Although varied, the musculoskeletal shoulder disorders that presented to a physician can include fractures, overuse injuries, and instability.

This article has 2 aims: (1) to evaluate the causes of musculoskeletal shoulder pain in the pediatric population, and (2) to present the mechanism of injury and treatment associated with the various causes of shoulder pain. To confirm historical findings, a retrospective chart review was performed after obtaining Institutional Review Board approval, on all children who met inclusion criteria for shoulder pain, treated between August of 2008 and 2009 at our tertiary care children's hospital. There were 613 individuals who met the inclusion criteria: 370 boys (60.4%) and 243 girls (39.6%). The mean age was 13.3 years (range 0.17–21.75 years). Patients outside the normal pediatric age range all presented with childhood comorbidities and were included.

Disclosures: None of the authors received financial support for this study.
[a] University of California, 9500 Gilman Drive, La Jolla, CA 92093, USA; [b] Orthopedic Research Department, Rady Children's Hospital, 3020 Childrens Way, Mailcode 5054, San Diego, CA 92123, USA; [c] Department of Orthopedics, Pediatric Orthopedic and Scoliosis Center, Rady Children's Hospital San Diego, University of California, 3030 Children's Way, Suite 410, San Diego, CA 92123, USA
* Corresponding author.
E-mail address: eedmonds@ucsd.edu

orthopedic.theclinics.com

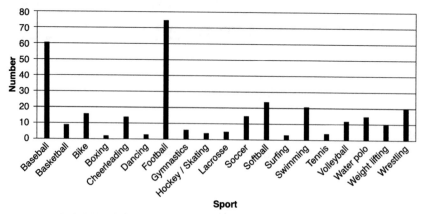

Fig. 1. Over a 1-year period, 54% of shoulder injuries presenting to our institution were sports related. Football, baseball, softball, swimming, wrestling, soccer, and water polo were leading causes.

FRACTURES (PROXIMAL HUMERUS AND CLAVICLE)
Introduction to Shoulder Fractures

The proximal humerus fracture in the skeletally immature represents about 0.45% of all pediatric fractures,[3] less than 5% in the adolescent age group,[1] and 4% to 7% of all epiphyseal fractures in children.[3] These injuries were reported to occur most commonly between the ages of 11 and 17 years in one study[1] and 10 to 14 years in another.[4]

Forces that act on the proximal humerus may:

- Result in fracture: forced extension, forced flexion, forced extension with lateral or medial rotation, and forced flexion with medial or lateral rotation.[5]
- Displace the epiphysis: muscular forces such as abduction, flexion, and slight external rotation.[3]

Ossification of the proximal humerus occurs in the following sequence:

- At birth, the epiphysis is cartilaginous.
- Ossification centers are first noticeable by 4 to 6 months of age.[3]
- Secondary ossification centers are present after 6 months of age.[4]
- Three ossification centers are seen: the humeral head, the greater tuberosity, and the lesser tuberosity (**Fig. 2**).[6]
- Greater tuberosity ossifies between 7 months and 3 years of age.
- Lesser tuberosity ossifies between 5 and 7 years of age.[3,4]
- The three ossification centers combine to create the proximal humeral epiphysis by 5 to 7 years of age.[3,4,6]
- Closure of the proximal humerus physis occurs at 14 to 17 of age in girls and 16 to 18

of age in boys (some reports suggest 19 and 22 years of age).[4,6] It is at this age range that this study distinguishes the skeletally immature from mature.

Certain age groups are prone to certain fracture patterns according to the growth of the proximal humerus:

- Neonates to 5 years old: Salter-Harris I injury
- From 5 to 11 years old: metaphyseal fractures
- From 10 to 11 years old: Salter-Harris II injuries[4,6]
- Adolescents: Salter-Harris II, III, and IV injuries[3]

It has been reported that about 20% of proximal humerus fractures in the skeletally immature are

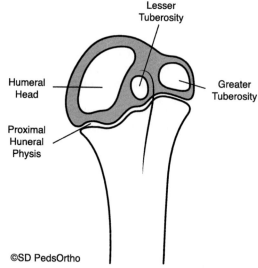

©SD PedsOrtho

Fig. 2. Ossification center locations on the proximal humerus.

associated with athletic activities.[1,4,6] During review of our own patient population, there were 190 fractures (40% of the cohort) and most of the fractures involved the proximal humerus. The mean age of the patients with fractures (9 ± 4 years) was significantly lower than the mean age of the patients with instability (16 ± 2 years, $P<.001$) (**Table 1**). Fractures were caused by the following:

- Falls (121 patients, 63.7%)
- Wheeled activities (32 patients, 16.8%)
- Sports (25 patients, 13.2%)

In contrast with the proximal humerus, the clavicle is a distinct long bone composed of cancellous material without a medullary cavity.[7] Clavicle fractures are the most common long bone fracture in children, representing 5% to 15% of fractures in this population.[1,7–9] They are unique in that they are the most common iatrogenic fractures, occurring in 1% to 7% of large babies (more than 4500 g), shoulder dystocias, or special instrumentation births.[7]

Ossification of the clavicle:

- Ossification centers are both medial and lateral
- The medial center provides 80% of the longitudinal growth of the clavicle[6]
- Ossification begins by 5 weeks of gestation
- Closure of the lateral growth center occurs from a few months of age to about 18 or

19 years of age, but is difficult to see on radiographs[6,10]
- Closure of the medial growth center occurs around 22 to 25 years of age[7,11]
- Eighty percent of the clavicle growth is completed by 9 years of age in girls and 12 years of age in boys[11]

Locations of clavicle fractures:

- The junction of the middle and lateral thirds accounts for 90% of midshaft fractures[1,7,9]
- The lateral third is the next most common, with 10% to 25%[9,10]
- Acromioclavicular (AC) separations are suspected, but AC dislocations are rare in children, with physeal injury being more common[10]
- The medial third of the clavicle is the location in 2% to 3%[9]
- As with AC separations, sternoclavicular joint injuries are rare in the pediatric population, with medial clavicle physeal fractures being more common[4]

Displacement of the clavicle fracture has the following characteristics: proximal fragment elevated superiorly because of spasm of the sternocleidomastoid or the trapezius muscles.[4] The mechanism of clavicle fractures includes:

- Most commonly, a direct fall onto the lateral aspect of the shoulder[1]
- A direct blow to the clavicle (10%)
- An indirect mechanism such as a fall on an outstretched hand (5%)[1,4]
- For sternoclavicular injury, an indirect force transmitted along the clavicle from a direct blow to the lateral shoulder[4]

As stated earlier, injury to the (open) clavicular physis is more common compared with AC or sternoclavicular joint dislocations, because the costoclavicular, sternoclavicular, and coracoclavicular ligaments are stronger than the physes.[7,9]

The work-up of any shoulder injury in a child should start with obtaining a good history, performing a physical examination, and initial plain films of the area of clinical suspicion.[4,7] Computed tomography imaging is occasionally required for complex comminuted fractures and/or for sternoclavicular injuries.[7]

Therapeutic Options for Shoulder Fractures

With a fracture diagnosis, treatment can be initiated based on the severity and location of the injury. For the clavicle, treatments may include:

Table 1
The mean age, standard deviation, and number of patients with each type of injury in our 1-year cohort

Injury	Mean Age (y)	Standard Deviation	N
Acromioclavicular separation	14.55	2.42	15
Fracture	9.05	4.63	190
Instability	15.51	2.27	158
Neurologic	8.74	9.04	8
Overhead	15.14	2.11	42
Pain	14.91	2.59	102
Post labrum	15.71	1.40	8
Rotator cuff	15.05	2.42	52
SLAP	16.58	1.77	28
Tumor	11.73	3.42	4
Weakness	14.17	2.96	6
Average	13.25	4.46	613

Abbreviation: SLAP, superior labral tear from anterior to posterior.

- Physeal clavicle injuries: conservative management with sling[9]
- Clavicle fractures less than 12 years old: conservative management with sling or figure-of-eight brace[1,10]
- Surgery

Indications for surgery on the clavicle in children are relative and controversial[4,7,10–12]:

- Open fractures
- Risk of skin perforation caused by skin tenting
- Fracture with shortening
- Floating shoulder injuries
- A clavicle fracture in the settling of multitrauma
- Pathologic fractures
- Cosmetic (unappealing bump with shortening or great displacement)
- Established painful nonunions and possibly comminuted fractures

Treatment options for the proximal humerus include:

- Sling immobilization, less than 11 years old, for any displacement[1]
- Sling immobilization, more than 11 years old, with less than 50% displacement and less than 20° to 40° angulation[1,3]
- However, most investigators recommend at least attempting a closed reduction in all cases[1]
- Percutaneous pinning and closed reduction for those with displacement or angulation outside the acceptable range for age[1,4]
- Open reduction and internal fixation, if closed reduction fails[3,13]

Indications for surgery on the proximal humerus include[3]:

- Irreducible fragment
- Insufficient reduction in patients near skeletal maturity
- Displaced or unstable fractures in those who do not tolerate immobilization
- Open or neurovascular lesions

In our series of patients, those found to have a fracture around the shoulder were treated with:

- Immobilization (84%)
- Physical therapy (11%)
- Surgery (5%)

Outcomes and Complications of Shoulder Fractures

Children seem to do well with proximal humerus fractures overall, but no prospective studies have been completed to date.[1,3] The healing time of a fracture can vary significantly based on age, with young patients healing faster than those who are closer to skeletal maturity. The proximal humerus in particular has great remodeling potential, accounting for 80% of longitudinal growth of the humerus[1,3] and allowing even severely displaced fractures to do well with conservative management. With regard to clavicle fractures, neonates can heal within weeks and teenagers may require up to 10 weeks.[1] Operative treatment has been associated with less disability of the upper extremity, earlier union, fever nonunions, and no malunions.[11] In adults, there is a 15% risk of nonunion in the nonoperative group compared with 2.2% in the operative group.[1] The same rate was seen with 100% displaced pediatric fractures treated conservatively with additional findings of chronic pain and functional loss,[7] but no prospective study has been completed on the skeletally immature clavicle to confirm these findings. Moreover, there is a report that skeletally immature individuals have a low rate of malunion and nonunion.[4] The surgical complication rate in clavicle fractures is 8%.[12] Complications of surgical intervention of the fractured clavicle include:

- Incisional numbness[8]
- An aesthetically unpleasing scar[7]
- Removal of implants[7]
- Pain from surgical implant[1]
- Neuroma from supraclavicular nerve laceration[12]
- K-wire migration causing pneumothorax[12]

With regard to the proximal humerus fracture, one of the biggest risks in children after physeal arrest seems to be nerve palsies, with the ulnar nerve most commonly affected, followed by radial and then medial nerves.[3] All resolved within 4 months.[3] If surgical intervention is required in young patients, it is important to avoid disturbing the periosteum so that an epiphysiodesis does not occur, resulting in iatrogenic disruption of the proximal humerus growth.[3] A growth arrest at this location could result in a reduction in humerus length of more than 1 cm per year (**Fig. 3**).

OVERUSE SHOULDER INJURIES
Introduction to Overuse Injuries

The most common overuse shoulder injury in children is Little League shoulder. This term refers to a traction physiolysis of the proximal humerus that is caused from rotational stress that occurs during overhead throwing[1,6] and should be considered a Salter-Harris I fracture to the proximal humerus physis.[1] Little League shoulder may be increasing

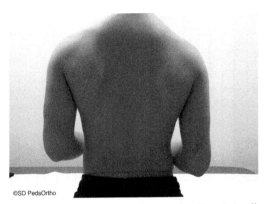

©SD PedsOrtho

Fig. 3. A 16-year-old boy who sustained a minimally displaced proximal humerus fracture 4 years earlier, which led to a limb length discrepancy. He continues to lead an active lifestyle, being on the high school varsity lacrosse team.

in frequency with year-round involvement in a single sport by adolescents.[6] There are a few reasons why the young adolescent is at particular risk for this proximal humerus overuse injury:

- Being skeletally immature, the physis is vulnerable to injury from torsional stresses.[1,6]
- Young adolescents have decreased muscular development and increased joint laxity in general, which allows more mechanical issues to arise.[6]
- The physis is particularly susceptible during rapid periods of growth such as puberty, so teenage athletes aged 11 to 16 years are most likely to sustain throwing overuse injuries.[4,6]

Another type of overuse injury seen at the shoulder in children is intra-articular disorders. The causes of this type of pain can be multifactorial but can be summarized by the term internal impingement of the shoulder. Internal impingement differs from external impingement in that the shape of the acromion plays no role in the injuries sustained. Instead, the impingement results from poor shoulder mechanics (weak rotator cuff and medial scapular stabilizer strength and glenohumeral internal rotation deficits) and results in partial articular supraspinatus tendon avulsions and posterosuperior labral tears.[14–16]

In the pediatric and adolescent population, the overall incidence of rotator cuff injury is low, with only small case series present in the literature.[17–20] Rotator cuff tears have typically been described in individuals more than 40 years old secondary to age-related changes from reduced mechanical properties of the shoulder (ie, degeneration of tendons).[18,21] However, with the increased

participation in overhead throwing sports seen over the past few decades, the incidence of overuse shoulder injuries in this younger cohort has increased substantially.[17] It has been reported that those younger than 20 years old comprise less than 1% of all rotator cuff tears in the general population with muscular imbalances that can predispose them to injury.[18,22] Our study found an incidence of 8.5% isolated rotator cuff disease and 6.9% of overhead spectrum disease (such as internal impingement, which may include rotator cuff disorders) among the 613 children in our childhood shoulder pain cohort.

Sporting activity accounted for 93% of injuries considered as overhead athlete overuse injuries in our study cohort. However, sports were only identified in 43% of the rotator cuff disorders in the cohort (**Figs. 4** and **5**). Adolescents sustain rotator cuff injuries from specific traumatic events, acute throwing events, or chronic repetitive motions such as rotator cuff tendinitis (so-called swimmer's shoulder).[18,23,24] Other possible causes include:

- Contact of the supraspinatus tendon with the acromion or superior glenoid, which can lead to degeneration of tendons and eventual failure.[24]
- Avulsion of the humeral tuberosity, with the lesser tuberosity being most commonly affected.[18]
- High tensional forces on the rotator cuff tendons, which become overloaded from a throwing motion.[18]
- Impingement causes, such as outlet syndromes or underlying instability in general.[20]
- Shoulder laxity eventually leading to rotator cuff tendinitis as a secondary phenomenon in overhead athletes.[23]

About 32% of young baseball pitchers have reported shoulder pain in a single season.[6] It has been noted in individuals 8 to 15 years old that 79% of those who are baseball pitchers have an increase in the physeal width in the dominant (throwing) proximal physis.[1] The risk factors of Little League shoulder are high pitch counts, the types of pitching, and poor pitching mechanics.[1,4,6]

Diagnosis of an overuse injury can be made with clinical findings and imaging. Patients may complain of progressive pain in the shoulder that is worsened by throwing.[1] For example, Little League shoulder can be diagnosed with tenderness directly over the proximal physis and evidence on radiographs of widening of the physis, metaphyseal sclerosis, osteopenia, and/or fragmentation.[1,4,6]

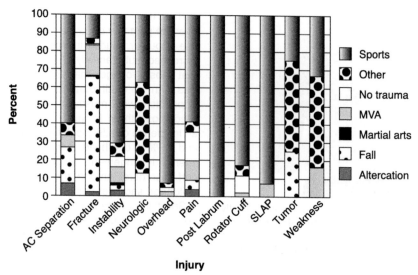

Fig. 4. One-hundred percent bar graph of the mechanisms of shoulder injuries. Sports were the most common mechanism of injury for the cohort. MVA, motor vehicle accident; SLAP, superior labral tear from anterior to posterior.

Therapeutic Options for Overuse Shoulder Injuries

Patients with Little League shoulder must rest their shoulders by not throwing and must work on activity modification.[1,6] Once children rest their arms for about 2 to 3 months and become pain free, they may progress back into their overhead sports by focusing on the following[1,4,6]:

- Stretching exercises of capsular structures (cross-arm and sleeper stretch)
- Strengthening exercises of the rotator cuff and other periscapular muscles
- A progressive throwing program that emphasizes proper throwing mechanics

For the intra-articular overuse injuries, treatment is more varied. In our study cohort, physical therapy was the initial treatment modality nearly 57% of the time. Surgery was not always successful, but was often required to relieve symptoms and restore function. Surgery was performed on 70% of superior labrum anterior-posterior tears, and 60% of internal impingement cases, which included partial rotator cuff injuries and posterosuperior labral tears.

Treatment of rotator cuff tears includes:

- Rest, nonsteroidal antiinflammatory drugs (NSAIDs), and rehabilitation.[4]
- Exercises focusing on range of motion and strengthening parascapular stabilizers and

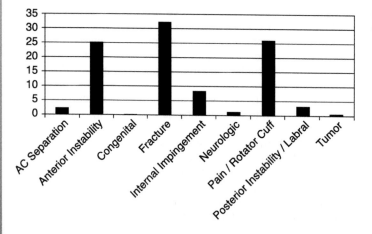

Fig. 5. The percentages of injuries in our 1-year cohort.

rotator cuff muscles to restore dynamic stability.[4]

- About one-third of partial-thickness tears treated conservatively can progress to full-thickness tears.[18] If conservative therapy fails, arthroscopy for debridement and/or repair should be performed.[4]

Outcomes and Complications for Overuse Shoulder Injuries

Treatment of Little League shoulder typically resolves the shoulder pain in 91% of pitchers.[6] Little is known about outcomes in children with regard to internal impingement, but there have been limited studies investigating specific injury patterns in several teenagers. About 43% of adolescent athletes with partial rotator cuff tears were shown to improve with a physical therapy program of at least 6 weeks' duration.[25] The same study found that those patients with magnetic resonance imaging (MRI) that diagnosed associated disorders with the rotator cuff tear were 1.8 times more likely to require surgery compared with those without MRI-identified associated disorders. Many isolated partial rotator cuff tears could be successfully treated with physical therapy; however, surgery for those patients who failed to improve with therapy alone could predictably improve pain and activities of daily living, albeit with risk for residual complaints during sports participation.

The primary complication seen for Little League shoulder is a physeal arrest caused by the continued stress on that growth plate, as seen in a Salter-Harris I injury (discussed earlier). Complications for internal impingement are not well described, other than an inability to return to the level of former play in sports.

SHOULDER INSTABILITY (ANTERIOR AND POSTERIOR)
Introduction to Shoulder Instability

The shoulder is the most commonly dislocated joint in the body, with traumatic anterior dislocations occurring more frequently than posterior dislocations.[1] It has been stated that 40% of primary shoulder dislocations occur in individuals younger than 22 years old, with anterior events representing 98% of the injuries and posterior events representing 2% to 12%.[1,6,26,27] Posterior instability has been shown to cause more morbidity than anterior instability. One study found that only 55% of throwing athletes with posterior instability returned to sports, compared with 71% returning for anterior instability.[26]

Because dislocations are often secondary to trauma, anterior dislocations are common in athletic injuries and occur in about 2% in the general population and 8% in younger patients.[28] In a study of rugby players, the nondominant shoulder was more likely to be affected, which was thought to be caused by a difference in strength and coordination between shoulders.[29] Instability injuries are difficult to diagnose because nonpathologic laxity is common in the general pediatric population.[23]

In our cohort study, the mean age of patients with instability injuries was significantly older (15–16 years) than the mean age of patients with fractures (11 years). This difference suggests that those who are skeletally immature may be more predisposed to fractures, whereas a closing physis at the proximal humerus is more likely to withstand injury and permit a soft tissue injury (Fig. 6).

Multidirectional instability is another possible injury in this population. The definition of multidirectional instability is symptomatic glenohumeral instability in more than one direction.[30–32] The distinction between multidirectional and unidirectional instability is difficult because there is a great deal of overlap between the two syndromes.[30] The inferior glenohumeral ligament complex plays an important role in the reciprocal tightening of anterior and posterior structures when the abducted arm is moved from external to internal rotation.[30] Repetitive strain of the inferior glenohumeral ligament can cause eventual failure and loosening, causing multidirectional instability.[30]

Anterior dislocation
The mechanism of injury for an anterior primary dislocation is typically a single traumatic event,[1,29,33] but this condition has also been seen with:

- Tackling, with the tackler more commonly injured[29]
- Fall onto an outstretched arm[29]
- Unexpected, unopposed anterior momentum caused by a missed punch[33]

Posterior dislocation
A direct load to the shoulder in a position of forward flexion, adduction, and internal rotation is the typical mechanism of injury. Other mechanisms include[1,26,27,34]:

- Baseball batting: in the lead shoulder caused by repetitive microtrauma from the rotational forces of a swing, which are magnified by a missed pitch[26]

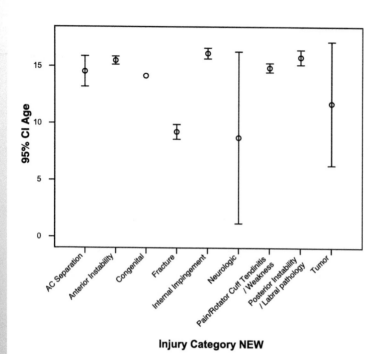

Fig. 6. The mean age with standard deviation at which specific injuries were sustained. CI, confidence interval.

- Wrestling: posterior axial loading or forced hyperadduction, horizontally adducted and flexed arm against the ground[27]
- Seizures
- Electric shocks

Multidirectional instability

Repetitive microtrauma as opposed to a discrete traumatic event:

- Nonsymptomatic laxity and/or instability in the contralateral shoulder[30]
- Capsular redundancy[31,32]
- Congenital diseases such as global ligamentous laxity, Ehlers-Danlos syndrome, Marfan syndrome[1,35,36]

Therapeutic Options for Shoulder Instability

Anterior dislocation

Conservative treatment options are acceptable for first-time anterior shoulder dislocations, although success varies.[1,6]

- Traditional treatment: internal rotation for 3 to 6 weeks to rest the arm[1]
- Immobilization in 35° of external rotation may lead to fewer recurrent dislocations, but there are issues with patient compliance[1,6]

Surgery has been helpful in preventing recurrent instability and dislocation, with possible indications including[1,28,37]:

- Good to excellent results in 88% to 100% of patients with open capsular plication, with only a 10% recurrence rate and similar results with arthroscopic intervention.
- High-level athletes, less than 35 years old and involved in high-risk sports, are good candidates for immediate surgical stabilization because these individuals are at a high risk for recurrence.
- Delaying a surgery until after a sports season after a primary anterior dislocation is acceptable for return to sports if strength symmetry and range of motion have been achieved.

Posterior dislocation

- Immobilization from 6 weeks to 3 months with physical therapy focusing on rotator cuff (especially the infraspinatus and teres minor to increase posterior stability) and scapular strengthening exercises with ice and NSAIDs.[1,27]
- If pain and instability persist, then proceed to surgical repair. Posterior labral repair and various capsulorrhaphy approaches with both arthroscopic and open techniques are acceptable.[1,4,27]

Multidirectional instability

The anterior surgical approach is suggested for major anterior instability and the posterior surgical approach for predominantly posterior instability.[30]

The goal should be to repair inferior instability, because this can help correct both anterior and posterior instability at the same time.[30]

Outcomes and Complications for Shoulder Instability

Long-term complaints with conservative treatment include dislocation recurrence, instability, pain, and stiffness.[1]

Anterior dislocation/subluxation has associated injuries including[1,33]:

- Bankart lesions, 87% to 100% (dislocations)
- Hill-Sachs lesions, 86% to 100% (dislocations)
- Bankart lesions, 49% (subluxations)
- Hill-Sachs lesions, 48% (subluxations)
- SLAP (superior labral tear from anterior to posterior) tears, 10% (dislocations)

Posterior dislocations have associated lesions including[27] posterior labral tears, posterior capsular laxity, or both.

The risk of reoccurrence approaches 100% in the population less than 20 years old, with athletes dislocating more commonly than nonathletes and older populations having fewer recurrences.[1,6,28,38-40] Some risk factors associated with recurrence are glenoid bone loss, anterior hyperlaxity, and Hill-Sachs lesions.[38] Recurrent dislocation by age are as follows[28,29]:

- Patients 21 to 30 years old: 79%
- Patients 31 to 40 years old: 50%
- Patients more than 40 years old: 14%
- In general, 90% in patients less than 20 years old and 50% in patients more than 25 years old

BRACHIAL PLEXUS INJURIES

Brachial plexus injuries in the pediatric population are rare and are typically caused by trauma or obstetric injuries, with the latter being more common.[41-43]

Trauma[42]:

- Brachial plexus injuries represent 0.1% of pediatric multitraumas (compared with 1% in adults, with motorcycle accidents as the cause in 77% of the cases)

One study found the cause of injury to be[42]:

- Passengers as motor vehicle accidents: 32%
- Pedestrian versus motor vehicle: 17%
- Gunshot injuries (gunshot injuries were 4 times more likely to cause brachial plexus injuries compared with the others in the population studied): 12%
- Sport injuries: 10%

Associated lesions[42]:

- Fractures about 54% of the time, with the bones around the brachial plexus most commonly affected 11% to 16% of the time
- Head injuries about 45% of the time
- Upper extremity vascular lesions 24% of the time
- Thoracic and abdominal injuries about 20% of the time

Brachial plexus injuries occur at a rate of 0.4 to 4 per 1000 live births, with most studies citing around 1 per 1000 live births and an incidence that has not changed over decades despite increased awareness.[43-47] Lateral traction during the birthing process may account for 4% to 47% of brachial plexus injuries.[44,48] This figure implies that half of all obstetric brachial plexus injuries occur without difficult deliveries and may be caused by atraumatic intrauterine forces.[48] Cesarean section is protective and reduces the risk of brachial plexus injury 10-fold.[46,49]

Diagnosis:

- Decreased arm movement on neonatal physical examination with the presence of first cervical rib or clavicle fracture[45]
- Electromyography can be used to help aid in diagnosis but can sometimes be misleading in the neonatal period (first few months of life)[43,44]

Risk factors include[44-46,48,49]:

- Shoulder dystocia (100 times increased risk)
- Diabetes gravida
- Excessive weight gain in pregnancy
- Macrosomia (14 times increased risk)
- Multiple pregnancies
- Prior births that resulted in brachial plexus injuries
- Breech delivery
- Instrument delivery (vacuum and forceps)

Specific lesions include[44,46,48,50]:

- Best prognosis (around 50% of cases): C5 to C6 involvement (Erb palsy), with function typically restored within 6 months
- Intermediate prognosis (around 25% to 30% of cases): C5 to C7 involvement, with recovery about 75%
- Worst prognosis (around 20% to 25% of cases): C5 to T1 involvement, with flail extremity and possible avulsion injury if Horner lesion present

Treatment guidelines[41,43,44,46]:

- Conservative treatment for about 3 months (range 6 weeks to 6 months), monitoring for antigravity biceps or shoulder movement
- Microsurgery is indicated if there is obvious global lesion and Horner syndrome or if no recovery after set time period

Microsurgical treatment goals and options[43,44,46]:

- Muscle and tendon transfers
- Neurotization of nearby muscles
- Nerve transfers with sural nerve as typical donor

REFERENCES

1. Taylor DC, Krasinski KL. Adolescent shoulder injuries: consensus and controversies. J Bone Joint Surg Am 2009;91(2):462–73.
2. Turkelson C, Zhao G. Musculoskeletal conditions and disorders: occurrence and healthcare use in the United States 2009. Available at: http://www.aaos.org/research/stats/patientstats.asp. Accessed July 8, 2011.
3. Di Gennaro GL, Spina M, Lampasi M, et al. Fractures of the proximal humerus in children. Chir Organi Mov 2008;92(2):89–95.
4. Kocher MS, Waters PM, Micheli LJ. Upper extremity injuries in the paediatric athlete. Sports Med 2000;30(2):117–35.
5. Hilton M, Yngve DA, Carmichael KD. Proximal humerus fractures sustained during the use of restraints in adolescents. J Pediatr Orthop 2006; 26(1):50–2.
6. Leonard J, Hutchinson MR. Shoulder injuries in skeletally immature throwers: review and current thoughts. Br J Sports Med 2010;44(5):306–10.
7. Shannon EG, Hart ES, Grottkau BE. Clavicle fractures in children: the essentials. Orthop Nurs 2009;28(5):210–4 [quiz: 215–6].
8. Namdari S, Ganley TJ, Baldwin K, et al. Fixation of displaced midshaft clavicle fractures in skeletally immature patients. J Pediatr Orthop 2011;31(5): 507–11.
9. van der Meijden OA, Gaskill TR, Millett PJ. Treatment of clavicle fractures: current concepts review. J Shoulder Elbow Surg 2012;21(3):423–9.
10. Nenopoulos SP, Gigis IP, Chytas AA, et al. Outcome of distal clavicular fracture separations and dislocations in immature skeleton. Injury 2011;42(4):376–80.
11. Caird MS. Clavicle shaft fractures: are children little adults? J Pediatr Orthop 2012;32(Suppl 1):S1–4.
12. Mehlman CT, Yihua G, Bochang C, et al. Operative treatment of completely displaced clavicle shaft fractures in children. J Pediatr Orthop 2009;29(8): 851–5.
13. Bahrs C, Zipplies S, Ochs BG, et al. Proximal humeral fractures in children and adolescents. J Pediatr Orthop 2009;29(3):238–42.
14. Paley KJ, Jobe FW, Pink MM, et al. Arthroscopic findings in the overhand throwing athlete: evidence for posterior internal impingement of the rotator cuff. Arthroscopy 2000;16(1):35–40.
15. Halbrecht JL, Tirman P, Atkin D. Internal impingement of the shoulder: comparison of findings between the throwing and nonthrowing shoulders of college baseball players. Arthroscopy 1999;15(3): 253–8.
16. Walch G, Boileau P, Noel E, et al. Impingement of the deep surface of the supraspinatus tendon on the posterosuperior glenoid rim: an arthroscopic study. J Shoulder Elbow Surg 1992;1:238–45.
17. Kleposki RW, Wells L, Wilson M, et al. Rotator cuff injuries in skeletally immature patients: prevention and indications for the orthopaedic nurse. Orthop Nurs 2009;28(3):134–8 [quiz: 139–40].
18. Tarkin IS, Morganti CM, Zillmer DA, et al. Rotator cuff tears in adolescent athletes. Am J Sports Med 2005;33(4):596–601.
19. Paschal SO, Hutton KS, Weatherall PT. Isolated avulsion fracture of the lesser tuberosity of the humerus in adolescents. A report of two cases. J Bone Joint Surg Am 1995;77(9):1427–30.
20. Battaglia TC, Barr MA, Diduch DR. Rotator cuff tear in a 13-year-old baseball player: a case report. Am J Sports Med 2003;31(5):779–82.
21. Feng S, Guo S, Nobuhara K, et al. Prognostic indicators for outcome following rotator cuff tear repair. J Orthop Surg (Hong Kong) 2003;11(2):110–6.
22. Stickley CD, Hetzler RK, Freemyer BG, et al. Isokinetic peak torque ratios and shoulder injury history in adolescent female volleyball athletes. J Athl Train 2008;43(6):571–7.
23. Rupp S, Berninger K, Hopf T. Shoulder problems in high level swimmers–impingement, anterior instability, muscular imbalance? Int J Sports Med 1995;16(8):557–62.
24. Burns TC, Reineck JR, Krishnan SG. Rotator cuff tears in adolescent female catchers. J Shoulder Elbow Surg 2009;18(6):e13–6.
25. Eisner EA, Roocroft JH, Edmonds EW. Underestimation of labral pathology in adolescents with anterior shoulder instability. J Pediatr Orthop 2012; 32(1):42–7.
26. Wanich T, Dines J, Dines D, et al. 'Batter's shoulder': can athletes return to play at the same level after operative treatment? Clin Orthop Relat Res 2012;470(6):1565–70.
27. Eckenrode BJ, Logerstedt DS, Sennett BJ. Rehabilitation and functional outcomes in collegiate wrestlers following a posterior shoulder

stabilization procedure. J Orthop Sports Phys Ther 2009;39(7):550–9.

28. Wheeler JH, Ryan JB, Arciero RA, et al. Arthroscopic versus nonoperative treatment of acute shoulder dislocations in young athletes. Arthroscopy 1989;5(3):213–7.

29. Sundaram A, Bokor DJ, Davidson AS. Rugby Union on-field position and its relationship to shoulder injury leading to anterior reconstruction for instability. J Sci Med Sport 2011;14(2):111–4.

30. Choi CH, Ogilvie-Harris DJ. Inferior capsular shift operation for multidirectional instability of the shoulder in players of contact sports. Br J Sports Med 2002;36(4):290–4.

31. Emery RJ, Mullaji AB. Glenohumeral joint instability in normal adolescents. Incidence and significance. J Bone Joint Surg Br 1991;73(3):406–8.

32. Alpert JM, Verma N, Wysocki R, et al. Arthroscopic treatment of multidirectional shoulder instability with minimum 270 degrees labral repair: minimum 2-year follow-up. Arthroscopy 2008;24(6):704–11.

33. Owens BD, Duffey ML, Nelson BJ, et al. The incidence and characteristics of shoulder instability at the United States Military Academy. Am J Sports Med 2007;35(7):1168–73.

34. Faustin CM, El Rassi G, Toulson CE, et al. Isolated posterior labrum tear in a golfer: a case report. Am J Sports Med 2007;35(2):312–5.

35. Monteiro GC, Ejnisman B, Andreoli CV, et al. Absorbable versus nonabsorbable sutures for the arthroscopic treatment of anterior shoulder instability in athletes: a prospective randomized study. Arthroscopy 2008;24(6):697–703.

36. Mather RC 3rd, Orlando LA, Henderson RA, et al. A predictive model of shoulder instability after a first-time anterior shoulder dislocation. J Shoulder Elbow Surg 2011;20(2):259–66.

37. Christoffersson M, Rydhstroem H. Shoulder dystocia and brachial plexus injury: a population-based study. Gynecol Obstet Invest 2002;53(1): 42–7.

38. Peleg D, Hasnin J, Shalev E. Fractured clavicle and Erb's palsy unrelated to birth trauma. Am J Obstet Gynecol 1997;177(5):1038–40.

39. Terzis JK, Kokkalis ZT. Pediatric brachial plexus reconstruction. Plast Reconstr Surg 2009;124(Suppl 6): e370–85.

40. Dorsi MJ, Hsu W, Belzberg AJ. Epidemiology of brachial plexus injury in the pediatric multitrauma population in the United States. J Neurosurg Pediatr 2010;5(6):573–7.

41. Kwazneski DR, Iyer RC, Panthaki Z, et al. Controversies in the diagnosis and treatment of pediatric brachial plexus injuries. J Craniofac Surg 2009; 20(4):1036–8.

42. Pham CB, Kratz JR, Jelin AC, et al. Child neurology: brachial plexus birth injury: what every neurologist needs to know. Neurology 2011;77(7): 695–7.

43. Alfonso DT. Causes of neonatal brachial plexus palsy. Bull NYU Hosp Jt Dis 2011;69(1):11–6.

44. Hale HB, Bae DS, Waters PM. Current concepts in the management of brachial plexus birth palsy. J Hand Surg Am 2010;35(2):322–31.

45. Walsh JM, Kandamany N, Ni Shuibhne N, et al. Neonatal brachial plexus injury: comparison of incidence and antecedents between 2 decades. Am J Obstet Gynecol 2011;204(4):324.e1–6.

46. Chauhan SP, Rose CH, Gherman RB, et al. Brachial plexus injury: a 23-year experience from a tertiary center. Am J Obstet Gynecol 2005;192(6): 1795–800.

47. Foad SL, Mehlman CT, Ying J. The epidemiology of neonatal brachial plexus palsy in the United States. J Bone Joint Surg Am 2008;90(6):1258–64.

48. Mollberg M, Lagerkvist AL, Johansson U, et al. Comparison in obstetric management on infants with transient and persistent obstetric brachial plexus palsy. J Child Neurol 2008;23(12):1424–32.

49. Malfait F, Wenstrup R, De Paepe A. Ehlers-Danlos syndrome, classic type. 2007 [updated 2011]. In: Pagon RA, Bird TD, Dolan CR, et al. editors. GeneReview. Seattle (WA): University of Washington; 1993. [Internet]. Available at: http://www.ncbi.nlm.nih. gov/books/NBK1244/. Accessed August 18, 2011.

50. Wolf JM, Cameron KL, Owens BD. Impact of joint laxity and hypermobility on the musculoskeletal system. J Am Acad Orthop Surg 2011;19(8):463–71.

Prevention of Overuse Sports Injuries in the Young Athlete

Mark V. Paterno, PT, PhD, SCS, ATC[a,b,c,*],
Jeffery A. Taylor-Haas, PT, DPT, OCS, CSCS[a,b],
Gregory D. Myer, PhD, CSCS[a,c,d,e],
Timothy E. Hewett, PhD[a,f,g,h,i]

KEYWORDS

- Overuse injury • Mechanism • Injury prevention • Sports specialization

KEY POINTS

- The prevalence of overuse injuries in young athletes in increasing.
- The mechanism of overuse injuries in young athletes is multi-factoral and can be classified as either intrinsic or extrinsically related.
- Identification of a mechanism unique to the individual athlete is important to apply targeted intervention strategies.
- Targeted neuromuscular interventions developed to prevent acute lower extremity injuries may also have a role in the reduction of certain overuse injuries, as well.

INTRODUCTION

Participation in organized sports is increasing in the United States. An estimated 30 to 45 million children participate in organized sports annually.[1,2] Concurrent with this increase in participation is an upward trend in year-round participation in athletics in either one or multiple sports. The benefits of athletic participation in children as a means to stay active and physically fit are well documented[3]; however, an increased prevalence of athletic injury in young athletes has raised concern regarding the safety of intense athletic participation at a young age.[4] Although many of these injuries may represent traumatic incidents, as many as one-third[5] to more than 50%[6,7] of these injuries are estimated to be a result of overuse.

Overuse injuries include a broad spectrum of injuries within sports medicine. Classically, they are defined as chronic injuries related to "constant levels of physiologic stress without sufficient recover time."[5] Globally, they can be perceived as the outcome of the difference between the volume

[a] Human Performance Lab, Division of Sports Medicine, Sports Medicine Biodynamics Center, Cincinnati Children's Hospital Medical Center, 3333 Burnet Avenue, MLC 10001, Cincinnati, OH 45229, USA; [b] Division of Occupational Therapy and Physical Therapy, Cincinnati Children's Hospital Medical Center, 3333 Burnet Avenue, MLC 10001, Cincinnati, OH 45229, USA; [c] Department of Pediatrics, University of Cincinnati College of Medicine, Cincinnati, OH, USA; [d] Department of Orthopaedic Surgery, University of Cincinnati College of Medicine, Cincinnati, OH, USA; [e] Athletic Training Division, School of Health and Rehabilitation Sciences, The Ohio State University, 2050 Kenny Road, Sports Medicine Suite 3100, Columbus, OH 43221, USA; [f] Department of Physiology and Cell Biology, The Sports Health and Performance Institute, The Ohio State University, 2050 Kenny Road, Sports Medicine Suite 3100, Columbus, OH 43221, USA; [g] Department of Orthopaedic Surgery, The Sports Health and Performance Institute, The Ohio State University, 2050 Kenny Road, Sports Medicine Suite 3100, Columbus, OH 43221, USA; [h] Department of Family Medicine, The Sports Health and Performance Institute, The Ohio State University, 2050 Kenny Road, Sports Medicine Suite 3100, Columbus, OH 43221, USA; [i] Department of Biomedical Engineering, The Sports Health and Performance Institute, The Ohio State University, 2050 Kenny Road, Sports Medicine Suite 3100, Columbus, OH 43221, USA
* Corresponding author. Cincinnati Children's Hospital, 3333 Burnet Avenue, MLC 10001, Cincinnati, OH 45229.
E-mail address: mark.paterno@cchmc.org

Orthop Clin N Am 44 (2013) 553–564
http://dx.doi.org/10.1016/j.ocl.2013.06.009
0030-5898/13/$ – see front matter © 2013 Elsevier Inc. All rights reserved.

of the stress or force applied to the body and the ability of the body to dissipate this stress or force. Injury may result from repetitive microtrauma imposed on otherwise healthy tissue or the repeated application of lesser magnitudes of force to pathologic tissue. Either scenario can lead to the sequelae of tissue breakdown. Unfortunately, the mechanism by which this stress ultimately leads to overuse injuries is not consistent among young athletes.

In the absence of a well-defined mechanism, the development of targeted intervention strategies is more difficult. Traumatic injuries, such as ligament tears, are typically the result of a single macrotrauma on otherwise healthy tissue, which results in tissue failure. Many injury-prevention programs attempt to develop the athlete's neuromuscular control mechanisms to help dampen these external forces and reduce the likelihood of traumatic tissue failure.[8,9] In the case of overuse injuries, there is significantly less evidence regarding the most efficacious program to reduce the incidence of these injuries. Therefore, current intervention programs that attempt to address potential underlying mechanisms or target specific risk factors that may contribute to abnormally high stress with repeated activities are still in development. The purpose of this article is to highlight the prevailing theories of overuse injury mechanisms as well as review the best available evidence for the implementation of prevention strategies designed to target overuse injuries in both endurance and pivoting/cutting sports.

MECHANISM OF OVERUSE INJURY

Factors that increase the likelihood of overuse injuries can be classified as either intrinsic or extrinsic risk factors. Intrinsic factors are categorized as implicit or unique to the individual that may increase the likelihood of sustaining an injury.[3] Maturational status, body mass index (BMI), gender, anatomic variations, and biomechanical movement patterns are all examples of intrinsic risk factors.[10] Theoretically, these factors can affect the ability of the athlete's tissue to dampen or respond to stress. For example, if an athlete possess a varus knee alignment, he or she is more likely to experience an increase load on the medial compartment of the knee. Over time, this may lead to more articular cartilage breakdown in the medial compartment. Anatomic variants, such as knee alignment, in the absence of a surgical intervention to realign the knee, are unmodifiable risk factors. Conversely, intrinsic risk factors, such as BMI, strength deficits, or altered movement patterns, would generally be considered

modifiable risk factors, which have the potential to improve with an injury-prevention intervention.

Extrinsic risk factors are those factors that, when applied to the athlete, may increase the risk of injury. These factors may include training methods, equipment, and environment[3] and may have an effect on the magnitude, stress, or force applied to the body. Training regimes are often implicated as a potential mechanism of overuse injury. Hogan and Gross[5] identified 3 scenarios that may increase an individual's likelihood of developing an overuse injury. The first scenario involves the athlete who attempts to rapidly increase his or her training load after a period of inactivity or decreased activity. In this situation, the body has an insufficient adaptation period to respond to a higher level of stress and, therefore, is not adequately prepared to dissipate repetitive forces. Investigations of the high incidence of stress fractures during the initial stages of training in the military[5,11] support this theory of overuse injury caused by rapid increases in activity.

A second category of extrinsic risk factors includes athletes who attempt to participate at a level that exceeds their individual skill level.[5] In theory, this mismatch of individual skill or fitness level to imposed stress and physical demands can lead to tissue breakdown. Finally, consistent participation at an exceptionally high level is theorized to lead to overuse injury. This group may suffer from excessive microtrauma over time with insufficient rest, ultimately leading to tissue breakdown. Athletes who continuously participate in sports without rest[12] or who specialize in one sport throughout the year[4] are anecdotally thought to be included in this high-risk category; however, the current evidence is sparse.[12]

In summary, overuse injuries are generally a product of the application of an applied load to the body and the body's ultimate inability to dampen the applied load. This inability may be caused by intrinsic factors that limit the body's ability to dampen the load or extrinsic factors that increase the load that is applied. Using this theory, programs designed to prevent overuse injuries should target impairments that decrease the individual's ability to dampen forces applied to the body and encourage participation in appropriate progressions of training to increase the individual's ability to dampen the applied load.

PREVENTING OVERUSE INJURIES IN YOUNG ENDURANCE ATHLETES

Running is an endurance sport that continues to grow in popularity among middle school and high school athletes; more than 450,000 young athletes participated in cross country during 2010 to 2011.[13] Concomitant with an increase in running participation comes an associated increase in injuries. The annual incidence rate among high school cross-country runners is reported to be as high as 17.0 per 1000 athletic exposures (AEs).[14] Unfortunately, the literature on running-related injury prevention is sparse and often contradictory. In addition, the potential confounding effects of growth and maturation on running biomechanics and injury risk in children may also limit the generalizability of adult literature to the pediatric running population. Although these challenges exist, focusing on known factors that contribute to pediatric running-related injuries, recognizing the hallmark signs and symptoms of these injuries, as well as having a strong understanding of the underlying biomechanics of distance running may serve to guide clinicians interested in the prevention of these injuries in a young population.

Common Pediatric Running-Related Injuries

The most common location of pediatric running-related injuries is shin injuries for girls and knee injuries for boys.[14] The 2 most common shin injuries are medial tibial stress syndrome (MTSS) and tibial stress fractures. In adolescent runners, the most common knee injuries are patellofemoral syndrome, iliotibial band syndrome, and injuries to the apophysis, such as Osgood-Schlatter disease (OSD).

MTSS is characterized as "an exercise-induced, localized pain along the distal two thirds of the posterior-medial tibia"[15] and affects more female than male long-distance runners. The risk factors for sustained MTSS include reduced running experience,[16] a previous history of MTSS,[16] and a higher BMI.[15] Although runners with a history of MTSS are more likely to report orthoses use than those runners without a history of MTSS,[15] the evidence supporting an association between a pronatory foot type and MTSS is mixed.[15,17,18] Adult athletes diagnosed with MTSS have significantly reduced plantar flexor muscle endurance compared with uninjured athletes.[19] Although retrospective in nature, this adds support to the theory that a lack of endurance of the plantar flexor muscle group may lead to a higher force transfer to the tibia.[20]

Stress fractures occur along a continuum of repetitive loading, bone remodeling, and microdamage accumulation[21] and can be classified as either fatigue or insufficiency fractures. A fatigue stress fracture occurs in healthy bone as the result of repetitive loading and mechanical stress,[22] whereas an insufficiency fracture is the result of normal loading on pathologic bone.[22] Most stress fractures that occur in pediatric long-distance runners can be classified as fatigue stress fractures, with tibial stress fractures as the most common type of stress fracture.[23]

Of all running injuries, patellofemoral syndrome (PFPS) is the most common[24,25] and the cause is still unclear.[26] Also known as runner's knee or anterior knee pain, PFPS is typically described as pain to the peripatellar region that increases with activities, such as running, stair ambulation, squatting, jumping, and/or prolonged sitting with the knees flexed.[27] Although many etiologic theories exist, 2 biomechanical pathways have received the most attention. First, a lack of proximal stability caused by impaired hip strength and/or hip muscular activation leads to excessive patellofemoral joint stress by increasing the dynamic quadriceps angle acting on the patellofemoral joint.[28] Second, excessive and/or mistimed pronation may lead to alterations in frontal and transverse plane mechanics at the patellofemoral joint resulting in patellofemoral compression, overuse, and pain.[28]

Proximally, the gluteus medius and gluteus maximus function to eccentrically stabilize the femur in the frontal and transverse planes, respectively, while running.[29] Recent systematic reviews suggest adolescent and young adult women with PFPS demonstrate deficits in hip strength[30] and adult runners with PFPS exhibit delayed and shorter muscle activation of the gluteus medius.[31] Together, these studies indicate an association between the lack of proximal pelvic girdle stability and PFPS. Furthermore, interventions targeted at improving the strength and neuromuscular control of the hip abductor, hip extensor, and hip external rotator musculature may be efficacious as part of an injury-prevention program. Distally, as the foot and ankle complex pronates the tibia internally rotates because of the anatomic wedging of the talus in the distal tibia-fibular mortise.[32] Some investigators theorize that excessive or mistimed pronation would lead to excessive patellofemoral stress because of the disruptions in transverse and frontal plane timing of the transverse plane tibiofemoral joint.[33] However, there is mixed evidence regarding the association between excessive foot pronation and PFPS.[34–37]

Iliotibial band syndrome (ITBS) is the most common cause of lateral knee pain in runners,[24] with an annual incidence rate of up to 12%.[38] Although originally thought of as a sagittal plane disorder secondary to a tight ITB fractioning over the lateral femoral epicondyle,[38,39] more recent evidence supports the theory that ITB occurs as a result of a lack of frontal and transverse plane control of the femur and tibia.[40–43] Antiinflammatory treatment is thought to be effective in the acute treatment of patients with ITBS,[38,44] whereas hip abductor strengthening has been shown to be effective at improving hip strength and returning injured runners back to function.[39,45]

OSD is the most common apophyseal disorder affecting adolescents[46] and presents as anterior knee pain, swelling, and tenderness to palpation over the tibial tubercle.[47] OSD typically occurs during a growth spurt and is seen most often in adolescents' participation in sports involving repetitive running and/or jumping.[47,48] Tightness to the rectus femoris is associated with OSD.[48] Interventions typically include relative rest, gentle quadriceps stretching, and quadriceps strengthening.[47–49] Because OSD is associated with recent growth, these athletes may benefit in the reduction of total running volume as part of an injury-prevention effort.

Risk Factors for Sustaining a Pediatric Running-Related Injury

Intrinsic risk factors

The intrinsic risk factors most often associated with running-related injuries in a pediatric population include sex, anatomic morphology, running mechanics, hip strength, and nutrition. Epidemiologic evidence of sex differences is sparse. Rauh and colleagues[14] prospectively tracked high school cross-country runners and noted that female runners had a higher injury rate as compared with boys (19.6 per 1000 AEs vs 15.0 per 1000 AEs) and sustained more injuries causing more than 15 days lost from running than boys. Compared with boys, the total injury rate for girls was significantly higher than boys for all injuries except those resulting in 5 to 14 days lost.[14] Retrospectively, Tenforde and colleagues[50] assessed a large cohort of long-distance runners and noted that girls had a higher overall injury rate than boys. The investigators noted the following most common injuries: tibial stress injuries, ankle sprain, patellofemoral pain, ITBS, and plantar fasciitis.

The risk factors related to anatomic morphology in runners include a quadriceps angle (Q angle) at the knee and foot morphology. Rauh and colleagues[51] report that high school cross country athletes with a standing Q angle of more than 20° were 1.7 times more likely to sustain a running-related injury compared with a standing Q angle of 10° to less than 15°. Runners with more than a 4° absolute right-left Q angle difference were at a 1.8 times greater risk compared with runners with a smaller difference. Runners with a Q angle of more than 20° were more likely

to injure their knee, whereas runners with more than a 4° Q angle difference were more likely to injure their shin.[51]

Anatomic variations related to foot morphology are often theorized to contribute to pediatric running-related injuries. Many investigators postulate that a pes planus foot type results is a more mobile foot leading to an increase in pronation excursion and excessive strain to medial soft tissue structures, whereas a pes cavus foot type results in a stiffer foot that is less well equipped to dampen ground reaction force (GRF) at the foot and ankle resulting in excessive bone stresses and lateral column injuries.[52] Although multiple investigators cite structural deviations of the arch as either indirectly or directly contributing to the running injury incidence in both adult civilian and military runners,[53–56] others have found no association.[57–59] Further, few studies have prospectively assessed the effect of foot structure on the incidence of pediatric running-related injuries (PRRI) with contradictory conclusions.[15,17,60,61] This contrary finding has lead one investigator to state that efforts to optimally "aligning the skeleton" with shoes and orthoses designed to mitigate anatomic variants should be reconsidered.[62] Thus, further high-quality prospective studies are warranted to help delineate the effect of arch structure on the risk of sustaining a running-related injury.

Altered running mechanics are theorized to lead to injury. Recently, primary biomechanical faults cited for an increased risk of sustaining a running-related injury are excessive rearfoot eversion[56,63–66] and altered stance phase impact forces.[56,67–72] Although limited work has been undertaken in pediatric running athletes, some prospective evidence exists correlating dynamic pronation excursion with the occurrence of exercise-related lower limb pain in a heterogeneous cohort of college-aged physical education students.[73]

Two studies have demonstrated altered running mechanics in adult women who have sustained tibial stress fractures.[56,66] In separate cross-sectional, retrospective studies comparing 3-dimensional mechanics of female runners with a history of tibial stress fracture to an uninjured cohort, it was noted that the tibial-stress-fracture groups demonstrated increased peak rearfoot eversion, a component of pronation, compared with controls.[56,66] Further, Milner and colleagues[66] reported that the tibial-stress-fracture group also demonstrated significantly higher peak hip adduction, whereas Pohl and colleagues[56] noted the variables of peak rearfoot eversion, peak hip adduction, and free moment (a measure of impact force) correctly classified 83% (50 out of 60) of runners into the tibial-stress-fracture or control group. Taken together, this suggests efforts aimed at reducing pronation and/or hip adduction may reduce the likelihood of developing a tibial stress fracture; however, caution must be noted because a cause-and-effect relationship cannot be ascertained from retrospective studies.

More recently, emphasis has shifted toward assessing hip strength, hip muscular activation, and running gait mechanics to assess the relative impact these variables may have on the development of a running-related injury. A lack of hip strength has been associated with multiple injuries, including PFPS,[27,29,30,74–79] ITBS,[39] and tibial stress fracture.[80] A lack of strength to the hip abductor, hip extensor, and hip external rotator musculature is theorized to place the femur into excessive amounts of adduction and internal rotation leading to alterations in joint coupling and mechanics to the knee, shank, and foot-ankle complex distally.[28] Indeed, there is limited evidence to suggest that altered hip strength affects running mechanics in a healthy population[81,82] and in a population of adult female runners with PFPS.[83] However, although improving hip strength has led to reductions in pain and improvement in function, particularly in patients with PFPS and ITBS,[27,39,84] they have not directly led to changes in running gait mechanics.[85,86] This seeming contradiction has, in part, caused some investigators to assess the effect of alterations in hip muscular activation and running gait mechanics on the relative risk of sustaining a running-related injury.

Proper nutrition is important for maintaining health and reducing the risk of sustaining a pediatric running-related injury. High School cross-country runners with a higher BMI have a higher risk of sustaining MTSS than those runners with a lower BMI.[15] Conversely, in a cohort of female collegiate track-and-field athletes, reduced nutritional fat intake was associated with an increased risk of sustaining a stress fracture.[87] This finding speaks to the intrinsic risk factors unique to female athletes, such as delayed age of menarche and irregular menstruation. Both menstrual irregularity, such as oligomenorrhea and amenorrhea, as well as a delayed age of attaining the first menstrual cycle are associated with increased risk of sustaining a bony stress-related injury.[87–90] Further, female long-distance runners who demonstrate signs or symptoms of disordered eating are at an increased risk of reduced bone mineral density than those runners with more typical eating habits.[88]

Extrinsic risk factors

Extrinsically, improper training is identified as a contributor to pediatric running-related injuries. Progressive training regimes with a focus on a gradual increase in running to help acclimate the body to the rigors of running, thereby reducing the likelihood of sustaining a running-related injury, are common. Unfortunately, little evidence exists to support this widely held belief. A randomized controlled trial did not find a protective effect for a preconditioning program at reducing running-related injury rates (RRIR) in novice adult runners.[91] This finding is in agreement with Buist and colleagues[92] who found no difference on the RRIR of adult novice runners using a 13-week graded training program that followed "the 10% rule" for mileage increase when compared with an 8-week control group. Because many pediatric runners can be considered novice runners or runners who have been running for 2 years or less, these results may provide some insight into the effect of training on the PRRI rate.

The type and duration of previous sports participation may alter the risk of sustaining a running-related injury. In novice adult men training for a 4-mile race, those runners who had participated in sports without axial loading before training, such as swimming and cycling, were more than twice as likely to sustain an running-related injury than those men who had participated in sports such as basketball or soccer.[93] This finding is in agreement with Fredericson and colleagues[94] who noted that youth participation in basketball or soccer was protective against the future risk of sustaining a stress fracture in collegiate track athletes. Taken together, these studies impart 2 valuable clinical pearls. First, participation in sports that induce axial loading in a 3-dimensional fashion may enhance bone mass and, thereby reduce the likelihood of sustaining a stress-related running-related injury. Second, participation in sports whereby athletes are required to perform sprinting, cutting, and jumping maneuvers may enhance an athlete's neuromuscular control capabilities, which might impart a reduced likelihood of sustaining a running-related injury.

Potential Interventions to Target Altered Mechanics and Reduce Injury Risk

Although attempts to reduce the incidence of running-related injuries in adults through graded training programs[91,92] or by matching shoe wear to foot type[95] have proven to be ineffective, a careful review of the literature on risk factors for sustaining a PRRI as well as treatments for the most common PRRI suggests a pathway toward prevention. The key variables to this pathway may include the following:

1. Identifying at-risk populations
2. The application of a preseason and in-season hip strengthening program
3. Assessment of running biomechanics

Based on the epidemiologic reports of Rauh and colleagues[14,96] and Tenforde and colleagues[50] as well as the application of the reports on risk factors for novice runners,[91–93,97,98] the following characteristics of pediatric and adolescent long-distance runners should be taken into consideration and can be broken down between intrinsic and extrinsic measures. The assessments of 4 intrinsic measures are recommended. First, measuring the standing Q angle is recommended based on the aforementioned studies by Rauh and colleagues.[14,51,99] Specifically, runners with a Q angle of more than 20° and/or runners with a right-left difference of more than 4° should be noted and the application of modified training programs and/or targeted hip and quadriceps strengthening programs is recommended.[14,51] Second, measuring the BMI should be considered because an increased BMI is associated with MTSS,[15] whereas a reduced BMI may serve as a warning to coaches, parents, and health care professionals that the runner may be at risk for bony stress-related injuries, such as stress reaction and stress fractures.[100] Third, the navicular drop test should be considered, but caution should be noted in interpreting the results because of the conflicting reports noting its association with MTSS,[15,17,18] exertion-related lower limb pain[101] (a condition that encompasses pain between the knee and ankle that occurs with exercise[102]), and stress fractures.[24] Fourth, preseason measures of hip abductor, hip extensor, and hip external rotator strength should be considered because of the fair to strong evidence noting the relationship between hip muscle weakness and conditions such as PFPS[30] and ITBS.[39] Additionally, indirect evidence suggests a possible biomechanical link between hip muscle weakness and tibial stress fractures[56,66,80,81]; however, further prospective studies are warranted. Finally, with regard to female athletes, it is strongly recommended to regularly measure menstrual cycle status and regularity to reduce the likelihood of incurring bony stress-related injuries.[87–89,100]

Dynamics evaluation of altered gait mechanics, with the potential for targeted gait retraining, is viewed as a potential new avenue in the evaluation, treatment, and perhaps prevention of pediatric running-related injuries. With regard to stress fractures, multiple investigators have noted that adult female runners who have sustained a tibial stress fracture demonstrate altered running kinetics, specifically increases in loading rate[69,70] and ground reaction forces.[68,71] This finding had led some investigators to attempt to retrain running gait mechanics of at-risk and/or injured runners to reduce these variables of impact shock that may be associated with injury. Techniques such as real-time visual feedback,[72,103] mirror gait retraining,[104,105] and increasing step rate[106] have been used to target altered running mechanics. Taken together, both visual and auditory gait retraining provide clinicians with emerging interventions to address the high incidence of pediatric running-related injuries. However, future prospective research in a pediatric population is warranted to determine the effect of gait retraining on the reduction of injuries in at-risk populations.

With regard to modifiable extrinsic factors, 3 steps are recommended. First, cataloging an athlete's preseason activity level by using such valid and reliable tools as the Tegner Activity Scale[99,100] may be warranted to both determine the athlete's readiness to run as well as his or her relative risk for sustaining a running-related injury. Based on weak to fair evidence in the adult population, determining the fitness level before running,[96,107] the length of time running,[108] the type and severity of prior running-related injuries,[93] as well as the types of previous sporting activities[93] are recommended. Second, modifying training volumes and intensity for runners who have recently undergone a growth spurt are recommended to reduce stressors to the apophysis.[47,48] Finally, early and continued participation in ball sports and/or sports involving a 360° playing field are recommended based on weak to fair evidence.[94] Providing runners individualized training programs that take into account their fitness level, growth and maturation, and prior running-related injuries and that afford runners an opportunity to perform cross-training activities that challenges their coordination and neuromuscular control are recommended to help modify the extrinsic risk factors associated with pediatric running-related injuries.

In conclusion, more high-quality prospective research is warranted to better illuminate the intrinsic and extrinsic risk factors associated with sustaining a running-related injury. Further, high-quality randomized controlled trials assessing the effects of preseason interventions on the incidence and severity of these injuries are necessary to help guide coaches, parents, student-athletes, and health care professionals in making quality decisions regarding evidence-based steps to reduce the likelihood of sustaining a running-related injury.

Although these challenges remain, the continued participation in endurance sports, such as long-distance running, by pediatric and adolescent youths is recommended as a means of promoting a healthy and well-rounded lifestyle.

PREVENTING OVERUSE INJURIES IN PIVOTING AND CUTTING SPORTS

Team sports, such as basketball, handball, soccer, and volleyball, demonstrate an increased acute and overuse injury risk relative to individual sports.[109] Injuries to the anterior cruciate ligament (ACL) result in the greatest time lost from sport and recreational participation by young athletes who compete in running and cutting team sports. However, chronic conditions, such as patellofemoral pain, are the most common disorders of the knee, with their greatest incidence in young, physically active girls.[110–114] There is a similar sex disparity in both conditions because adolescent girls and young women who participate in pivoting and cutting sports are affected by PFPS and ACL injuries 2 to 10 times more often than their male counterparts.

Altered Mechanics That may Predispose to Overuse Injury

Altered or reduced motor control during physical activities may result in frontal plane dysfunction during running and cutting sports. This frontal plane dysfunction seems to be similar to those described in endurance sports, which may underlie injury risk. For example, in long-distance runners, the predictive factor that lead to chronic knee pain was increased knee frontal plane impulse moment during the single support stance phase of running.[115] Similarly, as previously noted, Rauh and colleagues[51] reported that high school cross-country runners with abnormal frontal plane static alignments (Q angle measures of 20° or more) were more likely to miss practice or competition from an injury to their knee. Increased frontal plane anatomic alignments and dynamic knee loads are associated with patellofemoral pain, and knee injury incidence has been noted previously with strong evidence in endurance runners, although this association has not been reported previously in other populations. However, recent evidence indicates that similar neuromuscular dysfunction, such as frontal plane alignment and control of the knee, also seems to increase the risk of both acute injury and chronic injury in young girls who play competitive team sports.[116,117]

Current Evidence of Neuromuscular Interventions That Reduce Incidence of Overuse Injury

It is acknowledged that the volume, intensity, and number of competitions vary among both team and individual sports. In addition, overscheduling and other factors, such as nutrition and lack of sleep, can contribute to overuse injury risk in youth.[6] A recent report indicates that early sport specialization during youth may be associated with an increased risk of patellofemoral pain compared with multisport athletes.[118] These data further indicate that the variety in sport and exercise may limit the risk of overuse injuries in this population. In addition, participation in a variety of sports may help prevent the development of neuromuscular deficits that likely underlie chronic injury in sports.[119] Although extrinsic factors likely contribute to chronic injury risk in running and cutting sports, the current evidence indicates that neuromuscular deficits, such as ligament dominance and quadriceps dominance, are the primary determinant of both acute and chronic injury risk. If neuromuscular dysfunction underlies both chronic and acute injury risk, this may provide a mechanism to target risk factors that increase the injury risk across all sport types and possibly prevent them in the future.[109]

Neuromuscular training focused on frontal plane dysfunction has been effective to reduce deficits that may increase the risk of injury.[120–123] In addition, neuromuscular training that is focused on increasing hip abduction strength and recruitment may improve the ability of young growing athletes to better control for the increased height of their center of mass and improve dynamic lower extremity alignments to reduce loads that may contribute to the chronic injuries.[124,125] Accordingly, a similar preseason neuromuscular training protocol was administered to young female athletes and found a reduced prevalence of chronic knee pain at the postseason follow-up.[126] Young athletes who have missed a critical window to prevent the development of movement deficits that increase the injury risk may be more responsive to specially designed neuromuscular training.[123] Current projects aimed toward the utilization of outlined neuromuscular screening techniques to identify potential high-risk young athletes and to target identified factors that put them at high risk with the most appropriate neuromuscular training for their specific observed deficits are well underway.[123,127,128] Recent evidence indicates that young athletes categorized as high risk based on previous coupled biomechanical and epidemiologic studies are more responsive to neuromuscular training.[116] Through the identification of young athletes at a greater risk for chronic injury, prevention strategies may be substantially improved; however, as recently suggested, variety and initiation of training during the younger years before playing competitive years with residual neuromuscular deficits may be the *best* approach to prevent chronic injury in youth.[129–132]

Strengths and Limitations of This Work and Future Directions

There are multiple strengths and limitations to the previously published work in the areas of overuse injuries in young athletes during pivoting and cutting sports,[110–114] the biomechanics that may predispose children to these injuries,[115] and the current evidence regarding interventions that may reduce the incidence of these overuse injuries.[129–132] One major limitation with this body of work is that most of this work is retrospective in nature. This limitation is a major limitation because of a questionable cause-and-effect scenario: did the identified factors underlie the onset of the overuse injury or were they the result of it? However, the more recent studies reported in the literature have been prospective in nature.[115] In addition, many of the prior reported studies are underpowered to draw valid conclusions from their work. Large, multicenter trials are needed to recruit and retain the large numbers of young athletes in longitudinal, prospective cohort studies in order to fully power these level I and level II experimental designs. There are multiple qualified multidisciplinary groups currently developing such powerful predictive studies.

SUMMARY

The prevalence of overuse injuries in a young athletic population is increasing, and the evidence related to risk factors in both endurance and cutting sports is lacking. However, the evidence that exists supports the potential for specific targeted prevention programs to reduce the injury risk. The assessment of the risk factors underlying the mechanisms of overuse injuries indicates a potential link between acute injury prevention and overuse injury prevention. In addition, preliminary attempts to use targeted neuromuscular training to reduce the incidence of overuse injury shows promise in small cohorts. Future research is warranted to investigate the potential for targeted neuromuscular training to reduce overuse injury rates or to investigate whether underlying risk factors need to be addressed before more significant reductions in overuse injury incidence rates are seen.

REFERENCES

1. Adirim TA, Cheng TL. Overview of injuries in the young athlete. Sports Med 2003;33(1):75–81.
2. Pate RR, Trost SG, Levin S, et al. Sports participation and health-related behaviors among US youth. Arch Pediatr Adolesc Med 2000;154(9):904–11.
3. Caine D, Maffulli N, Caine C. Epidemiology of injury in child and adolescent sports: injury rates, risk factors, and prevention. Clin Sports Med 2008; 27(1):19–50, vii.
4. Jayanthi N, Pinkham C, Dugas L, et al. Sports specialization in young athletes: evidence-based recommendations. Sport Health 2013;5(3):251–7.
5. Hogan KA, Gross RH. Overuse injuries in pediatric athletes. Orthop Clin North Am 2003;34(3): 405–15.
6. Luke A, Lazaro RM, Bergeron MF, et al. Sports-related injuries in youth athletes: is overscheduling a risk factor? Clin J Sport Med 2011;21(4):307–14.
7. Pommering TL, Kluchurosky L. Overuse injuries in adolescents. Adolesc Med State Art Rev 2007; 18(1):95–120, ix.
8. Hewett TE, Ford KR, Myer GD. Anterior cruciate ligament injuries in female athletes: part 2, a meta-analysis of neuromuscular interventions aimed at injury prevention. Am J Sports Med 2006;34(3): 490–8.
9. Renstrom P, Ljungqvist A, Arendt E, et al. Non-contact ACL injuries in female athletes: an International Olympic Committee current concepts statement. Br J Sports Med 2008;42(6):394–412.
10. McGuine T. Sports injuries in high school athletes: a review of injury-risk and injury-prevention research. Clin J Sport Med 2006;16(6):488–99.
11. Margulies JY, Simkin A, Leichter I, et al. Effect of intense physical activity on the bone-mineral content in the lower limbs of young adults. J Bone Joint Surg Am 1986;68(7):1090–3.
12. Cuff S, Loud K, O'Riordan MA. Overuse injuries in high school athletes. Clin Pediatr (Phila) 2010; 49(8):731–6.
13. National Federation of High Schools survey of participation. Available at: http://www.nfhs.org/ Participation/.
14. Rauh MJ, Koepsell TD, Rivara FP, et al. Epidemiology of musculoskeletal injuries among high school cross-country runners. Am J Epidemiol 2006;163(2):151–9.
15. Plisky MS, Rauh MJ, Heiderscheit B, et al. Medial tibial stress syndrome in high school cross-country runners: incidence and risk factors. J Orthop Sports Phys Ther 2007;37(2):40–7.
16. Hubbard TJ, Carpenter EM, Cordova ML. Contributing factors to medial tibial stress syndrome: a prospective investigation. Med Sci Sports Exerc 2009;41(3):490–6.

17. Bennett JE, Reinking MF, Pluemer B, et al. Factors contributing to the development of medial tibial stress syndrome in high school runners. J Orthop Sports Phys Ther 2001;31(9):504–10.

18. Raissi GR, Cherati AD, Mansoori KD, et al. The relationship between lower extremity alignment and medial tibial stress syndrome among non-professional athletes. Sports Med Arthrosc Rehabil Ther Technol 2009;1(1):11.

19. Madeley LT, Munteanu SE, Bonanno DR. Endurance of the ankle joint plantar flexor muscles in athletes with medial tibial stress syndrome: a case-control study. J Sci Med Sport 2007;10(6):356–62.

20. Clement DB. Tibial stress syndrome in athletes. J Sports Med 1974;2(2):81–5.

21. Pepper M, Akuthota V, McCarty E. The pathophysiology of stress fractures. Clin Sports Med 2006; 25(1):1–16.

22. Egol KA, Koval KJ, Kummer F, et al. Stress fractures of the femoral neck. Clin Orthop Relat Res 1998;(348):72–8.

23. Bennell KL, Malcolm SA, Thomas SA, et al. The incidence and distribution of stress fractures in competitive track and field athletes. A twelve-month prospective study. Am J Sports Med 1996; 24(2):211–7.

24. Taunton JE, Ryan MB, Clement DB, et al. A retrospective case-control analysis of 2002 running injuries. Br J Sports Med 2002;36(2): 95–101.

25. Taunton JE, Ryan MB, Clement DB, et al. A prospective study of running injuries: the Vancouver Sun Run "In Training" clinics. Br J Sports Med 2003;37(3):239–44.

26. Wilson T, Carter N, Thomas G. A multicenter, single-masked study of medial, neutral, and lateral patellar taping in individuals with patellofemoral pain syndrome. J Orthop Sports Phys Ther 2003; 33(8):437–43 [discussion: 444–8].

27. Earl JE, Hoch AZ. A proximal strengthening program improves pain, function, and biomechanics in women with patellofemoral pain syndrome. Am J Sports Med 2011;39(1):154–63.

28. Powers CM. The influence of altered lower-extremity kinematics on patellofemoral joint dysfunction: a theoretical perspective. J Orthop Sports Phys Ther 2003;33(11):639–46.

29. Souza RB, Powers CM. Differences in hip kinematics, muscle strength, and muscle activation between subjects with and without patellofemoral pain. J Orthop Sports Phys Ther 2009;39(1):12–9.

30. Prins MR, van der Wurff P. Females with patellofemoral pain syndrome have weak hip muscles: a systematic review. Aust J Physiother 2009;55(1): 9–15.

31. Barton CJ, Lack S, Malliaras P, et al. Gluteal muscle activity and patellofemoral pain syndrome: a systematic review. Br J Sports Med 2013;47(4): 207–14.

32. Ferber R, Davis IM, Williams DS 3rd. Effect of foot orthotics on rearfoot and tibia joint coupling patterns and variability. J Biomech 2005;38(3):477–83.

33. Tiberio D. The effect of excessive subtalar joint pronation on patellofemoral mechanics: a theoretical model. J Orthop Sports Phys Ther 1987;9(4): 160–5.

34. Powers CM, Chen PY, Reischl SF, et al. Comparison of foot pronation and lower extremity rotation in persons with and without patellofemoral pain. Foot Ankle Int 2002;23(7):634–40.

35. Thijs Y, Van Tiggelen D, Roosen P, et al. A prospective study on gait-related intrinsic risk factors for patellofemoral pain. Clin J Sport Med 2007;17(6):437–45.

36. Eng JJ, Pierrynowski MR. Evaluation of soft foot orthotics in the treatment of patellofemoral pain syndrome. Phys Ther 1993;73(2):62–8 [discussion: 68–70].

37. McPoil TG, Vicenzino B, Cornwall MW. Effect of foot orthoses contour on pain perception in individuals with patellofemoral pain. J Am Podiatr Med Assoc 2011;101(1):7–16.

38. Ellis R, Hing W, Reid D. Iliotibial band friction syndrome–a systematic review. Man Ther 2007;12(3): 200–8.

39. Fredericson M, Cookingham CL, Chaudhari AM, et al. Hip abductor weakness in distance runners with iliotibial band syndrome. Clin J Sport Med 2000;10(3):169–75.

40. Noehren B, Davis I, Hamill J. ASB clinical biomechanics award winner 2006 prospective study of the biomechanical factors associated with iliotibial band syndrome. Clin Biomech (Bristol, Avon) 2007;22(9):951–6.

41. Ferber R, Noehren B, Hamill J, et al. Competitive female runners with a history of iliotibial band syndrome demonstrate atypical hip and knee kinematics. J Orthop Sports Phys Ther 2010;40(2): 52–8.

42. Hamill J, Miller R, Noehren B, et al. A prospective study of iliotibial band strain in runners. Clin Biomech (Bristol, Avon) 2008;23(8):1018–25.

43. Miller RH, Lowry JL, Meardon SA, et al. Lower extremity mechanics of iliotibial band syndrome during an exhaustive run. Gait Posture 2007;26(3): 407–13.

44. Gunter P, Schwellnus MP. Local corticosteroid injection in iliotibial band friction syndrome in runners: a randomised controlled trial. Br J Sports Med 2004;38(3):269–72 [discussion: 272].

45. Beers A, Ryan M, Kasubuchi Z, et al. Effects of multi-modal physiotherapy, including hip abductor strengthening, in patients with iliotibial band friction syndrome. Physiother Can 2008;60(2):180–8.

46. Maffulli N, Wong J, Almekinders LC. Types and epidemiology of tendinopathy. Clin Sports Med 2003;22(4):675–92.

47. Seto C, Statuta S, Solari I. Pediatric running injuries. Clin Sports Med 2010;29(3):499–511.

48. de Lucena GL, dos Santos Gomes C, Guerra RO. Prevalence and associated factors of Osgood-Schlatter syndrome in a population-based sample of Brazilian adolescents. Am J Sports Med 2011; 39(2):415–20.

49. Wall EJ. Osgood-Schlatter disease: practical treatment for a self-limiting condition. Phys Sportsmed 1998;26(3):29–34.

50. Tenforde AS, Sayres LC, McCurdy ML, et al. Overuse injuries in high school runners: lifetime prevalence and prevention strategies. PM R 2011;3(2): 125–31 [quiz: 131].

51. Rauh MJ, Koepsell TD, Rivara FP, et al. Quadriceps angle and risk of injury among high school cross-country runners. J Orthop Sports Phys Ther 2007; 37(12):725–33.

52. Razeghi M, Batt ME. Biomechanical analysis of the effect of orthotic shoe inserts: a review of the literature. Sports Med 2000;29(6):425–38.

53. Korpelainen R, Orava S, Karpakka J, et al. Risk factors for recurrent stress fractures in athletes. Am J Sports Med 2001;29(3):304–10.

54. Williams DS 3rd, McClay IS, Hamill J. Arch structure and injury patterns in runners. Clin Biomech (Bristol, Avon) 2001;16(4):341–7.

55. Cowan DN, Jones BH, Robinson JR. Foot morphologic characteristics and risk of exercise-related injury. Arch Fam Med 1993;2(7):773–7.

56. Pohl MB, Mullineaux DR, Milner CE, et al. Biomechanical predictors of retrospective tibial stress fractures in runners. J Biomech 2008;41(6):1160–5.

57. Nakhaee Z, Rahimi A, Abaee M, et al. The relationship between the height of the medial longitudinal arch (MLA) and the ankle and knee injuries in professional runners. Foot (Edinb) 2008;18(2):84–90.

58. Wen DY, Puffer JC, Schmalzried TP. Injuries in runners: a prospective study of alignment. Clin J Sport Med 1998;8(3):187–94.

59. Wen DY, Puffer JC, Schmalzried TP. Lower extremity alignment and risk of overuse injuries in runners. Med Sci Sports Exerc 1997;29(10):1291–8.

60. Reinking MF, Austin TM, Hayes AM. Exercise-related leg pain in collegiate cross-country athletes: extrinsic and intrinsic risk factors. J Orthop Sports Phys Ther 2007;37(11):670–8.

61. Reinking MF, Hayes AM. Intrinsic factors associated with exercise-related leg pain in collegiate cross-country runners. Clin J Sport Med 2006; 16(1):10–4.

62. Nigg BM. The role of impact forces and foot pronation: a new paradigm. Clin J Sport Med 2001;11(1): 2–9.

63. McClay I, Manal K. A comparison of three-dimensional lower extremity kinematics during running between excessive pronators and normals. Clin Biomech (Bristol, Avon) 1998;13(3):195–203.

64. McClay I, Manal K. The influence of foot abduction on differences between two-dimensional and three-dimensional rearfoot motion. Foot Ankle Int 1998; 19(1):26–31.

65. McClay I, Manal K. Three-dimensional kinetic analysis of running: significance of secondary planes of motion. Med Sci Sports Exerc 1999;31(11): 1629–37.

66. Milner CE, Hamill J, Davis IS. Distinct hip and rearfoot kinematics in female runners with a history of tibial stress fracture. J Orthop Sports Phys Ther 2010;40(2):59–66.

67. Creaby MW, Dixon SJ. External frontal plane loads may be associated with tibial stress fracture. Med Sci Sports Exerc 2008;40(9):1669–74.

68. Crossley K, Bennell KL, Wrigley T, et al. Ground reaction forces, bone characteristics, and tibial stress fracture in male runners. Med Sci Sports Exerc 1999;31(8):1088–93.

69. Milner CE, Davis IS, Hamill J. Free moment as a predictor of tibial stress fracture in distance runners. J Biomech 2006;39(15):2819–25.

70. Zadpoor AA, Nikooyan AA. The relationship between lower-extremity stress fractures and the ground reaction force: a systematic review. Clin Biomech (Bristol, Avon) 2011;26(1):23–8.

71. Zifchock RA, Davis I, Hamill J. Kinetic asymmetry in female runners with and without retrospective tibial stress fractures. J Biomech 2006;39(15): 2792–7.

72. Crowell HP, Milner CE, Hamill J, et al. Reducing impact loading during running with the use of real-time visual feedback. J Orthop Sports Phys Ther 2010;40(4):206–13.

73. Willems TM, Witvrouw E, De Cock A, et al. Gait-related risk factors for exercise-related lower-leg pain during shod running. Med Sci Sports Exerc 2007;39(2):330–9.

74. Baldon Rde M, Nakagawa TH, Muniz TB, et al. Eccentric hip muscle function in females with and without patellofemoral pain syndrome. J Athl Train 2009;44(5):490–6.

75. Bolgla LA, Malone TR, Umberger BR, et al. Comparison of hip and knee strength and neuromuscular activity in subjects with and without patellofemoral pain syndrome. Int J Sports Phys Ther 2011;6(4):285–96.

76. Boling MC, Padua DA, Alexander Creighton R. Concentric and eccentric torque of the hip musculature in individuals with and without patellofemoral pain. J Athl Train 2009;44(1):7–13.

77. Cichanowski HR, Schmitt JS, Johnson RJ, et al. Hip strength in collegiate female athletes with

patellofemoral pain. Med Sci Sports Exerc 2007; 39(8):1227–32.

78. Ireland ML, Willson JD, Ballantyne BT, et al. Hip strength in females with and without patellofemoral pain. J Orthop Sports Phys Ther 2003; 33(11):671–6.

79. Souza RB, Powers CM. Predictors of hip internal rotation during running: an evaluation of hip strength and femoral structure in women with and without patellofemoral pain. Am J Sports Med 2009;37(3):579–87.

80. Niemuth PE, Johnson RJ, Myers MJ, et al. Hip muscle weakness and overuse injuries in recreational runners. Clin J Sport Med 2005;15(1):14–21.

81. Snyder KR, Earl JE, O'Connor KM, et al. Resistance training is accompanied by increases in hip strength and changes in lower extremity biomechanics during running. Clin Biomech (Bristol, Avon) 2009;24(1):26–34.

82. Heinert BL, Kernozek TW, Greany JF, et al. Hip abductor weakness and lower extremity kinematics during running. J Sport Rehabil 2008;17(3):243–56.

83. Dierks TA, Manal KT, Hamill J, et al. Proximal and distal influences on hip and knee kinematics in runners with patellofemoral pain during a prolonged run. J Orthop Sports Phys Ther 2008;38(8):448–56.

84. Tyler TF, Nicholas SJ, Mullaney MJ, et al. The role of hip muscle function in the treatment of patellofemoral pain syndrome. Am J Sports Med 2006; 34(4):630–6.

85. Ferber R, Kendall KD, Farr L. Changes in knee biomechanics after a hip-abductor strengthening protocol for runners with patellofemoral pain syndrome. J Athl Train 2011;46(2):142–9.

86. Willy RW, Davis IS. The effect of a hip-strengthening program on mechanics during running and during a single-leg squat. J Orthop Sports Phys Ther 2011; 41(9):625–32.

87. Bennell KL, Malcolm SA, Thomas SA, et al. Risk factors for stress fractures in track and field athletes. A twelve-month prospective study. Am J Sports Med 1996;24(6):810–8.

88. Cobb KL, Bachrach LK, Greendale G, et al. Disordered eating, menstrual irregularity, and bone mineral density in female runners. Med Sci Sports Exerc 2003;35(5):711–9.

89. Koenig SJ, Toth AP, Bosco JA. Stress fractures and stress reactions of the diaphyseal femur in collegiate athletes: an analysis of 25 cases. Am J Orthop (Belle Mead NJ) 2008;37(9):476–80.

90. Bennell KL, Brukner PD, Malcolm SA. Effect of altered reproductive function and lowered testosterone levels on bone density in male endurance athletes. Br J Sports Med 1996;30(3):205–8.

91. Bredeweg SW, Zijlstra S, Bessem B, et al. The effectiveness of a preconditioning programme on preventing running-related injuries in novice runners: a randomised controlled trial. Br J Sports Med 2012;46(12):865–70.

92. Buist I, Bredeweg SW, van Mechelen W, et al. No effect of a graded training program on the number of running-related injuries in novice runners: a randomized controlled trial. Am J Sports Med 2008; 36(1):33–9.

93. Buist I, Bredeweg SW, Lemmink KA, et al. Predictors of running-related injuries in novice runners enrolled in a systematic training program: a prospective cohort study. Am J Sports Med 2010; 38(2):273–80.

94. Fredericson M, Ngo J, Cobb K. Effects of ball sports on future risk of stress fracture in runners. Clin J Sport Med 2005;15(3):136–41.

95. Ryan MB, Valiant GA, McDonald K, et al. The effect of three different levels of footwear stability on pain outcomes in women runners: a randomised control trial. Br J Sports Med 2011;45(9):715–21.

96. Rauh MJ, Macera CA, Trone DW, et al. Epidemiology of stress fracture and lower-extremity overuse injury in female recruits. Med Sci Sports Exerc 2006;38(9):1571–7.

97. Thijs Y, De Clercq D, Roosen P, et al. Gait-related intrinsic risk factors for patellofemoral pain in novice recreational runners. Br J Sports Med 2008;42(6):466–71.

98. Van Ginckel A, Thijs Y, Hesar NG, et al. Intrinsic gait-related risk factors for Achilles tendinopathy in novice runners: a prospective study. Gait Posture 2009;29(3):387–91.

99. Rauh MJ, Margherita AJ, Rice SG, et al. High school cross country running injuries: a longitudinal study. Clin J Sport Med 2000;10(2):110–6.

100. Bennell K, Brukner P. Preventing and managing stress fractures in athletes. Phys Ther Sport 2005; 6(4):171–80.

101. Reinking MF. Exercise-related leg pain in female collegiate athletes: the influence of intrinsic and extrinsic factors. Am J Sports Med 2006;34(9): 1500–7.

102. Reinking MF. Exercise related leg pain (ERLP): a review of the literature. N Am J Sports Phys Ther 2007;2(3):170–80.

103. Crowell HP, Davis IS. Gait retraining to reduce lower extremity loading in runners. Clin Biomech (Bristol, Avon) 2011;26(1):78–83.

104. Noehren B, Scholz J, Davis I. The effect of real-time gait retraining on hip kinematics, pain and function in subjects with patellofemoral pain syndrome. Br J Sports Med 2011;45(9):691–6.

105. Willy RW, Scholz JP, Davis IS. Mirror gait retraining for the treatment of patellofemoral pain in female runners. Clin Biomech (Bristol, Avon) 2012;27(10): 1045–51.

106. Heiderscheit BC, Chumanov ES, Michalski MP, et al. Effects of step rate manipulation on joint

mechanics during running. Med Sci Sports Exerc 2011;43(2):296–302.

107. Shaffer RA, Rauh MJ, Brodine SK, et al. Predictors of stress fracture susceptibility in young female recruits. Am J Sports Med 2006;34(1):108–15.

108. van Mechelen W. Running injuries. A review of the epidemiological literature. Sports Med 1992;14(5): 320–35.

109. Theisen D, Frisch A, Malisoux L, et al. Injury risk is different in team and individual youth sport. J Sci Med Sport 2013;16(3):200–4.

110. Heintjes E, Berger M, Bierma-Zeinstra S, et al. Exercise therapy for patellofemoral pain syndrome. The Cochrane Collaboration. Hobken (NJ): John Wiley & Sons Ltd; 2005.

111. Louden JK, Gajewski B, Goist-Foley HL, et al. The effectiveness of exercise in treating patellofemoral-pain syndrome. J Sport Rehabil 2004;13:323–42.

112. Natri A, Kannus P, Jarvinen M. Which factors predict the long-term outcome in chronic patellofemoral pain syndrome? A 7-yr prospective follow-up study. Med Sci Sports Exerc 1998;30(11):1572–7.

113. Witvrouw E, Lysens R, Bellemans J, et al. Intrinsic risk factors for the development of anterior knee pain in an athletic population. A two-year prospective study. Am J Sports Med 2000;28(4):480–9.

114. Kannus P, Aho H, Jarvinen M, et al. Computerized recording of visits to an outpatient sports clinic. Am J Sports Med 1987;15(1):79–85.

115. Stefanyshyn DJ, Stergiou P, Lun VM, et al. Knee angular impulse as a predictor of patellofemoral pain in runners. Am J Sports Med 2006;34(11): 1844–51.

116. Hewett TE, Myer GD, Ford KR, et al. Biomechanical measures of neuromuscular control and valgus loading of the knee predict anterior cruciate ligament injury risk in female athletes: a prospective study. Am J Sports Med 2005;33(4):492–501.

117. Myer GD, Ford KR, Barber Foss KD, et al. The incidence and potential pathomechanics of patellofemoral pain in female athletes. Clin Biomech (Bristol, Avon) 2010;25(7):700–7.

118. Hall R, Barber Foss KB, Hewett TE, et al. Sports specialization is associated with an increased risk of developing patellofemoral pain in adolescent female athletes. Presented at the 2013 AMSSM National Meeting, San Diego, CA. 2013.

119. Mostafavifar AM, Best TM, Myer GD. Early sport specialization, does it lead to long term problems? Br J Sports Med 2012.

120. Myer GD, Ford KR, Palumbo JP, et al. Neuromuscular training improves performance and lower-extremity biomechanics in female athletes. J Strength Cond Res 2005;19(1):51–60.

121. Myer GD, Ford KR, McLean SG, et al. The effects of plyometric versus dynamic stabilization and balance training on lower extremity biomechanics. Am J Sports Med 2006;34(3):445–55.

122. Myer GD, Ford KR, Brent JL, et al. The effects of plyometric versus dynamic balance training on power, balance and landing force in female athletes. J Strength Cond Res 2006;20(2):345–53.

123. Myer GD, Ford KR, Brent JL, et al. Differential neuromuscular training effects on ACL injury risk factors in "high-risk" versus "low-risk" athletes. BMC Musculoskelet Disord 2007;8(39):39.

124. Myer GD, Chu DA, Brent JL, et al. Trunk and hip control neuromuscular training for the prevention of knee joint injury. Clin Sports Med 2008;27(3): 425–48, ix.

125. Myer GD, Brent JL, Ford KR, et al. A pilot study to determine the effect of trunk and hip focused neuromuscular training on hip and knee isokinetic strength. Br J Sports Med 2008;42(7):614–9.

126. LaBella CR, Huxford MR, Smith TL, et al. Preseason neuromuscular exercise program reduces sports-related knee pain in female adolescent athletes. Clin Pediatr (Phila) 2009;48(3):327–30.

127. Myer GD, Ford KR, Brent JL, et al. An integrated approach to change the outcome part I: neuromuscular screening methods to identify high ACL injury risk athletes. J Strength Cond Res 2012;26(8): 2265–71.

128. Myer GD, Ford KR, Brent JL, et al. An integrated approach to change the outcome part II: targeted neuromuscular training techniques to reduce identified ACL injury risk factors. J Strength Cond Res 2012;26(8):2272–92.

129. LaBella CR, Huxford MR, Grissom J, et al. Effect of neuromuscular warm-up on injuries in female soccer and basketball athletes in urban public high schools: cluster randomized controlled trial. Arch Pediatr Adolesc Med 2011;165(11):1033–40.

130. Myer GD, Faigenbaum AD, Chu DA, et al. Integrative training for children and adolescents: techniques and practices for reducing sports-related injuries and enhancing athletic performance. Phys Sportsmed 2011;39(1):74–84.

131. Myer GD, Faigenbaum AD, Ford KR, et al. When to initiate integrative neuromuscular training to reduce sports-related injuries and enhance health in youth? Curr Sports Med Rep 2011; 10(3):157–66.

132. Myer GD, Sugimoto D, Thomas S, et al. The influence of age on the effectiveness of neuromuscular training to reduce anterior cruciate ligament injury in female athletes: a meta-analysis. Am J Sports Med 2013;41(1):203–15.

Advances in the Orthopedic Management of Osteogenesis Imperfecta

Dominique Laron, MD, Nirav K. Pandya, MD*

KEYWORDS

- Osteogenesis imperfecta • Advances • Medical • Surgical • Orthopedic • Bisphosphonates
- Intramedullary fixation

KEY POINTS

- Osteogenesis imperfecta (OI) can be a debilitating disease with a wide range of phenotypic manifestations.
- The Sillence subtypes of OI can be explained by different variations in genetic mutations.
- Bisphosphonate therapy augments bone turnover and increases bone density in OI patients, although its efficacy in preventing fracture, reducing pain, and improving function is controversial.
- Recommendations for indications, duration, and type of bisphosphonate therapy in children have not been agreed upon.
- Fassier-Duval rodding systems show great promise in decreasing fracture rates while requiring less revision and causing fewer complications traditionally seen with older systems.

THE SCIENCE AND GENETICS OF OSTEOGENESIS IMPERFECTA
History

The first scientific documentation of osteogenesis imperfecta (OI) by army surgeon Olaus Jacob Elkman dates back to 1788. He detailed observational reports of bone fragility and fractures in 3 familial generations afflicted with "congenital osteomalacia."[1,2] OI was later given its name by Dutch professor Willem Vrolik in 1849.[3] The varying array of clinical manifestations grouped under this broad diagnosis sparked a field of study that aimed to classify and determine the root cause of this debilitating disease (**Fig. 1**). David Sillence developed his classification system in the 1970s, that has since been added to and modified, but is still widely used today (**Table 1**).[4]

Past Discovery

Electron microscopy research in OI patients in the 1970s led to the discovery of altered collagen structure in these patients compared with that of normal histologic controls.[5] This collagen was branded Type I, as it was the first discovery of altered connective tissue leading to clinical disease. In the 1980s, a gene deletion coding for the pro-α1 collagen chain steered the discovery of poor collagen synthesis and inspired further research detailing the underlying genetic causes of OI.[6,7] As a result, it was thought for a long time that mutations in collagen type I genes (COLA1 or COLA2) were the sole cause of OI, and that it was an autosomal dominant disorder.

The authors have no conflicts of interest or funding sources to report.
Department of Orthopedic Surgery, University of California San Francisco, Children's Hospital and Research Center Oakland, 747 52nd Street, Oakland, CA 94609, USA
* Corresponding author.
E-mail address: PandyaN@orthosurg.ucsf.edu

Orthop Clin N Am 44 (2013) 565–573
http://dx.doi.org/10.1016/j.ocl.2013.06.010
0030-5898/13/$ – see front matter © 2013 Elsevier Inc. All rights reserved.

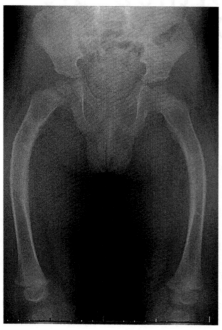

Fig. 1. Anteroposterior (AP) radiograph of a 2-year-old male infant with OI, with bowing deformity of the bilateral femurs and a history of multiple prior femur fractures.

Table 1
Types of osteogenesis imperfecta (OI), gene defect, and inheritance

OI Type	Gene Defect	Inheritance
I	COLA1	AD
II	COLA1/COLA2	AD
III	COLA1/COLA2	AD
IV	COLA1/COLA2	AD
V	Not known	AR
VI	SERPINF1	AR
VII	CRTAP	AR
VIII	LEPRE1	AR
IX	PPIB	AR
X	SERPINH1	AR
XI	FKB910	AR
N/A	PLOD2	AR
N/A	LRP5	AR
N/A	SP7	AR

Abbreviations: AD, autosomal dominant; AR, autosomal recessive; N/A, not yet classified.

Data from Morello R, Esposito PW. Osteogenesis imperfect. In: Lin Y, editor. Osteogenesis. Rijeka (Croatia):InTech; 2012. Chapter 9:223–52.

Current Genetics

In the early 1990s, Wallis and colleagues[8] described cases of OI not caused by mutations in COLA1 or COLA2. Stemming from this study, there has been the discovery of multiple new forms of OI not originally described by Sillence. These forms involve various other genetic defects that manifest in an autosomal-recessive fashion. These genetic defects involve CRTAP,[9] LEPRE1,[10] PPIB,[11] SERPINH1,[12] SERPINF1,[13] PLOD2,[14] FKBP10,[15] LRP5,[16] and SP7[17] (see **Table 1**).

DIAGNOSIS OF OI
Prenatal

Our understanding of this disease from a genetic level has not only allowed for more accurate diagnosis of the disease using collagen molecular testing,[18] but also has allowed us to understand the manifestations of the disease, even as early as the prenatal period.[19] Features that can be seen on prenatal ultrasonography usually between 14 and 18 weeks of gestation (for Types II and III OI; Type I cannot be easily diagnosed) include increased nuchal translucency,[20] reduced echogenicity of bones,[21] multiple fractures of the long bones, ribs, and skull at various stages of healing,[21] and bowing of the long bones (+/− shortening).[22] Once there is a concern for OI via prenatal ultrasonography, the diagnosis can be made via either (1) chorionic villus sampling demonstrating abnormal type I collagen via electrophoresis, or (2) amniocentesis, which obtains fetal DNA for molecular analysis.[18] As the majority of mutations will involve COLA1/COLA2 genes, testing is centered around the identification of these genes followed by examination of the other aforementioned genes.

Postnatal

In the postnatal period, positive clinical findings (multiple fractures, blue sclera, and so forth) and the exclusion of other metabolic causes of osteoporosis can then warrant confirmation of the diagnosis via dermal biopsy and/or DNA analysis. Dermal biopsy has been shown to be about 90% positive in suspected OI cases,[23] whereas DNA analysis has been able to identify COLA1/COLA2 mutations in 95% of cases of OI, with the remaining percentage having CRTAP/LEPRE1 mutations.[9,24] As a result, it may be suggested that DNA testing should be utilized because it is more sensitive for disease diagnosis. Best-practice guidelines exist for the laboratory diagnosis of OI.[18]

TREATMENT OF OI

An understanding of the genetics of OI allows for an insight into the current molecular methods of disease diagnosis, which have evolved tremendously since the clinical descriptors of pathology used initially. Once the diagnosis has been made, the treating team (including the orthopedic surgeon) must formulate the appropriate treatment plan for the patient. These interventions include both pharmacologic and surgical interventions.

Pharmacologic Treatment

Basic science

The primary objective of OI therapy revolves around decreasing the number of pathologic fractures, decreasing pain, increasing growth, improving bone metabolism, and optimizing function. The current mainstay of pharmacologic treatment has been centered on bisphosphonate (BP) therapy, which serves to decrease bone turnover and inhibit bone resorption. Within the adult population receiving treatment for osteoporosis, it is clear that BPs slow down bone resorption by shortening osteoclast life. This fact creates a dilemma in the child treated with OI: although less bone is resorbed, osteoblasts may still be producing defective collagen. In turn, this leads to several quandaries regarding the treatment of pediatric OI patients with BPs: the potential long-term side effects in children, whether changes in bone mineral density (BMD) can lead to improved bone strength and/or bone matrix, the most effective dosing/duration/mode of administration for the various forms of OI and varying ages, and whether fracture risk and function are improved with treatment. Although current guidelines do not exist, there have been several key studies in the literature detailing the results of BP therapy in children with OI.

Clinical systematic reviews

In a Cochrane review, Phillipi and colleagues[25] examined the results of BP treatment of OI. The investigators looked specifically at BMD, fracture reduction, and improvement in clinical function, reflective of the knowledge surrounding BP and OI treatment. Only 8 quality studies were identified. From these studies, it was concluded that both oral and intravenous bisphosphonate therapy increased BMD in children and adults with OI. However, this increase in BMD was not shown to translate into decreased fracture risk or improvement in clinical parameters (pain, growth, and/or mobility).

These findings were also supported by the work of Castillo and colleagues[26] in their own systematic review. Whereas improvement in BMD was found with BP treatment, decreased fracture rate and improved growth once again could not be found. In addition, the reviewed studies were lacking in their examination of the effect of treatment on deformity, need for surgery, pain, function, and quality of life. Further recommendations regarding dosing regime and treatment duration were also unclear, as was the impact of therapy on patients with mild OI or infants.

Even with the aforementioned limitations, several studies have attempted to answer these questions, and these need to be examined specifically to aid in understanding the best pharmacologic treatment options, with further high-quality study still being necessary in the future.

Oral BP treatment

Oral treatment was initially the mode of BP delivery for patients with bone disorders. Sakkers and colleagues[27] examined 34 pediatric patients with OI who were randomly assigned to placebo or oral olpadronate for 2 years. The investigators found that olpadronate treatment was associated with a 31% reduction in the relative risk of long-bone fracture and an increase in spinal bone mineral content and density. However, there was no difference in functional outcome, anthropometrics, vertebral height, or urinary markers of bone resorption.

Furthermore, Ward and colleagues[28] examined alendronate for the treatment of OI in a randomized, placebo-controlled study. In this multicenter study, 130 children with Types I, III, or IV OI were randomized to placebo or alendronate for 2 years. Alendronate was found to increase bone mineral density by 51% as opposed to 12% by placebo ($P<.001$), and bone turnover (measured by urinary N-telopeptide of collagen I) decreased by 62% in the alendronate group versus 32% in the placebo group ($P<.001$). However, the incidence of long-bone fracture, bone pain, and physical activity were similar between the alendronate and placebo groups, similar to the findings of the systematic reviews already cited.

Intravenous BP treatment

Intravenous treatment developed as an alternative to oral BP, with potential increased potency and speed of action. Barros and colleagues[29] compared the safety and efficacy of zoledronic acid and pamidronate in children with OI. Pamidronate has been proposed as the standard treatment in children with OI. In 23 patients with OI over a 1-year period, intravenous infusion was used for these medications. Both groups had statistically significant increases in BMD (67.6% and 51.8% respectively) with minimal side effects.

Intravenous BP treatment versus oral BP therapy

In one of the few studies comparing intravenous BPs with oral BPs, DiMeglio and Peacock[30] compared oral alendronate and intravenous pamidronate in children with OI in a 2-year randomized controlled trial. Eighteen children participated in the study, which found that total body and lumbar spine BMD increased, turnover markers decreased, and linear growth increased equally in both groups. Fracture incidence was not significantly different between both groups. These studies still leave the question unanswered as to the best method of treatment for OI patients, and the potential short-term and long-term consequences of the particular mode of treatment chosen by the clinician.

Role of growth hormone with BP therapy

Some investigators have postulated that the use of BP with recombinant human growth hormone (GH) may be a feasible treatment for some forms of OI, particularly as GH may increase the production of type I collagen in patients who have a collagen synthesis defect. Antoniazzi and colleagues[31] performed a randomized controlled trial comparing children who underwent neridronate treatment alone or neridronate with GH. Patients who underwent combined treatment had greater improvement in BMD and growth velocity, although there was no difference in fracture risk.

BP treatment, orthopedic intervention, and quality of life

One of the main concerns regarding BP treatment is that although it has been shown to reliably increase BMD, the translation of this increased BMD into improved quality of life and a decreased need for orthopedic intervention has not been definitively established. Looking at a more clinically relevant set of outcomes, de Graaff and colleagues[32] examined outpatient visits and operative interventions in patients who underwent BP therapy. The investigators retrospectively examined OI patients undergoing BP therapy from 1988 to 2009 to determine the clinical efficacy and outcomes of pharmacologic intervention. Of the 201 OI patients in this study, 118 were treated with BP along with vitamin D and calcium supplementation. The primary end points were the number of outpatient visits by each patient; this rate decreased from 3.35 to 2.14 per year. There was also a decrease in operative fracture interventions, from 0.73 per year to 0.38 per year. Regarding the

overall group, clinic visits naturally decreased with age (also in the nontreatment group). However, after the age of 7, visits decreased significantly with BP therapy.

Quality of life was also examined by Kok and colleagues,[33] whose results differed from those of de Graaff and colleagues.[32] In this study, 34 children with OI were randomized to olpadronate or placebo. Quality of life was measured using the Self-Perception Profile for Children and the Health-Utility Index. The investigators found only slightly significant improvements in quality of life from BP treatment, with no significant differences with regard to pain.

These studies once again raise the concern of BP treatment being able to translate microstructural changes (increased BMD) into macro–clinically relevant outcomes.

Treatment of infants and mild OI patients with BP

Although BP treatment is used in older severely affected patients, it is unclear whether patients at the extremes, infants who are severely affected with OI, or older patients with mild OI can benefit from BP treatment.

Regarding the treatment of young children, Antoniazzi and colleagues[34] prospectively examined the efficacy of BP treatment in infants with severe OI (Type III). Five children who started treatment with intravenous neridronate at birth, 5 children who started intravenous treatment at 6 months of age, and a historical control group of 10 children with OI who were untreated were compared. The investigators found that patients who were started with intravenous treatment after birth had a lower incidence of fractures than the other 2 groups in the first 6 months of treatment. In addition, the birth-treated group had the highest improvement in vertebral body area and structure.

The long-term deleterious effects of BP treatment are unknown; therefore, BP treatment of "mild" OI is still controversial. Rauch and colleagues[35] examined the use of BPs in patients with mild OI. Twenty-six children with mild OI (type I) were randomized to oral risedronate or placebo for 2 years. The investigators found that the risedronate group had decreased levels of bone-resorption markers (35% vs 6%), and increased lumbar spine BMD Z-scores (increase of 0.65 vs a decrease of 0.15). However, there was no difference in the number of new fractures or bone mass and density of the total body.

Further study is necessary to determine the role of treatment with BPs in the various forms of OI, with consideration of their potential clinical utility and long-term side effects in children.

Surgical Management

Along with the ever-expanding knowledge of the genetic basis of OI and pharmacologic treatments, there have also been major advancements in surgical technique and technology addressing fracture treatment and intervention in OI. Among the constellation of symptoms and maladies that plague patients with OI, the principal issue from an orthopedic standpoint remains pathologic fractures and deformities of long bones (see **Fig. 1**). With poor bone stock and decreased quality of collagenous tissues, patients can experience fractures starting in utero and later in life from otherwise benign falls or minor injuries. There has been a continual evolution of the fixation options for these patients.

Early treatment modalities

In 1959, Sofield and Millar introduced the concept of osteotomies secured with intramedullary nails to treat fractures and deformity in patients with OI.[36] Treatment involved complete subperiosteal exposure of the bone with multiple osteotomies fixed around an intramedullary pin. Although leading to excellent correction of deformity and fracture prevention, this procedure was fraught with complications including devascularization of bone via a wide subperiosteal exposure, bone thinning, decreased ambulatory capacity, hardware failure, and multiple revisions because of growth.[37–40]

As a result, this led to the development of expanding rod systems, most notably developed by Bailey and Dubow[41,42] (**Fig. 2**). These rods had fixation in the epiphyses (via a T-piece) and grew as the child grew. These early telescoping systems, however, had high complication and failure rates. Lang-Stevenson and Sharrard[43] examined the results of 28 patients who underwent fixation with Bailey-Dubow extensible rods and found 10 instances of proximal migration of the distal end of the rod, 1 incorrect placement in the proximal femur, 4 instances of loosening of a

T-piece, and 3 infections in the area of the rods. Similar complications were noted by Jerosch and colleagues[44] in their review of 107 long-bone fixations with Bailey-Dubow rods. Here there was a 63.5% complication rate, most commonly rod migration combined with perforation of the joint, bone, and soft tissues.

Likewise, Gamble and colleagues[45] examined 108 intramedullary rod placements in patients with OI (42 Bailey-Dubow rods and 66 nonelongating rods). The investigators' overall complication rate was 60% to 69% for the Bailey-Dubow rods and 55% for the nonelongating rods. The Bailey-Dubow rods had a 19% reoperation rate and a 12% replacement rate, whereas nonelongating rods had a 29% reoperation rate and a 24% replacement rate. The migration rate in the Bailey-Dubow group was 26% (mainly due to T-piece complications) as opposed to 42.0% for the nonelongating group (**Fig. 3**).

As a result of problems with T-piece fixation, the Sheffield telescoping rod system was developed in the 1980s. This system had a fixed T-piece on either end that could be rotated during the procedure for better epiphyseal fixation.[46,47] Wilkinson and colleagues[47] examined 60 long bones treated with the Sheffield system and found an increase in

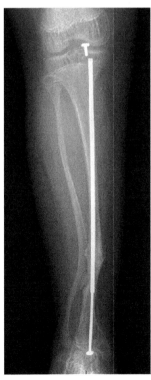

Fig. 3. AP radiograph of a 9-year-old girl with OI after treatment of a tibia fracture with a Bailey-Dubow rod, with disengagement of the proximal T-piece.

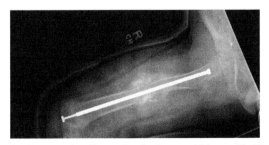

Fig. 2. Lateral radiograph of a 5-year-old boy with OI after treatment of a mid-shaft femur fracture with a Bailey-Dubow rod.

ambulatory capacity, no evidence of epiphyseal damage, and only a 7% rate of complications requiring rod revision.

Nicolaou and colleagues[48] examined retrospective data on 22 OI patients who had previously undergone Sheffield telescoping rod insertion for fracture stabilization and prevention. With an average 19-year follow-up, the rods had a success rate of 32% as determined by no further fractures with rod stabilization. The system did show overall inadequate fracture prevention, with 41% of patients having 1 or 2 fractures and 27% having 3 or more fractures. Further complications of the Sheffield system included the need for rod exchange as patients outgrew their rods; 35% required exchange because of both outgrowth and rod bending, with an overall rod survival rate of 80%. As with standard nailing systems, 15% needed exchange for infectious complications, rod subsidence, or rod migration. Physeal damage was not seen following surgery, and all rods elongated with growth.

Current techniques

One of the concerns regarding the Sheffield system related to the insertion technique of the 2 telescoping components, which requires a knee arthrotomy for femoral rod insertion and knee and ankle arthrotomies for tibial rod insertion. As a result, the Fassier-Duval (FD) Telescopic IM System (Pega Medical, Quebec, Canada) was developed, with initial reports of only a 14% reoperation rate (**Fig. 4**).[49–51] The advantage of this system is a single proximal entry point and improved "screw-in" fixation in the epiphyses without the need for a large arthrotomy. This system protected the peri-rod joint, reduced migration, and aimed to be less invasive with reduced mechanical complications. Using principles used in traditional adult trauma and standard intramedullary nailing, FD rods are introduced through the greater trochanter of the femur and the area anterior to the tibial spines of the proximal tibia.

There are a select few studies regarding this technique in the literature beyond what has been reported at national meetings. Birke and colleagues[52] examined 24 consecutive patients (15 with OI) with FD insertions with a minimum of 1 year of follow-up. There was a 13% reoperation rate in OI patients for proximal rod migration, and a 40% complication rate (rod migration and limited telescoping in 5 patients, intraoperative joint extrusion in 1 patient). Of note, in the non-OI patients (neurofibromatosis, epidermal nevus syndrome, hypophosphatemic rickets) there were several reoperations for nonunion, loss of fixation, shortening, migration, and joint extrusion. The

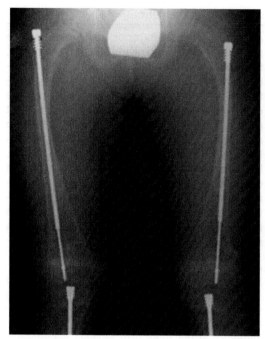

Fig. 4. AP radiograph of a 5-year-old boy with OI treated with Fassier-Duval rods in the long bones. (*Modified from* Birke O, Davies N, Latimer M, et al. Experience with the Fassier-Duval telescopic rod: first 24 consecutive cases with a minimum of 1-year follow-up. J Pediatr Orthop 2011;31:462; with permission.)

investigators concluded that the FD rod is a good choice for OI patients with longitudinal stability and good bone-healing potential. In cases lacking stability or bone-healing potential, other options may be beneficial.

In another study, Ruck and colleagues[53] examined the functional outcomes of children with OI treated with FD rodding of the femur at 1 year. Sixty children (also undergoing BP treatment) who underwent initial FD rodding (101 rods) were reviewed. Outcomes on the Gillette Functional Assessment Questionnaire (FAQ) Ambulation Scale, the Gross Motor Function Measure (GMFM), and the Pediatric Evaluation of Disability Inventory (PEDI) were compared preoperatively and at 1 year after surgery. The investigators found statistically significant improvements from baseline to 1 year on the FAQ; crawling, standing, walking and running, and total domains of the GMFM; and PEDI mobility and self-care. These results indicate that initial FD rodding can result in improved ambulation, gross motor function, self-care, and mobility for OI patients with femoral deformities.

FD rods seem to have addressed many of the concerns regarding surgical fixation of long bones in OI patients, with minimal surgical exposure, progressive growth of the implant, diminished need for revision, and ease of insertion.

Combination treatments

Regardless of the type of surgical technique used, the use of BP in the perioperative period still remains controversial. Munns and colleagues[54] examined 197 lower limb fractures in 82 OI patients as well as 200 intramedullary rodding procedures in 79 OI patients. In the fracture patients, improved mobility status (not pamidronate therapy) was predictive of delayed fracture healing. By contrast, in the osteotomy group, delayed healing was more frequent in osteotomy patients who had been started on pamidronate therapy before surgery, compared with osteotomy patients with no prior BP treatment. On the other hand, Pizones and colleagues[55] examined 24 bones of OI patients who underwent surgical intervention while being treated with BPs. The investigators found only an 8% rate of reoperation for fracture below primary fixation, and only 1 case of pseudarthrosis, suggesting that the rate of fracture healing was typical for an OI population regardless of BP treatment. Furthermore, El Sobky and colleagues[56] compared OI patients who received both surgery and BP with those who underwent surgery alone (20 in each group). The investigators found 3 good, 9 fair, and 8 poor results in the surgery group in comparison with 11 excellent, 4 good, and 5 fair results in the combined treatment group. The combined group had an average increase in BMD of 35.2%, with a decreased refracture rate. This study suggests that a multifaceted approach combining pharmacologic and surgical intervention is important and potentially more favorable.

SUMMARY

OI is a complex disease encompassing a vast range of clinical presentations. This wide spectrum has led to the discovery of multiple causative genetic mutations that have increased our understanding of the underlying mechanisms. These discoveries have led to newer and more effective pharmacologic treatments and more advanced surgical interventions. If we are to fully understand and combat this debilitating disease it is clear that more research must be done, and we must increase our efforts to develop more effective pharmacologic and surgical techniques.

REFERENCES

1. Peltier LF. The classic: congenital osteomalacia. Olaus Jacob Ekman. Clin Orthop Relat Res 1981;(159):3–5.

2. Baljet B. Aspects of the history of osteogenesis imperfecta (Vrolik's syndrome). Ann Anat 2002; 184:1–7.

3. Baljet B. Willem Vrolik as a teratologist. Ned Tijdschr Geneeskd 1984;128:1530–4 [in Dutch].

4. Sillence DO, Senn A, Danks DM. Genetic heterogeneity in osteogenesis imperfecta. J Med Genet 1979;16:101–16.

5. Teitelbaum SL, Kraft WJ, Lang R, et al. Bone collagen aggregation abnormalities in osteogenesis imperfecta. Calcif Tissue Res 1974;17:75–9.

6. Barsh GS, David KE, Byers PH. Type I osteogenesis imperfecta: a nonfunctional allele for pro alpha 1 (I) chains of type I procollagen. Proc Natl Acad Sci U S A 1982;79:3838–42.

7. Chu ML, Williams CJ, Pepe G, et al. Internal deletion in a collagen gene in a perinatal lethal form of osteogenesis imperfecta. Nature 1983;304:78–80.

8. Wallis GA, Sykes B, Byers PH, et al. Osteogenesis imperfecta type III: mutations in the type I collagen structural genes, COL1A1 and COL1A2, are not necessarily responsible. J Med Genet 1993;30: 492–6.

9. Morello R, Bertin TK, Chen Y, et al. CRTAP is required for prolyl 3-hydroxylation and mutations cause recessive osteogenesis imperfecta. Cell 2006;127:291–304.

10. Cabral WA, Chang W, Barnes AM, et al. Prolyl 3-hydroxylase 1 deficiency causes a recessive metabolic bone disorder resembling lethal/severe osteogenesis imperfecta. Nat Genet 2007;39: 359–65.

11. Barnes AM, Carter EM, Cabral WA, et al. Lack of cyclophilin B in osteogenesis imperfecta with normal collagen folding. N Engl J Med 2010;362: 521–8.

12. Christiansen HE, Schwarze U, Pyott SM, et al. Homozygosity for a missense mutation in SERPINH1, which encodes the collagen chaperone protein HSP47, results in severe recessive osteogenesis imperfecta. Am J Hum Genet 2010;86:389–98.

13. Becker J, Semler O, Gilissen C, et al. Exome sequencing identifies truncating mutations in human SERPINF1 in autosomal-recessive osteogenesis imperfecta. Am J Hum Genet 2011;88:362–71.

14. Ha-Vinh R, Alanay Y, Bank RA, et al. Phenotypic and molecular characterization of Bruck syndrome (osteogenesis imperfecta with contractures of the large joints) caused by a recessive mutation in PLOD2. Am J Med Genet A 2004;131:115–20.

15. Alanay Y, Avaygan H, Camacho N, et al. Mutations in the gene encoding the RER protein FKBP65 cause autosomal-recessive osteogenesis imperfecta. Am J Hum Genet 2010;86:551–9.

16. Gong Y, Slee RB, Fukai N, et al. LDL receptor-related protein 5 (LRP5) affects bone accrual and eye development. Cell 2001;107:513–23.

17. Lapunzina P, Aglan M, Temtamy S, et al. Identification of a frameshift mutation in Osterix in a patient with recessive osteogenesis imperfecta. Am J Hum Genet 2010;87:110–4.

18. van Dijk FS, Byers PH, Dalgleish R, et al. EMQN best practice guidelines for the laboratory diagnosis of osteogenesis imperfecta. Eur J Hum Genet 2012;20:11–9.

19. Tsai PY, Chang CH, Yu CH, et al. Three-dimensional ultrasound in the prenatal diagnosis of osteogenesis imperfecta. Taiwan J Obstet Gynecol 2012;51:387–92.

20. Viora E, Sciarrone A, Bastonero S, et al. Increased nuchal translucency in the first trimester as a sign of osteogenesis imperfecta. Am J Med Genet 2002;109:336–7.

21. Morgan JA, Marcus PS. Prenatal diagnosis and management of intrauterine fracture. Obstet Gynecol Surv 2010;65:249–59.

22. Marini JC, Forlino A, Cabral WA, et al. Consortium for osteogenesis imperfecta mutations in the helical domain of type I collagen: regions rich in lethal mutations align with collagen binding sites for integrins and proteoglycans. Hum Mutat 2007;28:209–21.

23. Körkkö J, Annunen S, Pihlajamaa T, et al. Conformation sensitive gel electrophoresis for simple and accurate detection of mutations: comparison with denaturing gradient gel electrophoresis and nucleotide sequencing. Proc Natl Acad Sci U S A 1998;95:1681–5.

24. Bodian DL, Chan TF, Poon A, et al. Mutation and polymorphism spectrum in osteogenesis imperfecta type II: implications for genotype–phenotype relationships. Hum Mol Genet 2009;18:463–71.

25. Phillipi CA, Remmington T, Steiner RD. Bisphosphonate therapy for osteogenesis imperfecta. Cochrane Database Syst Rev 2008;(4):CD005088.

26. Castillo H, Samson-Fang L, American Academy for Cerebral Palsy and Developmental Medicine Treatment Outcomes Committee Review Panel. Effects of bisphosphonates in children with osteogenesis imperfecta: an AACPDM systematic review. Dev Med Child Neurol 2009;51:17–29.

27. Sakkers R, Kok D, Engelbert R, et al. Skeletal effects and functional outcome with olpadronate in children with osteogenesis imperfecta: a 2-year randomised placebo-controlled study. Lancet 2004;9419:1427–31.

28. Ward LM, Rauch F, Whyte MP, et al. Alendronate for the treatment of pediatric osteogenesis imperfecta: a randomized placebo-controlled study. J Clin Endocrinol Metab 2011;96:355–64.

29. Barros ER, Saraiva GL, de Oliveira TP, et al. Safety and efficacy of a 1-year treatment with zoledronic acid compared with pamidronate in children with osteogenesis imperfecta. J Pediatr Endocrinol Metab 2012;25(5–6):485–91.

30. DiMeglio LA, Peacock M. Two-year clinical trial of oral alendronate versus intravenous pamidronate in children with osteogenesis imperfecta. J Bone Miner Res 2006;21:132–40.

31. Antoniazzi F, Monti E, Venturi G, et al. GH in combination with bisphosphonate treatment in osteogenesis imperfecta. Eur J Endocrinol 2010;163:479–87.

32. de Graaff F, Verra W, Pruijs J, et al. Decrease in outpatient department visits and operative interventions due to bisphosphonates in children with osteogenesis imperfecta. J Child Orthop 2011;5:121–5.

33. Kok DH, Sakkers RJ, Janse AJ, et al. Quality of life in children with osteogenesis imperfecta treated with oral bisphosphonates (Olpadronate): a 2-year randomized placebo-controlled trial. Eur J Pediatr 2007;166:1155–61.

34. Antoniazzi F, Zamboni G, Lauriola S, et al. Early bisphosphonate treatment in infants with severe osteogenesis imperfecta. J Pediatr 2006;149:174–9.

35. Rauch F, Munns CF, Land C, et al. Risedronate in the treatment of mild pediatric osteogenesis imperfecta: a randomized placebo-controlled study. J Bone Miner Res 2009;24:1282–9.

36. Sofield HA, Millar EA. Fragmentation, realignment, and intramedullary rod fixation of deformities of the long bones in children: a ten year appraisal. J Bone Joint Surg Am 1959;41:1371–91.

37. Abulsaad M, Abdelrahman A. Modified Sofield-Millar operation: less invasive surgery of lower limbs in osteogenesis imperfecta. Int Orthop 2009;33:527–32.

38. Li YH, Chow W, Leong JC. The Sofield-Millar operation in osteogenesis imperfecta. A modified technique. J Bone Joint Surg Br 2000;82:11–6.

39. Khoshhal KI, Ellis RD. Effect of lower limb Sofield procedure on ambulation in osteogenesis imperfecta. J Pediatr Orthop 2001;21:233–5.

40. Dal Monte A, Manes E, Capanna R, et al. Osteogenesis imperfecta: results obtained with the Sofield method of surgical treatment. Ital J Orthop Traumatol 1982;8:43–52.

41. Bailey RW, Dubow HI. Studies of longitudinal bone growth resulting in an extensible nail. Surg Forum 1963;14:455–8.

42. Bailey RW. Further clinical experience with the extensible nail. Clin Orthop Relat Res 1981;(159):171–6.

43. Lang-Stevenson AI, Sharrard WJ. Intramedullary rodding with Bailey-Dubow extensible rods in osteogenesis imperfecta. An interim report of results and complications. J Bone Joint Surg Br 1984;66:227–32.

44. Jerosch J, Mazzotti I, Tomasevic M. Complications after treatment of patients with osteogenesis

imperfecta with a Bailey-Dubow rod. Arch Orthop Trauma Surg 1998;117:240–5.

45. Gamble JG, Strudwick WJ, Rinsky LA, et al. Complications of intramedullary rods in osteogenesis imperfecta: Bailey-Dubow rods versus nonelongating rods. J Pediatr Orthop 1988;8:645–9.

46. Stockley I, Bell MJ, Sharrard WJ. The role of expanding intramedullary rods in osteogenesis imperfecta. J Bone Joint Surg Br 1989;71:422–7.

47. Wilkinson JM, Scott BW, Clarke AM, et al. Surgical stabilisation of the lower limb in osteogenesis imperfecta using the Sheffield Telescopic Intramedullary Rod System. J Bone Joint Surg Br 1998;80: 999–1004.

48. Nicolaou N, Bowe JD, Wilkinson JM, et al. Use of the Sheffield telescopic intramedullary rod system for the management of osteogenesis imperfecta: clinical outcomes at an average follow-up of nineteen years. J Bone Joint Surg Am 2011;93:1994–2000.

49. Fassier F, Duval P. New concept for telescoping rodding in osteogenesis imperfecta: preliminary results. In: Proceedings of the Annual Meeting of the Pediatric Orthopaedic Society of North America (POSNA). Cancun (Mexico): 2001.

50. Fassier F, Esposito P, Sponsellor P, et al. Multicenter radiological assessment of the Fassier-Duval femoral rodding. In: Proceedings of the Annual Meeting of the Pediatric Orthopaedic

Society of North America (POSNA). San Diego (CA): 2006.

51. Fassier F, Halloran JP, Allam N. Fassier-Duval tibial rodding in patients with osteogenesis imperfecta. In: Proceedings of the Annual Meeting of the Pediatric Orthopaedic Society of North America (POSNA). Waikoloa (HI): 2010.

52. Birke O, Davies N, Latimer M, et al. Experience with the Fassier-Duval telescopic rod: first 24 consecutive cases with a minimum of 1-year follow-up. J Pediatr Orthop 2011;31:458–64.

53. Ruck J, Dahan-Oliel N, Montpetit K, et al. Fassier-Duval femoral rodding in children with osteogenesis imperfecta receiving bisphosphonates: functional outcomes at one year. J Child Orthop 2011;5:217–24.

54. Munns C, Rauch F, Zeitlin L, et al. Delayed osteotomy but not fracture healing in pediatric osteogenesis imperfecta patients receiving pamidronate. J Bone Miner Res 2004;19:1779–86.

55. Pizones J, Plotkin H, Parra-Garcia J, et al. Bone healing in children with osteogenesis imperfecta treated with bisphosphonates. J Pediatr Orthop 2005;25:332–5.

56. El Sobky M, Zaky H, Atef A, et al. Surgery versus surgery plus pamidronate in the management of osteogenesis imperfecta patients: a comparative study. J Pediatr Orthop B 2006;15:222–8.

Femoroacetabular Impingement
Current Concepts and Controversies

Wudbhav N. Sankar, MD[a],[*], Travis H. Matheney, MD[b],
Ira Zaltz, MD[c]

KEYWORDS

- Femoroacetabular impingement • CAM lesions • Pincer lesions • Osteoarthritis • Impingement

KEY POINTS

- Femoroacetabular impingement (FAI) is a clinical syndrome of hip pain, limitation in movement, and joint damage from abnormal mechanical contact of the acetabular rim and the proximal femur.
- There is a high prevalence of morphologic abnormalities associated with FAI in asymptomatic individuals.
- Cross-sectional and longitudinal studies support FAI playing a causative role in the development of osteoarthritis and need for total hip arthroplasty in certain patients.
- Surgical treatment approaches for FAI include hip arthroscopy, anterior mini-arthrotomy with/ without arthroscopic assistance, and surgical dislocation of the hip.

WHAT IS FEMOROACETABULAR IMPINGEMENT?

The modern concept of femoroacetabular impingement (FAI), especially its causal relation to acetabular labral and cartilage damage, emerged following the observation that FAI can be precipitated by acetabular reorientation and can produce new labral damage.[1] Following this observation, interest in the association between chondrolabral damage and variations in femoral and acetabular anatomy has established a causal relationship between mechanical aberration in the function of the hip joint and the development of labral and cartilage damage.[2,3] The resulting modern accepted definition of FAI is that it is characterized by abnormal mechanical contact between the rim of the acetabulum and the upper femur. Certain anatomic femoral or acetabular morphologies,

hip-specific supraphysiologic flexion or rotational movements, repetition, and forceful motions may damage the acetabular labrum and the cartilage around the rim of the acetabulum, leading to a clinical syndrome of hip pain, limitation of movement, and joint damage now known as FAI.

CLASSIFICATION

Two distinct hip morphotypes have been described that are associated with intracapsular, mechanical FAI. The CAM morphotype of FAI is an aspherical epiphyseal extension that produces a characteristic bump at the junction of the femoral head and femoral neck (**Fig. 1**). The origin is thought to be caused by an extension of the upper femoral epiphysis along the anterolateral femoral neck junction[4]; however, the pathogenesis of this bump is not well understood and may represent

[a] Division of Orthopaedic Surgery, The Children's Hospital of Philadelphia, 2nd Floor Wood Building, 34th and Civic Center Boulevard, Philadelphia, PA 19104, USA; [b] Department of Orthopaedic Surgery, Boston Children's Hospital, 300 Longwood Avenue, Boston, MA 02115, USA; [c] Department of Orthopaedic Surgery, William Beaumont Hospital, 3535 West 13 Mile Road, Royal Oaks, MI 48073, USA
* Corresponding author.
E-mail address: sankarw@email.chop.edu

Orthop Clin N Am 44 (2013) 575–589
http://dx.doi.org/10.1016/j.ocl.2013.07.003
0030-5898/13/$ – see front matter © 2013 Elsevier Inc. All rights reserved.

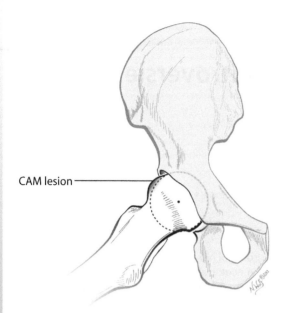

CAM lesion

Fig. 1. Lateral view of the hip shows the typical appearance and location of a CAM lesion. As the hip comes into flexion and internal rotation, this prominence can abut the acetabular rim and labrum, causing impingement.

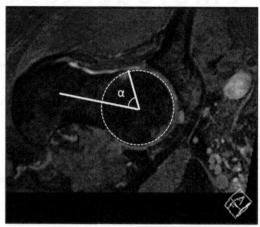

Fig. 2. Image from a radial sequence MRI showing reduced offset at the femoral head-neck junction. The degree of asphericity can be quantified using the alpha angle of Nötzli.[6] A best-fit circle is first drawn around the femoral head. The alpha angle is the angle formed between a line drawn down the axis of the femoral neck and a line drawn to the point at which the contour of the femoral head-neck junction deviates from the perfect circle. The larger the alpha angle, the greater the degree of asphericity.

a distinct type of upper femoral chondroepiphyseal maturation.[5] Because the size, location, and extension of the deformity are unique for each hip, the ability to visualize the prominence using plain radiographs is variable. Frog-lateral, cross-table lateral, or Dunn-lateral views may be used; however, the reliability depends on the location of the deformity and the rotation of the limb during the radiograph. Because of this variability, radial magnetic resonance imaging (MRI) reconstructions are often used to more accurately assess the morphology of the head-neck junction and minimize the chance of missing CAM lesions (**Fig. 2**). On either plain radiographs or radial sequences, the severity of deformity can be characterized by the alpha angle of Nötzli.[6] The alpha angle estimates the degree at which the radius of curvature of the femoral head begins to increase. Thus, larger alpha angle measurements indicate a more aspherical femoral head.

Acetabular-sided deformity or pincer impingement includes global overcoverage, focal overcoverage, and retroversion of the acetabulum, and results in premature contact between the femoral neck and acetabular rim when the hip is flexed (**Fig. 3**). These features are recognizable radiographically using an anteroposterior (AP) pelvis radiograph. The coverage of the acetabulum relative to the femoral head is traditionally assessed using the lateral center-edge angle (LCE). There is general agreement that a normal LCE is

between 25° and 35° and that hips with an LCE greater than 40° are at risk for impingement in flexion. Focal overcoverage can be assessed using the crossover sign that is observed when the anterior acetabular wall crosses over the posterior acetabular wall on a properly oriented AP pelvis radiograph (**Fig. 4**). There is conflicting information regarding the sensitivity of the crossover sign. Although the crossover sign may represent true focal acetabular overcoverage in some cases, in others it may be artifactually caused by the orientation of the anterior inferior iliac spine.[7–9] In addition, when a crossover sign is accompanied by a posterior wall sign, which occurs when the posterior wall of the acetabulum is located medial to the center of the femoral head, the acetabulum may be retroverted and the posterosuperior femoral coverage may be insufficient. A crossover sign accompanied by a posterior wall sign may be associated with anterior impingement when the hip is flexed and posterosuperior instability when the hip is in extension.[10]

Many hips are thought to have features of both CAM-type femoral morphology and acetabular overcoverage, resulting in so-called mixed-type impingement.

PATHOPHYSIOLOGY

The mechanics of impingement limit the degree of sagittal plane hip motion, diminishing the degree

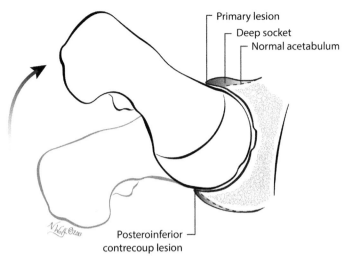

Fig. 3. Pincer morphology from an excessively deep hip socket. With motion, the femoral head-neck junction prematurely abuts the edge of the deep acetabulum, causing primary injury to the labrum and peripheral articular cartilage. This impingement can also cause levering of the femoral head away from the joint, resulting in posterior shear and contrecoup chondrolabral lesions.

to which an affected individual is able to squat.[11] Normal mechanical gait parameters are altered in patients affected by CAM-type FAI, with demonstrated decrease in hip abduction and frontal plane motion compared with control hips.[12]

Chegini and colleagues[13] used computational models to analyze stresses along the acetabular rim in simulated dysplastic and impinging joints. Impingement was modeled by increasing the alpha angle and the acetabular depth using a

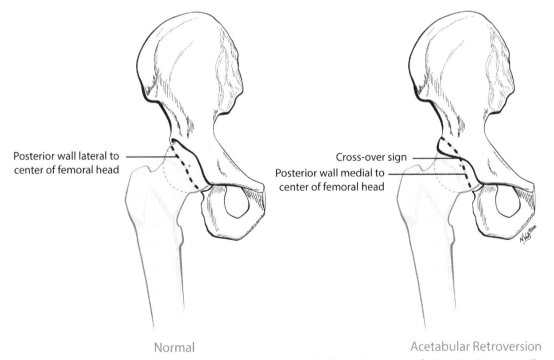

Fig. 4. Radiographic signs suggesting acetabular retroversion, which can be a cause of pincer impingement. The crossover sign is formed when the anterior acetabular wall crosses over the posterior acetabular wall. The posterior wall sign is formed when the edge of the posterior wall lies medial to the center of the femoral head. The presence of both signs on a properly oriented AP pelvic radiograph suggests acetabular retroversion.

standing-to-sitting motion and was shown to cause distortion and shearing at the bone-tissue interface, a calculated conclusion that is consistent with damage observed clinically in impinging joints at the time of surgery.[13] These mechanical studies support theories developed by observing patterns of chondral injury at the time of surgical treatment.[2]

CAM-type impingement, in which an aspherical bump enters the acetabular fossa during flexion, causes labral distortion and shear forces within the peripheral acetabulum that can cause detachment of the labrum from the rim of the acetabulum and full-thickness or partial-thickness delamination injuries of the hyaline cartilage within the joint.[2,3,14–16] In contrast, the damage pattern in hips with pincer-type mechanics is more peripheral. These hips often have a characteristic trough located in the femoral neck, thought to be related to remodeling caused by chronic and repetitive contact between the acetabular rim and femoral neck. The labrum is therefore crushed between the bony acetabular rim and femoral neck and the peripheral-most acetabular cartilage may become detached and frayed. In addition, contrecoup chondrolabral lesions in the posterior acetabulum, thought to result from anterior levering of the femur causing posterior shear, have been observed clinically.[2] The two major differences between CAM-type and pincer-type injury patterns are the increased depth of chondral injury associated with the CAM mechanism, and confinement of damage to the rim and peripheral acetabulum in pincer-type impingement.

CLINICAL PRESENTATION

The presentation of patients with symptomatic anterior FAI has been described by multiple investigators.[17–19] Patients usually present with insidious-onset pain about the hip that is characteristically localized to the groin but may be experienced in the buttock, lower back, trochanteric region, or the anterior thigh and knee. Pain may be precipitated by athletic activity or activities that require flexion, such as crouching or sitting. The pain pattern often goes unrecognized by primary physicians, leading to missed diagnosis or misdirected treatment.[19] Because the symptoms caused by FAI are not disease specific, careful patient history is essential when entertaining the diagnosis of FAI.

The physical examination of a patient with symptomatic FAI is characterized by painful limitation of hip flexion. In patients with highly irritable hip joints, hip guarding and compensatory lumbar

motion may confound the physical examination. Range of motion is usually limited in hips that are morphologically prone to symptomatic FAI, with average flexion reportedly slightly greater than 90°. The classic provocative maneuver is the anterior impingement test, which is pain elicited by flexion, adduction, and internal rotation of the affected hip (**Fig. 5**). Other provocative tests include the resisted straight-leg raise and the posterior impingement test. Clinical symptoms and physical examination signs must be correlated with radiographic data to firmly establish the diagnosis of FAI.

PREVALENCE OF DISEASE

The prevalence of clinically significant FAI remains unknown. The reported prevalence of FAI varies widely depending on the parameters used to define the condition. Ochoa and colleagues[20] reviewed 155 patients with a mean age of 32 years (range, 18–50 years) who presented to primary care or orthopedic clinics with a chief complaint of hip pain. Based on radiographic signs of FAI (herniation pits, pistol grip deformity, crossover sign, center-edge angle >39°, and/or alpha angle >50°), the investigators reported that 87% of the patients had at least 1 finding consistent with FAI, and 81% had at least 2 findings.

However, several recent studies have established a high prevalence of morphologic abnormalities associated with FAI in asymptomatic individuals as well:

- Reichenbach and colleagues[21] reported on 1,080 asymptomatic military recruits in Sumiswald, Switzerland, of whom 430 were

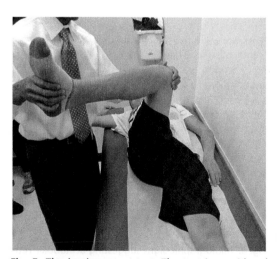

Fig. 5. The impingement test. The test is considered positive if pain is elicited by flexion, adduction, and internal rotation of the affected hip.

randomly selected, and 244 agreed, to undergo a radial sequence MRI looking for abnormal morphology at the femoral head-neck junction.

○ Mean age was 19.9 years
○ Adjusted overall prevalence of CAM-type deformity was 24% [95% CI 19, 30].[21]

• Jung and colleagues[22] evaluated 838 asymptomatic hips in 419 randomly selected patients aged 25 to 92 years who underwent abdominal or pelvic computed tomography (CT) for medical diseases unrelated to the hip. AP scout views of CT scans were used to measure asphericity of the femoral head-neck junction using the alpha angle as described by Nötzli and colleagues.[6] Study participants were classified according to criteria defined by Gosvig and colleagues[23] based on the Copenhagen Osteoarthritis Study.

○ For men, the three categories for α-angle ranges were:
  1. Pathological ($\geq 83°$)
  2. Borderline ($69°$ to $82°$)
  3. Normal ($\leq 68°$).
○ For women, the three categories for α-angle ranges were:
  1. Pathological ($\geq 57°$)
  2. Borderline ($51°$ to $56°$)
  3. Normal ($\leq 50°$).
○ Ages ranged 25 to 92 years
○ Men <50 years of age: mean α-angle was 57.2° with 14% demonstrating pathologic α-angles.
○ Women <50 years of age: mean α-angle was 45.3° with 7% demonstrating pathologic α-angles

• Hack and colleagues[24] studied 200 asymptomatic volunteers using radial MRI reformats.

○ Ages ranged 21.4 to 50.6 years; mean 29.4 years
○ α-angles were measured at both the 3 o'clock and 1:30 position with CAM deformity defined as an angle exceeding 50.5°.
○ At the 1:30 position, 53% of the volunteers had evidence of CAM morphology
○ At the 3 o'clock position, 14% had elevated α-angles.

These prevalence data in patients with minimal or no symptoms show the importance of clinical correlation during the diagnostic work-up for FAI. The presence of imaging findings consistent with FAI alone is not sufficient to warrant intervention. The treating clinician must rely on the history, physical examination, and imaging findings to determine whether a symptomatic patient is symptomatic because of FAI.

CAUSATIVE ROLE IN OSTEOARTHRITIS

The contemporary theory of FAI as a causative factor in the development of osteoarthritis has been championed by Ganz and colleagues,[25] and holds that the morphologic abnormalities of the femoral head and/or acetabulum result in abnormal contact between the femoral neck/head and the acetabular margin. This abnormal contact leads to supraphysiologic stress causing tearing of the labrum and avulsion of the underlying cartilage region (**Fig. 6**).[26,27] The continued abnormal contact results in further deterioration and wear of the articular cartilage, with eventual onset of arthritis. However, questions remain as to whether FAI is a cause or a result of osteoarthritis and whether joint deformities in FAI are congenital, developmental, or the reaction to the arthritic process (osteophytes).

Recent epidemiologic studies have attempted to clarify the role of FAI in the pathogenesis of osteoarthritis:

• The Nottingham United Kingdom Genetics of Osteoarthritis and Lifestyle (GOAL) study examined the morphology of the hip in 566 persons with unilateral hip osteoarthritis and compared this to the contralateral asymptomatic hip to non-osteoarthritic control hips from 1,100 subjects who had undergone intravenous urograms.[28]

○ All patients were ≥ 45 years of age or older; mean age was 66 years.
○ 48% of the subjects were women.
○ CAM morphology was defined as a ratio of head to neck diameter less than 1.27.

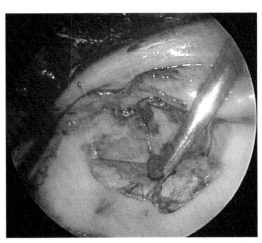

Fig. 6. Articular cartilage injury secondary to CAM-type FAI.

o Based on this criterion, the investigators reported a 5.5% risk of developing osteoarthritis in the contralateral non-osteoarthritic hip compared to a 3% risk in the control group.

o A pistol grip deformity conferred an 8.3% risk of developing osteoarthritis in the contralateral non-osteoarthritic hip compared to a 3.6% risk in the control group.

o Both factors were strongly and significantly associated with an increased risk of developing hip osteoarthritis after adjusting for age, body mass index, and gender.

In addition to this representative cross-sectional study, longitudinal studies of FAI have established the temporal relationship of cause to effect, by measuring proximal femoral morphology before it is altered by osteoarthritis:

- A prospective study of FAI in the Cohort Hip and Cohort Knee (CHECK) study reported on a Dutch national sample of 723 patients presenting for the first time with recent onset of hip or knee pain.[29] Initial AP pelvic radiographs were measured to determine the α-angle, and subjects were followed for 5 years to determine the risk of developing end-stage osteoarthritis.
  o Ages ranged 45 to 65 years
  o 80% of the cohort was female
  o Subjects had no osteoarthritis at baseline with either a Kellgren-Lawrence osteoarthritic grade of 0 (76%) or grade 1 (24%).
  o Hips with a baseline AP α-angle >83° had a 25% risk of developing end-stage osteoarthritis within 5 years compared to a less than 2% risk of end-stage osteoarthritis in hips with an α-angle less than 83° (odds ratio of 9.7 adjusted for age, sex, BMI and baseline Kellgren-Lawrence grade).
  o Hips with both an α-angle >83° and decreased internal rotation ≤20° had a 53% risk of developing end-stage osteoarthritis within 5 years.
- The Chingford cohort provides another recent longitudinal study of the relationship between hip morphology and the development of osteoarthritis.[30] 1003 healthy female subjects were enrolled after undergoing a baseline AP radiograph of the pelvis, which was measured the presence of CAM and pincer deformity. At 19 year follow-up, these radiographs were repeated. Of those patients who went on to THA, the baseline hip morphology was compared to a random sample of 243 hips that did not require THA.

o Ages ranged 44 to 67 years
o Median AP α-angle in those who required THA was 62.4° at baseline compared to 45.8° in controls ($P = .001$).
o The odds ratio of needing a THA increased 1.05 for each 1° increase in initial α-angle.

Recent evidence also suggests that FAI morphology may result from early exposure to high-impact sports, and may therefore be developmental in origin rather than a reaction to the arthritic process. Kapron and colleagues[31] reported that 95% of 134 hips in collegiate football players had at least one radiographic sign of CAM or pincer impingement, which exceeds the reported prevalence in asymptomatic members of the general population. Siebenrock and colleagues[32] showed a 10-fold increase in the prevalence of CAM morphology in a cohort of elite basketball players compared with nonactive age-matched controls. In addition, the investigators showed increasing alpha angles in the athletes during skeletal maturation, and suggested that repeated high-stress activities during childhood may modulate growth of the proximal femur toward an abnormal shape via subclinical physeal injury.

Based on the previously mentioned studies in which FAI morphology was studied before the presence of radiographic osteoarthritis and the prevalence studies in young, asymptomatic persons it is clear that FAI, and its morphologic risk factors, are common in young adult hips and predisposes to the later development of osteoarthritis in certain patients. Longitudinal studies also support that, in both men and women aged 45 to 65 years, the presence of CAM deformities at baseline substantially increases the risk of developing osteoarthritis and the need for a THA. However, in most hips the presence of a CAM lesion is not sufficient in isolation to lead to the development of clinically significant and symptomatic osteoarthritis. At this point, there is insufficient evidence from longitudinal population studies to confirm a similar association between the presence of a pincer deformity and the development of clinical or radiographic osteoarthritis.

TREATMENT

Treatment of FAI has evolved greatly over the past decade, in large part because of an increased recognition of the different morphologic factors that contribute to FAI as well as the development of new surgical techniques for reshaping the proximal femur and acetabular rim.[27]

The successful treatment of FAI demands:

- Accurate diagnosis. Is the pain caused by FAI, a nonarticular cause, or both?
  - A clear understanding of the possible pathomorphologies that can lead to arthrosis
  - A concomitant understanding of other possible causes of hip pain and arthrosis (eg, soft tissue impingement/inflammation, concomitant developmental dysplasia of the hip)
- Assessment of patient-based factors
  - Age
  - Demands. Can patients change their lives to mitigate their symptoms?
  - Expectations
- Knowledge of the surgeon's surgical skill set: can clinicians gain adequate access to address all disorders through open approaches, arthroscopy, or a combination of the two?

NONOPERATIVE MANAGEMENT

Because of the high prevalence of FAI morphology in asymptomatic hips, conservative management is usually warranted as an initial step, depending on the patient and the clinical picture.[24,31] Modalities including physical therapy to alleviate symptoms associated with periarticular causes, antiinflammatories, and activity/lifestyle modification can all be used. Medical and/or conservative management may also be of particular benefit when there is evidence of advanced arthrosis for which a joint-preserving procedure is not indicated.

SURGICAL MANAGEMENT

Since the initial description of his surgical dislocation approach to the hip, Ganz and colleagues[33] noted that, with improved familiarity with the vascular anatomy of the proximal femur, it has become safe to gain access to the hip joint without concern for avascular necrosis. This ability has laid the groundwork for the expansion in surgical treatment options for FAI. As previously noted, the first critical step is the accurate diagnosis of the cause of pain and arthrosis. Following this, a thorough understanding of the three-dimensional anatomy of the hip and the surgical techniques available to address its pathomorphology are paramount to ensure that any procedure remains safe as well as being efficacious.

In general, there are 3 surgical techniques currently used to treat FAI pathomorphology: surgical dislocation of the hip; anterior mini arthrotomy, with or without arthroscopic assistance; and arthroscopy. For the purposes of discussing and comparing these techniques, the following terminology is used to describe the regions around the hip joint:

- Central compartment: the area within the acetabulum, including the cotyloid notch, articular surface of the acetabulum, and ligamentum teres
- Peripheral compartment: the area outside the acetabulum, including the acetabular rim, labrum, femoral neck, joint capsule, iliopsoas, and the inferior portion of anterior inferior iliac spine

Surgical Dislocation

- Technique: performed through a lateral Gibson approach to the hip with a digastric trochanteric osteotomy and anterior-based arthrotomy. Once all portions of the hip joint are exposed, acetabular lesions are addressed, including rim resection, labral repair, acetabular chondroplasty, followed by femoral osteochondroplasty as needed **(Fig. 7)**. The capsule is repaired and the trochanteric fragment reattached with screws. Some surgeons favor postoperative

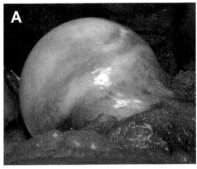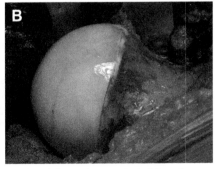

Fig. 7. (A) Intraoperative appearance of a CAM lesion visualized through a surgical dislocation approach. (B) Intraoperative view of femoral head-neck osteoplasty shows improved contour and restoration of offset.

abduction precautions. Such precautions are most likely not necessary because it is a digastric osteotomy and under compression in abduction. However, it may be more susceptible to rotational forces and therefore hip-strengthening exercises may need to be limited until there is trochanteric union.

- Regions accessible within the hip: central and complete peripheral compartment.
- Pros: complete visualization and access to both the acetabulum and femoral head, especially beneficial for treating posterior acetabular rim and posterior hip joint lesions. Allows easy repair of the joint capsule, which may be of benefit in preventing later hip instability.
- Cons: more invasive surgery, longer course of recovery, and potential for trochanteric nonunion and painful screws.

Anterior Mini Arthrotomy, With or Without Arthroscopic Assistance

- Technique: when used, arthroscopy is typically performed first under traction to assess the central compartment and perform chondroplasty and labral debridement as needed. This step is followed by an anterior arthrotomy performed through a standard anterior approach to perform the femoral osteochondroplasty and possibly labral debridement and limited acetabular rim resection.
- Regions accessible within the hip: central (limited central with arthrotomy alone) and limited peripheral compartment.
- Pros: less soft tissue dissection and no osteotomy but still able to visualize the central compartment to treat chondral injuries (with arthroscopy) as well as providing access to treat CAM lesions. Beneficial for the surgeon

who may be comfortable with arthroscopy for chondral debridement but not osteochondroplasty, rim resection, or labral repair through the arthroscope. Proponents of arthrotomy alone think that they can attain adequate access to the anterior acetabular rim, labrum, and femoral neck.

- Cons: treatment of acetabular rim lesions with rim resection and labral repair is difficult. There is also incomplete access and visualization of the posterior hip joint and acetabular rim.

Arthroscopy

- Technique: typically performed with the patient either supine or in a lateral position and a combination of portals including the peritrochanteric, midanterior, and anterior. Traction is used while assessing the central compartment, then released to perform femoral osteochondroplasty and assess range of motion/adequacy of femoral neck resection (**Fig. 8**).
- Regions accessible within the hip: central and limited peripheral compartment (poor access to posterior regions of the hip joint and acetabular rim).
- Pros: potentially the smallest amount of surgical dissection of superficial tissues and no trochanteric osteotomy. Without trochanteric osteotomy, patients can be mobilized with physical therapy more aggressively without concern for affecting osteotomy healing.
- Cons: to properly address all possible lesions within the hip with FAI morphology demands an advanced arthroscopic skill set that allows the surgeon to correct acetabular rim lesions and perform labral repair and femoral osteochondroplasty. In addition, there is increasing emphasis on the ability to perform a capsular repair.

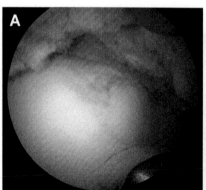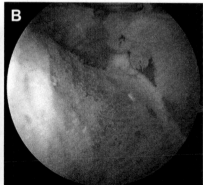

Fig. 8. (A) Arthroscopic view of the peripheral compartment shows prominence and injury of the head-neck junction from CAM-type FAI. (B) Arthroscopic view after femoral head-neck osteochondroplasty.

OUTCOMES

The outcome of the surgical treatment of FAI is variable. Patient-related factors such as lifestyle, work and sport demands, patient expectations, and duration of symptoms can all play a role.[2,27,34–55] Most studies reporting surgical outcome are single-surgeon experience, use a variety of outcome instruments, include mixed patient populations with variable types of impingement (CAM, pincer, both), use a variety of methods to describe the deformity, span a range of surgical experience, and have short-term (minimum 1 year) to midterm (average 5–6 year) follow-up (**Table 1**). Because the presentation can vary substantially, when this is combined with surgeon-related and surgery-related variables, the accurate determination of outcomes is difficult.

Nonoperative Management

Few outcome data exist for the nonoperative management of FAI. One investigator advocated an initial trial of conservative therapy and activity modification in symptomatic patients with prearthritic intra-articular hip disorder, stating that, provided there are ongoing follow-up evaluations, many patients may opt for continued conservative therapy.[40] In these cases and in the asymptomatic patient, continued close follow-up is critical because the rate of progression to advanced arthrosis is unpredictable and may lead to an inability to keep hip-preserving surgery as a viable option.[56]

Surgical Dislocation

Since its initial description by Ganz and colleagues,[33] surgical dislocation has remained the gold standard treatment of FAI. It has been used to treat a broad spectrum of deformity, across a wide spectrum of ages and causes (**Fig. 9**). Matsuda and colleagues[44] performed a systematic review of reported outcomes and, in general, short-term to mid-term results are good to excellent with few complications. Reported success rates across different studies ranged from 65% to 94%, whereas complication rates ranged from 0% to 20%, primarily from trochanteric nonunion. The conversion to THA as an end point for failure has been reported to be 0% to 30%.[46,49,55] Studies reporting higher rates of conversion to THA were earlier reports and in these initial patient cohorts the best indications for surgery had not been elucidated. These studies included older patients with more advanced arthrosis and concurrent dysplasia.[36,46] An argument can be made that more recent literature reflects outcomes

following refinement of surgical indication and technique in which the THA conversion rate is only 0% to 5%.[35,38,44,48]

Anterior Mini Arthrotomy, With or Without Arthroscopic Assistance

In groups that accessed the hip joint primarily via an anterior arthrotomy, with or without arthroscopic assistance, outcomes were similar to those obtained in the more recent surgical dislocation group (71%–92% success rate).[42,53,57–59] However, the incision lengths described for the mini open ranged from 2 to 12 cm. In the 4 reports cited by Matsuda and colleagues,[44] the complication rates ranged from 0% to 17% and included several inadequate resections requiring revision osteoplasty and/or labral fixation, transient lateral femoral cutaneous nerve injuries, and 1 femoral neck fracture treated nonoperatively.

Arthroscopy

With the advent of improved technique, several studies have evaluated the use of arthroscopy to treat FAI morphology rather than just labral debridement, the most commonly previously performed arthroscopic hip procedure. The published success rate ranged from 67% to 90%.[34,38,39,41,43,50,51,54,58,60–64] Most of these studies were short-term follow-up (1–2 years on average) and showed a conversion rate to THA of 0% to 9%. Complication rates were the lowest of the 3 surgical groups, ranging from 0% to 5%, with less frequent pudendal or lateral femoral cutaneous nerve palsy and (given the number of described cases in some series of more than 1000 arthroscopies) few reported revisions. A prominent point brought out in the current literature is that the learning curve for arthroscopic treatment is not well defined and may have an important effect on the individual surgeon's outcomes. Because most of these series were single-surgeon reports, the results may not be transferrable.

FUTURE DIRECTIONS

FAI as a clinical entity is in its infancy and understanding of the condition will undoubtedly increase in the years to come. Areas in need of further study include the natural history of FAI morphology, particularly pincer deformities, and other potentiating factors that explain why certain people with FAI become symptomatic and others do not. With regard to the deformity, more knowledge is needed about the importance of normal structures around the hip in the course of treating the more

Table 1
Selected outcome studies for FAI

Study	No. Hips	Mean FU (y)	Type of FAI	Outcome Measure	Outcomes	"Failures"	Predictors of Failure
Non-Operative Treatment							
Hunt et al,[40] 2012	58	1	Mixed	Satisfaction, need for surgery, others	44% satisfied	56% eventually chose surgery	Desire for "more active lifestyle"
Surgical Dislocation							
Beaulé et al,[35] 2007	37	3.1	CAM	WOMAC, UCLA, SF-12	↑ 20.2 pts ↑ 2.7 pts	16% dissatisfied	Advanced arthrosis
Beck et al,[36] 2004	19	4.7	CAM	Merle d'Aubigné	68% good to excellent	26%	Advanced (>Tönnis 1) arthrosis
Espinosa et al,[18] 2006	60	2	Pincer ± CAM	Merle d'Aubigné, Tönnis grade of arthrosis	76% good to excellent with labral debridement; 94% with labral refixation	4% with labral debridement	Results significantly better after rim trim with refixation of labrum vs debridement alone
Murphy et al,[46] 2004	23	5.2	Mixed	Conversion to THA	NR	30% converted to THA	Advanced arthrosis or combined impingement and instability
Peters et al,[49] 2010	96	2.2	Mixed	mHHS	↑ 24 pts	6% converted to THA	Advanced arthrosis
Yun et al,[55] 2009	15	>1	Mixed	mHHS	↑ 17 pts	0%	NR
Anterior arthrotomy ± Arthroscopy							
Laude et al,[58] 2009	100	4.9	CAM	NAHS	↑ 29.1 pts	11% converted to THA	NR
Lincoln et al,[43] 2009	16	2	CAM	mHHS	↑ 12.3 pts	6%	NR

Study	N	Follow-up	Type	Outcome	Results	Complications/Conversion	Prognostic factors
Nepple et al,[59] 2009 Arthroscopy (grp 1) vs arthroscopy with osteoplasty (Grp 2)	Grp 1: 36 Grp 2: 39	2.3 1.7	CAM	mHHS	74%–92% Good to Excellent; trend toward higher HHS in Group 2	Grp 1: 26% Grp 2: 4%	NR
Arthroscopy							
Ribas et al,[53] 2007	35	2.4	CAM	Merle d'Aubigné	↑ 3.1 pts	3%	Advanced (≥Tönnis 2) arthrosis
Ilizaliturri et al,[41] 2008	19	2.4	CAM	Clinical	84% reported improved symptoms	16% deteriorated	NR
Philippon et al,[50] 2009	112	2.3	Mixed	Satisfaction mHHS	Median 9/10 ↑ 26 pts	9% converted to THA	Increased age; decreased pre-op Harris Hip Score; minimum joint space <2 mm
Byrd & Jones,[60] 2009	207	1.3	Mixed	mHHS	↑ 24 pts	0.5% converted to THA	NR
Larson et al,[63] 2012 FAI correction plus (Grp 1: labral debridement) or (Grp 2: labral repair/refixation)	Grp 1: 44 Grp 2: 50	3.5	Pincer ± CAM	mHHS SF 12 VAS Pain	68% good to excellent results in Grp 1 vs 92% in Grp 2	Grp 1: 9.1% Grp 2: 8.0%	NR

Abbreviations: mHHS, modified Harris Hip Score; NAHS, Non arthritic hip score; NR, not reported; THA, total hip arthroplasty; UCLA, University of California Los Angeles activity score; WOMAC, Western Ontario and McMaster Universities Arthritis Index.

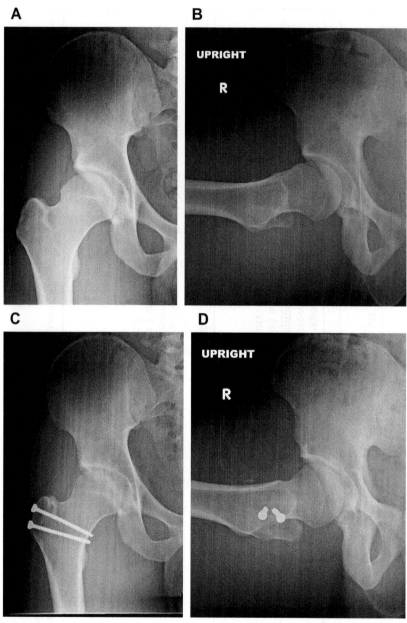

Fig. 9. (*A*) AP and (*B*) lateral view of the right hip showing a typical CAM lesion at the femoral head-neck junction. (*C, D*) AP and lateral view after osteochondroplasty was performed via an open surgical dislocation approach. Note the improvement in the head-neck contour and the screws used to repair the trochanteric osteotomy.

obvious disorders (eg, an intact labrum, importance of the ligamentum teres, capsular repair). In addition, the development of a comprehensive grading system for FAI would lay the foundation for comparative studies. In terms of treatment, longer follow-up studies with standardized outcome measures are necessary to determine the optimal treatment of particular patterns of disease.

REFERENCES

1. Myers SR, Eijer H, Ganz R. Anterior femoroacetabular impingement after periacetabular osteotomy. Clin Orthop Relat Res 1999;363:93–9.
2. Beck M, Kalhor M, Leunig M, et al. Hip morphology influences the pattern of damage to the acetabular cartilage: femoroacetabular impingement as a cause of early osteoarthritis of the hip. J Bone Joint Surg Br 2005;87(7):1012–8.

3. Pfirrmann CW, Mengiardi B, Dora C, et al. Cam and pincer femoroacetabular impingement: characteristic MR arthrographic findings in 50 patients. Radiology 2006;240:778–85.

4. Siebenrock KA, Wahab KH, Werlen S, et al. Abnormal extension of the femoral head epiphysis as a cause of cam impingement. Clin Orthop Relat Res 2004;(418):54–60.

5. Serrat MA, Reno PL, McCollum MA, et al. Variation in mammalian proximal femoral development: comparative analysis of two distinct ossification patterns. J Anat 2007;210:249–58.

6. Nötzli HP, Wyss TF, Sotecklin CH. The contour of the femoral head-neck junction as a predictor for the risk of anterior impingement. J Bone Joint Surg Br 2002;84:556–60.

7. Zaltz I, Kelly BT, Hestroni I, et al. The crossover sign overestimates acetabular retroversion. Clin Orthop Relat Res 2012;471(8):2463–70.

8. Jamali AA, Mladenov K, Meyer DC, et al. Anteroposterior pelvic radiographs to assess acetabular retroversion: high validity of the "cross-over-sign". J Orthop Res 2007;25:758–65.

9. Ezoe M, Naito M, Inoue T. Prevalence of acetabular retroversion among various disorders of the hip. J Bone Joint Surg Am 2006;88:372–9.

10. Dandachli W, Islam SU, Liu M, et al. Three-dimensional CT analysis to determine acetabular retroversion and the implications for the management of femoro-acetabular impingement. J Bone Joint Surg Br 2009;91:1031–6.

11. Lamontagne M, Kennedy MJ, Beaule PE. The effect of cam FAI on hip and pelvic motion during maximum squat. Clin Orthop Relat Res 2009;467: 645–50.

12. Kennedy MJ, Lamontagne M, Beaule PE. Femoroacetabular impingement alters hip and pelvic biomechanics during gait walking biomechanics of FAI. Gait Posture 2009;30:41–4.

13. Chegini S, Beck M, Ferguson SJ. The effects of impingement and dysplasia on stress distributions in the hip joint during sitting and walking: a finite element analysis. J Orthop Res 2009;27: 195–201.

14. Ito K, Leunig M, Ganz R. Histopathologic features of the acetabular labrum in femoroacetabular impingement. Clin Orthop Relat Res 2004;429: 262–71.

15. Leunig M, Podeszwa D, Beck M, et al. Magnetic resonance arthrography of labral disorders in hips with dysplasia and impingement. Clin Orthop Relat Res 2004;(418):74–80.

16. Anderson LA, Peters CL, Park BB, et al. Acetabular cartilage delamination in femoroacetabular impingement. Risk factors and magnetic resonance imaging diagnosis. J Bone Joint Surg Am 2009;91(2):305–13.

17. Beck M, Leunig M, Clarke E, et al. Femoroacetabular impingement as a factor in the development of nonunion of the femoral neck: a report of three cases. J Orthop Trauma 2004;18(7):425–30.

18. Espinosa N, Rothenfluh DA, Beck M, et al. Treatment of femoro-acetabular impingement: preliminary results of labral refixation. J Bone Joint Surg Am 2006;88(5):925–35.

19. Clohisy JC, Knaus ER, Hunt DM, et al. Clinical presentation of patients with symptomatic anterior hip impingement. Clin Orthop Relat Res 2009;467(3): 638–44.

20. Ochoa LM, Dawson L, Patzkowski JC, et al. Radiographic prevalence of femoroacetabular impingement in a young population with hip complaints is high. Clin Orthop Relat Res 2010;468:2710–4.

21. Reichenbach S, Juni P, Werlen S, et al. Prevalence of cam-type deformity on hip magnetic resonance imaging in young males: a cross-sectional study. Arthritis Care Res 2010;62:1319–27.

22. Jung KA, Restrepo C, Hellman M, et al. The prevalence of cam-type femoroacetabular deformity in asymptomatic adults. J Bone Joint Surg Br 2011; 93B:1303–7.

23. Gosvig KK, Jacobsen S, Palm H, et al. A new radiological index for assessing asphericity of the femoral head in cam impingement. J Bone Joint Surg Br 2007;89B:1309–16.

24. Hack K, Di Primio G, Rakhra K, et al. Prevalence of cam-type femoroacetabular impingement morphology in asymptomatic volunteers. J Bone Joint Surg Am 2010;92(14):2436–44.

25. Ganz R, Parvizi J, Beck M, et al. Femoroacetabular impingement: a cause of early osteoarthritis of the hip. Clin Orthop Relat Res 2003;417:112–20.

26. Parvizi J, Leunig M, Reinhold G. Femoroacetabular impingement. J Am Acad Orthop Surg 2007; 9:561–70.

27. Ganz R, Leunig M, Leunig-Ganz K, et al. The etiology of osteoarthritis of the hip: an integrated mechanical concept. Clin Orthop Relat Res 2008; 466(2):264–72.

28. Doherty M, Courtney P, Doherty S, et al. Nonspherical femoral head shape (pistol grip deformity), neck shaft angle, and risk of hip osteoarthritis. Arthritis Rheum 2008;58(10):3172–82.

29. Agricola R, Heijboer MP, Bierma-Zeinstra SM, et al. Cam impingement causes osteoarthritis of the hip: a nationwide prospective cohort study (CHECK). Ann Rheum Dis 2013;72(6):918–23.

30. Nicholls AS, Kiran A, Pollard TC, et al. The association between hip morphology parameters and nineteen-year risk of end-stage osteoarthritis of the hip: a nested case-control study. Arthritis Rheum 2011;63(11):3392–400.

31. Kapron AL, Anderson AI, Aoki SK, et al. Radiographic prevalence of femoroacetabular impingement in

collegiate football players: AAOS Exhibit Selection. J Bone Joint Surg Am 2011;93(19): e111(1–10).

32. Siebenrock KA, Ferner F, Noble PC, et al. The cam-type deformity of the proximal femur arises in childhood in response to vigorous sporting activity. Clin Orthop Relat Res 2011;469:3229–40.

33. Ganz R, Gill TJ, Gautier E, et al. Surgical dislocation of the adult hip a technique with full access to the femoral head and acetabulum without the risk of avascular necrosis. J Bone Joint Surg Br 2001;83(8):1119–24.

34. Bardakos NV, Vasconcelos JC, Villar RN. Early outcome of hip arthroscopy for femoroacetabular impingement: the role of femoral osteoplasty in symptomatic improvement. J Bone Joint Surg Br 2008;90(12):1570–5.

35. Beaulé PE, Le Duff MJ, Zaragoza E. Quality of life following femoral head-neck osteochondroplasty for femoroacetabular impingement. J Bone Joint Surg Am 2007;89(4):773–9.

36. Beck M, Leunig M, Parvizi J, et al. Anterior femoroacetabular impingement: part II. Midterm results of surgical treatment. Clin Orthop Relat Res 2004;(418):67–73.

37. Bedi A, Zaltz I, De La Torre K, et al. Radiographic comparison of surgical hip dislocation and hip arthroscopy for treatment of cam deformity in femoroacetabular impingement. Am J Sports Med 2011;39(Suppl):20S–8S.

38. Espinosa N, Beck M, Rothenfluh DA, et al. Treatment of femoro-acetabular impingement: preliminary results of labral refixation. Surgical technique. J Bone Joint Surg Am 2007;89(Suppl 2 Pt.1):36–53.

39. Fabricant PD, Heyworth BE, Kelly BT. Hip arthroscopy improves symptoms associated with FAI in selected adolescent athletes. Clin Orthop Relat Res 2012;470(1):261–9.

40. Hunt D, Prather H, Harris Hayes M, et al. Clinical outcomes analysis of conservative and surgical treatment of patients with clinical indications of prearthritic, intra-articular hip disorders. PM R 2012; 4(7):479–87.

41. Ilizaliturri VM Jr, Orozco-Rodriguez L, Acosta-Rodriguez E, et al. Arthroscopic treatment of cam-type femoroacetabular impingement: preliminary report at 2 years minimum follow-up. J Arthroplasty 2008;23(2):226–34.

42. Lincoln M, Johnston K, Muldoon M, et al. Combined arthroscopic and modified open approach for cam femoroacetabular impingement: a preliminary experience. Arthroscopy 2009;25(4):392–9.

43. Malviya A, Stafford GH, Villar RN. Impact of arthroscopy of the hip for femoroacetabular impingement on quality of life at a mean follow-up of 3.2 years. J Bone Joint Surg Br 2012;94(4): 466–70.

44. Matsuda DK, Carlisle JC, Arthurs SC, et al. Comparative systematic review of the open dislocation, mini-open, and arthroscopic surgeries for femoroacetabular impingement. Arthroscopy 2011;27(2):252–69.

45. Meftah M, Rodriguez JA, Panagopoulos G, et al. Long-term results of arthroscopic labral debridement: predictors of outcomes. Orthopedics 2011; 34(10):e588–92.

46. Murphy S, Tannast M, Kim YJ, et al. Debridement of the adult hip for femoroacetabular impingement: indications and preliminary clinical results. Clin Orthop Relat Res 2004;(429):178–81.

47. Nho SJ, Magennis EM, Singh CK, et al. Outcomes after the arthroscopic treatment of femoroacetabular impingement in a mixed group of high-level athletes. Am J Sports Med 2011;39(Suppl):14S–9S.

48. Peters CL, Erickson JA. Treatment of femoroacetabular impingement with surgical dislocation and debridement in young adults. J Bone Joint Surg Am 2006;88(8):1735–41.

49. Peters CL, Schabel K, Anderson L, et al. Open treatment of femoroacetabular impingement is associated with clinical improvement and low complication rate at short-term followup. Clin Orthop Relat Res 2010;468(2):504–10.

50. Philippon MJ, Briggs KK, Yen YM, et al. Outcomes following hip arthroscopy for femoroacetabular impingement with associated chondrolabral dysfunction: minimum two-year follow-up. J Bone Joint Surg Br 2009;91(1):16–23.

51. Philippon MJ, Yen YM, Briggs KK, et al. Early outcomes after hip arthroscopy for femoroacetabular impingement in the athletic adolescent patient: a preliminary report. J Pediatr Orthop 2008;28(7): 705–10.

52. Rebello G, Spencer S, Millis MB, et al. Surgical dislocation in the management of pediatric and adolescent hip deformity. Clin Orthop Relat Res 2009;467(3):724–31.

53. Ribas M, Marin-Pena OR, Regenbrecht B, et al. Hip osteoplasty by an anterior minimally invasive approach for active patients with femoroacetabular impingement. Hip Int 2007;17(2):91–8.

54. Tran P, Pritchard M, O'Donnell J. Outcome of arthroscopic treatment for cam type femoroacetabular impingement in adolescents. ANZ J Surg 2013;83(5):382–6.

55. Yun HH, Shon WY, Yun JY. Treatment of femoroacetabular impingement with surgical dislocation. Clin Orthop Surg 2009;1(3):146–54.

56. Beaule PE, Allen DJ, Clohisy JC, et al. The young adult with hip impingement: deciding on the optimal intervention. Instr Course Lect 2009;58: 213–22.

57. Clohisy JC, McClure JT. Treatment of anterior femoroacetabular impingement with combined hip

arthroscopy and limited anterior decompression. Iowa Orthop J 2005;25:164–71.

58. Laude F, Sariali E, Nogier A. Femoroacetabular impingement treatment using arthroscopy and anterior approach. Clin Orthop Relat Res 2009; 467(3):747–52.

59. Nepple JJ, Zebala LP, Clohisy JC. Labral disease associated with femoroacetabular impingement: do we need to correct the structural deformity? J Arthroplasty 2009;24(Suppl 6):114–9.

60. Byrd JW, Jones KS. Arthroscopic femoroplasty in the management of cam-type femoroacetabular impingement. Clin Orthop Relat Res 2009;467(3): 739–46.

61. Clohisy JC, St John LC, Schutz AL. Surgical treatment of femoroacetabular impingement: a systematic review of the literature. Clin Orthop Relat Res 2010;468(2):555–64.

62. Horisberger M, Brunner A, Herzog RF. Arthroscopic treatment of femoroacetabular impingement of the hip: a new technique to access the joint. Clin Orthop Relat Res 2010;468(1):182–90.

63. Larson CM, Giveans MR, Stone RM. Arthroscopic debridement versus refixation of the acetabular labrum associated with femoroacetabular impingement: mean 3.5-year follow-up. Am J Sports Med 2012;40(5):1015–21.

64. Philippon MJ, Weiss DR, Kuppersmith DA, et al. Arthroscopic labral repair and treatment of femoroacetabular impingement in professional hockey players. Am J Sports Med 2010;38(1): 99–104.

UPPER EXTREMITY

Preface

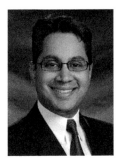

Asif M. Ilyas, MD
Editor

In this issue of the *Orthopedic Clinics of North America*, we present four interesting articles in the Upper Extremity section reviewing some common and uncommon pathologies:

Franko & Abrams present a summary of the most common infections of the hand and the latest anti-microbial and surgical management recommendations.

Limthongthang and coworkers have presented a detailed review of the evaluation and management of Adult Brachial Plexus Injuries. The successful management of these potentially devastating injuries requires accurate diagnosis of the site(s) of the lesion and both focused nonoperative and possibly operative management. The authors present a review of the most common patterns, detailed preoperative assessment, and surgical management options, including tendon, muscle, and nerve transfer options.

Namdari and colleagues have presented a review of the Spastic Shoulder, focusing on its proper evaluation and surgical treatment options. This diagnosis commonly presents after brain injury and its evaluation requires careful physical examination and possibly the use of electrodiagnostic testing and/or focused nerve blocks. A review of these diagnostic measures and the use of surgical options, such as tendon releases, muscle lengthening, arthrodesis, and arthroplasty, are reviewed.

Judson and Wolf have presented a review of injection treatments for Lateral Epicondylitis of the elbow, a common but often difficult complaint to manage. A thorough review of the literature on the role and efficacy of various injection therapies has been presented, including glucocorticoids, platelet-rich plasma, autologous blood, botulinum toxin, hyaluronic acid, prolotherapy, glycosaminoglycan, and saline.

Johnston and coworkers have presented a review of Os Acromiale of the shoulder and its surgical treatment options. This uncommon but well-recognized developmental defect presents in various forms and when symptomatic can be challenging to treat. The authors have presented a review of the most common forms and various treatment options, including their experience with Os Acromiale nonunion site excision.

Asif M. Ilyas, MD
Hand & Upper Extremity Surgery
Rothman Institute
Thomas Jefferson University
925 Chestnut Street
Philadelphia, PA 19107, USA

E-mail address:
asif.ilyas@rothmaninstitute.com

Orthop Clin N Am 44 (2013) xix
http://dx.doi.org/10.1016/j.ocl.2013.07.005
0030-5898/13/$ – see front matter © 2013 Published by Elsevier Inc.

orthopedic.theclinics.com

Adult Brachial Plexus Injury
Evaluation and Management

Roongsak Limthongthang, MD[a],*, Abdo Bachoura, MD[b],
Panupan Songcharoen, MD[a], A. Lee Osterman, MD[b]

KEYWORDS

- Adult brachial plexus injury • Pattern of injury • Preoperative evaluation • Intraoperative study
- Nerve transfer • Functioning free muscle transfer

KEY POINTS

- Brachial plexus injury involves damage to the C5-T1 spinal nerves. Common injury patterns include "upper arm type" (C5-6 ± C7) and "total arm type" (C5-T1).
- Preganglionic avulsion injury is suspected when the following observations are noted: Horner syndrome, winged scapula, absence of Tinel sign over the neck, hemidiaphragm paralysis, and pseudomeningocele. This type of injury infers poor potential for spontaneous recovery.
- The treatment of upper arm type injury involves the restoration of elbow flexion and shoulder control. Good results can be achieved by using nerve transfer surgery.
- The treatment of total arm type injury involves the re-establishment of shoulder, elbow, and hand function. The use of functioning free muscle transfers or nerve transfers may restore hand function.

INTRODUCTION

Traumatic brachial plexus injury (BPI) is regarded as one of the most devastating injuries of the upper extremity. Patients typically lose sensation, motor power, and may experience disabling neuropathic pain. Several decades ago, combined arm amputation, shoulder arthrodesis, and prosthetic replacement was a viable treatment option for patients with a flail arm, because this protocol resulted in superior functional results compared with other reconstructive procedures at that time, which included tenodesis, bone block, and arthrodesis.[1] However, advances in peripheral nerve surgery over the last few decades have significantly changed the image and outcomes of brachial plexus treatment. Today, one can expect good to excellent functional results in patients with upper arm deficits.[2] Although there remains much room for optimizing the functional results in patients with a flail arm, today's outcomes following reconstructive surgery have improved to a degree that renders amputation as an antiquated treatment option.

The treatment of BPI is based on a combination of evidence-based principles, practical feasibility, and the personal philosophy of the surgeon. In many instances, dogmatic practices flourish because of differences in the surgeon's approach, the patient's injuries and expectations, and the cultural environment. Over the past few decades, there has been a fair amount of trial and error in BPI surgery and some techniques have developed a reputation for consistent and encouraging results, whereas others have become of historical interest. This article provides an overview of the anatomy, diagnosis, and treatment of posttraumatic adult BPI. In addition, some of the controversial topics surrounding the management of this complex injury are addressed.

[a] Department of Orthopaedic Surgery, Faculty of Medicine Siriraj Hospital, Mahidol University, 2 Prannok Road, Bangkoknoi District, Bangkok 10700, Thailand; [b] The Philadelphia Hand Center, Thomas Jefferson University Hospital, 834 Chestnut Street, Suite G114, Philadelphia, PA 19107, USA
* Corresponding author.
E-mail addresses: droongsak@gmail.com; roongsak.lit@mahidol.ac.th

ANATOMY, FUNCTION, AND LOCALIZATION OF LESIONS

The brachial plexus is usually formed by the ventral rami of five spinal nerves (C5-T1), although some variations exist, which involve contributions from the C4 (prefixed) or T2 levels (postfixed). The small dorsal rami, which are not part of the plexus, supply the paraspinal muscles and skin of the posterior neck. After once the spinal nerves pass through the spinal foramina, they form the brachial plexus between the scalenus anterior and the scalenus medius muscles. The anatomy of the brachial plexus is normally divided into five segments: (1) spinal nerves or roots, (2) trunks, (3) divisions, (4) cords, and (5) terminal branches (**Figs. 1** and **2**).[3,4]

Spinal Nerves

Two terminal nerves emerge at the level of the spinal roots: the dorsal scapular nerve (C4-5), which supplies the levator scapulae and rhomboid muscles; and the long thoracic nerve (C5-7), which supplies the serratus anterior muscle. Injury to this nerve results in scapular winging.

The phrenic nerve (C3-5), considered an extraplexal nerve, lies on the scalenus anterior muscle. Therefore, plexus injury at the root level may cause paralysis and subsequent elevation of the diaphragm.

The sympathetic ganglion lies in close proximity to the brachial plexus at the T1 root level. Therefore, injury to the lower root may be associated with Horner syndrome, which consists of miosis, enophthalmos, ptosis, and anhydrosis (**Fig. 3**).

Trunks

Two terminal nerves emerge at the level of the trunks: the suprascapular (SSC) nerve (C5-6), which supplies the supraspinatus and infraspinatus muscles, arises from the superolateral aspect of the upper trunk, at a location referred to as Erb's point; and the nerve to the subclavius muscle (C5-6), which is smaller than its aforementioned counterpart and arises from the medial side of the upper trunk.

Divisions

The division level could be conceptualized as the equator of the brachial plexus. The all roots form the trunks that travel posterior to the clavicle and then split into anterior and posterior divisions that supply the flexor and extensor muscles respectively (see **Fig. 2**).

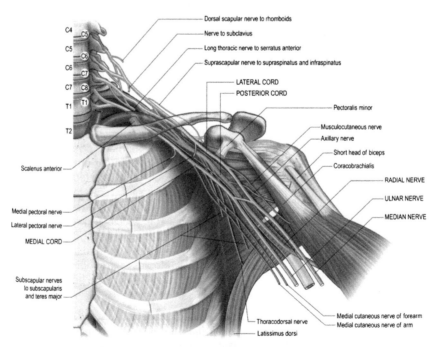

Fig. 1. The anatomy of the brachial plexus. The supraclavicular component includes the spinal nerves and trunks. The divisions form cords at a level approximately posterior to the clavicle. The infraclavicular component includes the cords and terminal nerve branches. These cords are named in reference to their anatomic relationship to the axillary artery, which is located posterior to the pectoralis minor muscle. (*From* Standring S. Gray's anatomy: the anatomic basis of clinical practice. 40th edition. Philadelphia: Elsevier; 2008.)

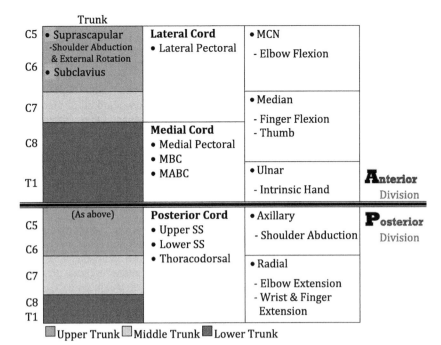

Trunk				
C5	• Suprascapular -Shoulder Abduction & External Rotation	**Lateral Cord** • Lateral Pectoral	• MCN - Elbow Flexion	
C6	• Subclavius			
C7			• Median - Finger Flexion - Thumb	
C8		**Medial Cord** • Medial Pectoral • MBC • MABC		
T1			• Ulnar - Intrinsic Hand	**A**nterior Division
C5	(As above)	**Posterior Cord** • Upper SS • Lower SS • Thoracodorsal	• Axillary - Shoulder Abduction	**P**osterior Division
C6			• Radial - Elbow Extension - Wrist & Finger Extension	
C7				
C8 T1				

☐ Upper Trunk ☐ Middle Trunk ■ Lower Trunk

Fig. 2. Structures of the brachial plexus. Five spinal nerve roots form three trunks and travel posterior to the clavicle, and then split into anterior and posterior divisions, which primarily supply the flexor and extensor muscles, respectively. The anterior divisions of the upper and middle trunks form the lateral cord, while the lower trunk becomes the medial cord. The posterior divisions of every trunk form the posterior cord by contributing various proportions of spinal nerve roots. •, indicates a terminal nerve branch; MABC, medial antebrachial cutaneous nerve; MBC, medial brachial cutaneous nerve; MCN, musculocutaneous nerve; upper and lower SS, upper and lower subscapular nerves. (*Reproduced from* Songcharoen P, Shin AY. Brachial plexus injury: acute diagnosis and treatment. In: Berger RA, Weiss AP, editors. Hand surgery. Philadelphia: Lippincott Williams & Wilkins; 2003. p. 1005–25.)

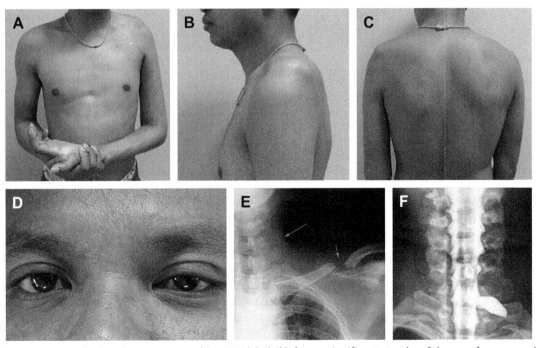

Fig. 3. Common findings in total root avulsion BPI. (*A*) Flail left arm, significant atrophy of the arm, forearm, and hand muscles are noted. (*B*) Lateral view demonstrating marked shoulder subluxation. (*C*) Atrophy of the supraspinatus, infraspinatus, and parascapular muscles on the left side. (*D*) Ptosis and enophthalmos are observed in this patient with Horner syndrome. (*E*) Transverse process fracture of the cervical spine and a widely gapped clavicle fracture (*arrows*). (*F*) Myelography demonstrates a pseudomeningocele at C8 and the absence of a nerve root sleeve at C7.

Cords

After the brachial plexus has traveled distal to the clavicle, or has become infraclavicular, it becomes invested by the axillary sheath. The anterior divisions of the upper and middle trunks form lateral cord, and lower trunk becomes medial cord. The posterior divisions of every trunk form the posterior cord by contributing various proportions of spinal nerve roots. These cords are named in reference to their anatomic relationship to the second part of the axillary artery, which is located posterior to the pectoralis minor muscle.

It should be noted that the aforementioned anatomic description characterizes an uninjured brachial plexus. During surgical exploration of BPI, however, the anatomy becomes more distorted and complicated because there is usually nerve retraction and associated fibrotic scar formation. Often, the chronically avulsed plexus is found to be retracted distally and located posterior to the clavicle. In addition, anatomic variations within the brachial plexus are not uncommon, and serve to further complicate anatomic exploration.

CLASSIFICATION, MECHANISM, AND PATTERNS OF THE INJURY

Previous reports have classified BPI according to a combination of injury mechanism, degree of nerve injury, location, and level of injury.[4–6]

Mechanism of Injury

An understanding of the mechanism of injury may help predict the type of brachial plexus lesion. Closed BPIs are usually associated with a traction mechanism where the arm and shoulder are forcefully distracted away from the neck or trunk. This mechanism mostly results in root avulsion lesions and 70% to 80% of these injuries have been found to occur in motorcycle accidents.[4,5] In these cases, spontaneous recovery rarely occurs. Other less common mechanisms include crush or compression caused by various mechanisms, such as compression of the clavicle against the rib cage secondary to seatbelt restraint, anterior shoulder dislocation, or iatrogenic surgical positioning. Crush or compression injury mechanisms tend to involve the infraclavicular part of the plexus, such as the cords or terminal braches, which may have some recovery potential.

Open BPI is usually a result of stab wounds, gunshot wounds, and sometimes open fractures of the shoulder girdle. In patients with gunshot wounds, the initial neurologic deficit is often extensive; however, one report showed that only 12% to 15% of patients sustained transected nerve lesions.[7] Open fractures of the shoulder girdle usually occur after high-energy injuries, in which the combination of nerve root avulsion and major vessel injury should be suspected (**Fig. 4**).

Degree of the Nerve Injury

The classification systems of peripheral nerve injury into neuropraxia, axonotmesis, and neurotmesis by Seddon[8] and first- to fifth-degree injury by Sunderland[9] are generally used to describe BPI. Neurapraxia, or Sunderland's first-degree injury, refers to localized myelin damage and conduction deficiencies. Complete recovery could be expected in 4 to 12 weeks. Axonotmesis or second-degree injury refers to a disruption of the nerve cell's axon, followed by wallerian degeneration. Complete axonal regeneration could be expected to occur at a rate of approximately 1 to 3 mm/day from the injury site to the target muscle.[9] During third-degree injury, internal derangement of the endoneurium and intrafascicular fibrosis precludes complete regeneration and results in partial recovery. In fourth-degree injury, owing to perineurial and fascicular disruption, neuroma in-continuity forms and spontaneous recovery is not expected. Neurotmesis, or fifth-degree injury, refers to complete nerve transection and the need for surgical intervention. MacKinnon and Dellon[10] added a sixth-degree injury as a combination of first- to fifth-degree fascicular injuries within the same nerve. This injury results in variable recovery and prognosis.

Location and Level of the Injury

Several terms and classification systems have been used to categorize the location and level of BPI.[5,6] In our experience, sometimes it is difficult to define the exact location of injury. Therefore, we prefer to use a simple and practical classification scheme that divides injury location into two groups: supraclavicular or infraclavicular lesions. Supraclavicular lesions imply injury at the spinal nerve and trunks levels. Similar to other authors, we have found that further subdivision into preganglionic and postganglionic lesions is beneficial during treatment planning and is of prognostic value. The signs that suggest a preganglionic injury are presented in **Table 1**. Infraclavicular lesions mostly occur at the cord and terminal branch levels (see **Fig. 4**). In Narakas' series, approximately 10% of patients had combined supraclavicular and infraclavicular lesions.[5] The common neurologic deficit patterns according to the level of the injury are presented in **Table 2**.

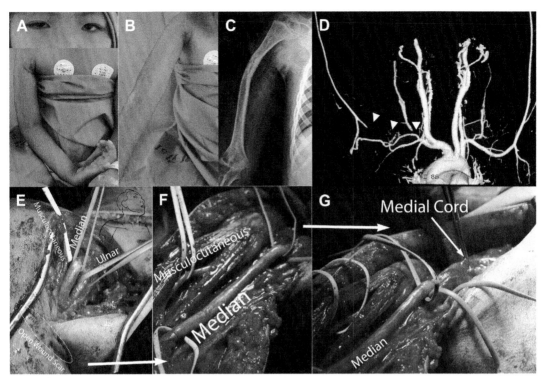

Fig. 4. This 6-year-old girl presented 4 months following open fracture of the proximal shaft of the humerus and infraclavicular BPI. (*A*) The patient lost all elbow, wrist, and hand function, and Horner syndrome was observed. (*B*) She could abduct her right shoulder to 30 degrees. (*C*) The x-ray showed union of the proximal shaft of the humerus. (*D*) The CT angiography revealed absence of right subclavian-axillary artery perfusion (*arrowheads*). (*E, F*) Adhesions were found extending all the way from the cord level to the area of the initial open wound scar. (*G*) An in-continuity lesion was found at the medial cord.

DIAGNOSIS
History Taking and Physical Examination

A detailed history of the mechanism of injury, associated injuries, and previous treatment is mandatory to guide lesion localization and treatment planning. The character and severity of pain should be documented. In addition to the motor and sensory examination of the injured limb, a global neurologic examination should be conducted, because associated cervical spine and spinal cord injury are not uncommon. A focused examination of the injured limb should be performed, including an assessment of the functional deficits secondary to BPI, and an evaluation of potential donor muscles and nerves, to ensure they meet the prerequisites required for subsequent transfer. The motor power of every muscle that is supplied by the brachial plexus should be documented according to the Medical Research Council system, between grades 0 and 5. Normal power of the trapezius muscle, innervated by cranial nerve (CN) XI (spinal accessory nerve), is required to allow CN XI transfer. Examination of the peripheral

vasculature is necessary especially during the planning of functioning free muscle transfers. Concomitant fractures and dislocations of the insensate paralytic limb are often missed or neglected, and if not addressed early, could lead to nonunion, malunion, or joint contracture. In this event, regardless of the reinnervation procedure, poor functional results develop because it is more difficult to rehabilitate weak, newly reinnervated muscles with stiff and deformed joints.

Plain Film

Chest radiographs may reveal hemidiaphragm elevation, which would indicate phrenic nerve palsy and raise suspicion about nerve root avulsion. First or second rib fractures may be associated with BPI. Knowledge of the presence or absence of additional rib fractures is important if intercostal nerve transfer is being considered. A transverse process fracture of the cervical spine may imply root avulsion injury, whereas a widely gapped clavicle fracture may indicate a traction mechanism of injury (see **Fig. 3**E).

Table 1
Signs and physical findings that suggest a preganglionic injury

Signs and Findings	Implications
Horner syndrome	Sympathetic ganglion injury (T1 level)
Winged scapula	Long thoracic nerve injury (C5-7)
Atrophy of parascapular muscle	Dorsal scapular nerve injury (C4-5)
Cervical paraspinal muscle weakness and loss of posterior neck sensation	Dorsal rami of cervical spinal nerve roots injury
Hemidiaphragm paralysis	Phrenic nerve injury (C3-5)
Absence of Tinel sign in neck area	Absence of proximal spinal nerve stump
Pseudomeningocele on myelogram	Development of meningeal diverticulum after healing of torn nerve root sleeve
Intact sensory nerve action potentials in the area of sensory deficit	Imply no wallerian degeneration of the sensory axons because the attached nerve cells reside in the dorsal root ganglion

Reproduced from Songcharoen P, Shin AY. Brachial plexus injury: acute diagnosis and treatment. In: Berger RA, Weiss AP, editors. Hand surgery. Philadelphia: Lippincott Williams & Wilkins; 2003. p. 1005–25.

Cervical Myelography or Computed Tomography Myelography

Cervical myelography has been used to demonstrate spinal nerve root lesions in BPI for more than 50 years and remains a useful tool.[11] Findings that suggest nerve root injury include the absence of a nerve root sleeve, a defect of the root sleeve shadow, and formation of a pseudomeningocele (see **Fig. 3**F).[4,12] Myelographic studies should be performed approximately 3 weeks or more after the injury to allow sufficient time for pseudomeningocele formation.

Current computed tomography (CT) myelography methods provide better resolution and more accurate categorization of nerve root status compared to plain film myelography, with a reported accuracy greater than 90%, especially when combined with the clinical examination.[13,14] The disadvantages of these techniques include their invasive nature and their inability to demonstrate lesions beyond the level of the intervertebral foramina.

Magnetic Resonance Imaging

Novel magnetic resonance imaging (MRI) techniques are increasing in popularity secondary to their noninvasive nature and the details they provide. Many evolving techniques, such as fast imaging using steady-state acquisition, MR neurography, and high-field 3-T MRI, are able to visualize spinal nerve root lesions with relatively high accuracy.[6,13] Doi and colleagues[14] reported a sensitivity and specificity of 92.9% and 81.3%, respectively, for overlapping coronal-oblique

Table 2
Common neurologic deficit patterns according to the level of the injury

Level	Patterns of Injury	Motor Deficits
Supraclavicular	Upper arm type (C5-6 nerve roots)	Shoulder abduction Elbow flexion
	Extended upper arm type (C5-7 nerve roots)	Shoulder abduction Elbow flexion and extension Wrist extension
	Total arm type (C5-T1 nerve roots)	Shoulder abduction Elbow flexion and extension Global hand function
Infraclavicular	Lateral cord (musculocutaneous nerve) Medial cord (medial and ulnar nerves)	Elbow flexion Finger flexion Intrinsic hand function
	Posterior cord (axillary and radial nerves)	Shoulder abduction (supraspinatus and infraspinatus muscles intact) Elbow and wrist extension

Reproduced from Spinner RJ, Shin AY, Hébert-Blouin M, et al. Traumatic brachial plexus injury. In: Wolfe SW, Hotchkiss RN, Pederson WC, editors. Green's operative hand surgery. 6th edition. Philadelphia: Churchill Livingstone Elsevier; 2010. p. 1235–92.

slices for detecting the presence of root avulsions. Moreover, MRI is capable of providing useful images of the entire brachial plexus. The disadvantages of MRI include false-positive interpretations.

Angiography

Major vessel injury associated with BPI has been reported to be as high as 23%.[5] The vessels most often damaged include the subclavian artery, subclavian vein, and the axillary artery in association with infraclavicular lesions. Conventional angiography, CT angiography (see **Fig. 4**D), or MR angiography should be considered in cases of suspected arterial damage, and cases that involve operative planning with consideration of functional free muscle transfer in order to demonstrate the status of the thoracoacromial trunk as a source of the arterial pedicle.

Electrodiagnostic Studies

Electrodiagnostic studies are useful during preoperative evaluation and intraoperative management. Preoperative evaluation usually consists of nerve conduction studies and needle electromyography. For nerve conduction studies, the preservation of the sensory nerve action potentials in the area of sensory deficit may indicate preganglionic nerve root avulsion injury at that given level. Electromyography may demonstrate the development of signs of muscle denervation (polyphasic, fibrillation, positive sharp wave) approximately 10 to 21 days after the injury has occurred.[15]

Intraoperative Studies

Intraoperative electrodiagnostic studies are very useful and could help guide operative decision-making, especially in cases of incomplete lesions, neuromas in-continuity, and the presence of nerve root stumps. During the treatment of partial injuries, intraoperative nerve action potential recordings across the lesion may help determine which fascicles should be resected and grafted, or which fascicles are intact or recovering.[16]

Various additional intraoperative techniques have been described to assess the functional condition and usefulness of spinal nerve stumps as donor tissue for nerve reconstruction. The techniques and their respective results are displayed in **Table 3**.

MANAGEMENT

Return to the preinjury functional status would be an ideal goal; however, the reconstructive options for the regain of C5-T1 function is limited secondary to the small number of available donor nerves. Sensate prehensile hand function may be the most required function for patients. However, whereas elbow flexion and shoulder abduction take priority as they have a higher likelihood of success.

Timing

The timing of surgery is one of the most important aspects of treatment. With too long of a delay, denervated muscles will undergo the process of

---

Table 3
Intraoperative diagnostic tests used to assess the condition of the nerve root stump

Authors	Techniques	Results
Oberle et al,[34] 2002	Evoked MEP and SSEP	Absence of MEP demonstrated a 100% sensitivity for anterior root lesions Absence of SSEP from the scalp demonstrated a 100% sensitivity for posterior root lesions
Flores,[33] 2008	Electrical stimulation of the long thoracic nerve, used for the C5 root stump grafted to the suprascapular nerve	Transfer of C5 root with positive electrical stimulation can achieve M3 (37%) and M4 (62%) of shoulder abduction
Malessy et al,[35] 1999	Frozen section of the C5-6 root stumps, used for the restoration of biceps muscle function	Prefer myelinated axons >50% Significant relation between biceps muscle strength and percentage of myelinated axons ($P = .02$)
Hattori et al,[36] 2001	Measurement of CAT activity of donor nerve for FFMT	All donors with CAT activity >2000 cpm provided all muscles with functional recovery by 3.2 mo

Abbreviations: CAT, choline acetyltransferase; cpm, counts per minute; FFMT, functioning free muscle transfer; MEP, muscle evoked action potentials; SSEP, somatosensory evoked potentials.

denervation atrophy, rendering them refractory to reinnervation. Furthermore, animal studies have demonstrated that recovered muscle force decreases by at least 30% to 50% if the nerve repair is delayed for a month or longer.[17] However, early or immediate nerve reconstruction may preclude the chance for spontaneous recovery, especially for hand function, which usually requires a lengthy time period.

Immediate or early (3–4 weeks postinjury) brachial plexus exploration and repair is generally accepted for sharp, open injuries. If the nerves are found to be ruptured or crushed and divided, tagging and re-exploration in 3 to 4 weeks is planned, because this time period allows for better identification of the nerve injury zone.[18]

Nerve reconstruction surgery within 6 to 9 months of injury is generally an acceptable timeframe for intervention.[7,19] This allows sufficient time for axonal regeneration to reach the target muscle before irreversible motor end plate degeneration occurs. In light of advanced neuroimaging techniques and more precise diagnoses, early nerve reconstruction is an attractive treatment option. Birch encouraged early plexus exploration for closed traction injuries within 3 months of injury, and recommended repair or reconstruction within 14 days of injury.[20] He pointed out that the benefit of early intervention allows identification and full assessment of the lesion and the usefulness of the nerve root stumps as a donor before the onset of fibrotic scar tissue, which are likely to distort the anatomy further. Kline found that 40% of C5-6 injuries spontaneously recovered in 3 to 4 months, whereas 15% of C5-7 injuries recovered in 3 to 4 months, and only 5% of flail arms (C5-T1) had functional recovery.[7] Thus, preganglionic total arm BPI seems to be the type of injury that may benefit most from earlier nerve reconstruction procedures, especially for hand function reconstruction, which is obstinate to treatment.

C5-6 Injury

The functional deficits of C5-6 injury include the loss of elbow flexion and shoulder control (stability, flexion, abduction, and external rotation). The terminal nerve branches that usually need to have their function restored are (1) the musculocutaneous nerve to re-establish elbow flexion, (2) SSC nerve, and (3) the axillary nerve to re-establish shoulder control.

The restoration of elbow flexion in C5-6 injury could be performed either by biceps reinnervation, or biceps and brachialis reinnervation. The locations of recipient nerves include the anterior division of the upper trunk, the musculocutaneous nerve, or

the motor branches that supply the biceps and brachialis muscles.[18] Reinnervation by the upper trunk or musculocutaneous nerve could restore function to the biceps and brachialis. Most of the time, however, these techniques require the interposition of nerve grafts and long recovery periods.[5,18,19] If when close-targeted intraplexal donors are available, transfer of an ulnar (or median) nerve fascicle to the motor branch of the biceps muscle could achieve more reliable functional results compared to the use of extraplexal donor nerves, such as the intercostal and spinal accessory nerves.[21] Today, the double fascicular nerve transfer to the biceps and brachialis' motor branches has become an attractive option that theoretically allows for a greater regain in elbow flexion strength.[22,23] A comparison of elbow flexion torque strength between single and double transfers, however, was not found to result in significant differences (single 16% vs double 21% of normal side).[24] In our practice, we do not use double fascicular transfers as routinely because we believe that this approach may increase the risk of donor site morbidity, in exchange for no additional gain in function. However, this is our own personal bias, and previous studies have indicated that double fascicular transfer is a safe procedure.[22,23]

In C5-6 injury, many combinations of nerve transfers to the SSC and axillary nerves could be performed to restore shoulder function. In one series that studied single nerve transfer of spinal accessory nerve (CN XI) to the SSC nerve, 80% motor recovery was observed, with 70 degree of shoulder abduction, 60 degree of shoulder flexion, and 30 degree of external rotation.[25] Whenever possible, double transfer of CN XI to the SSC nerve, along with transfer of the motor branches of the medial or long head of the triceps to the axillary nerve, is recommended because this has resulted in encouraging functional results (**Figs. 5 and 6**).[2] The phrenic nerve also allows direct coaptation of SSC nerve transfer.[25] Although adverse clinical consequences are rare, the measurable deficits in lung function[26] deter many surgeons from using phrenic nerve transfer. Other alternative donor nerves that have been used include the thoracodorsal nerve, intercostal nerves, and medial pectoral nerves.

C5-7 Injury

Patients with this type of BPI have deficits similar to patients with C5-C6 injury, in addition to loss of elbow extension and wrist extension as a result of C7 root involvement. The principles of nerve reconstruction are similar to those for patients with C5-6 injury. Additional problems include

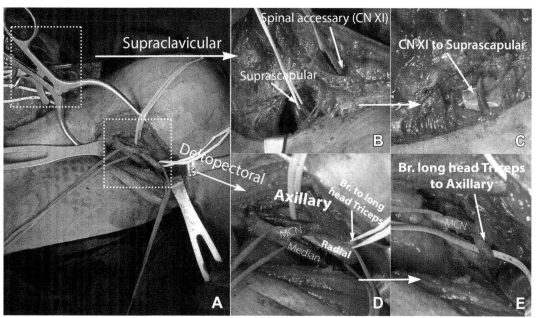

Fig. 5. (*A*) Restoration of shoulder function in C5-6 injury through the anterior approach. (*B, C*) The spinal accessory nerve has been transferred to the suprascapular nerve via the supraclavicular approach. (*D, E*) The motor branch to the long head of the triceps was transferred to the axillary nerve via the deltopectoral approach. The ulnar fascicular transfer to the motor branch of the biceps muscle was used to restore elbow flexion in this patient.

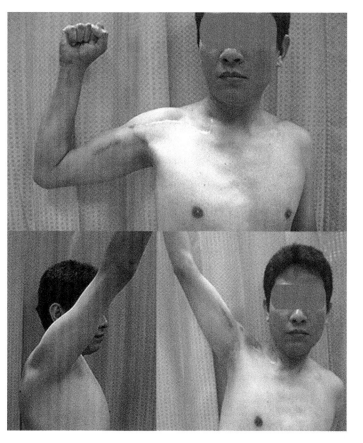

Fig. 6. The result of the patient with C5-6 injury 2 years after (1) spinal accessary transfer to suprascapular nerves, (2) branch of long head triceps transfer to the axillary nerve via the anterior approach, and (3) fascicles of ulnar transfer to the motor branch of the biceps muscle. The pictures demonstrate elbow flexion and shoulder external rotation, forward flexion, and abduction. (*Courtesy of* S. Wongtrakul, MD, Department of Orthopaedic Surgery, Faculty of Medicine Siriraj Hospital, Thailand.)

(1) the absence of a branch to the triceps that could be used for transfer to the axillary nerve; (2) loss of elbow extension, which restricts reach and the ability to position the hand in space; and (3) loss of wrist extension.

Restoration of the axillary nerve could be accomplished by the use of alternative donors, such as the intercostal nerve, or interposition nerve grafts from the C5-C6 nerve stump,[27] which could simultaneously restore radial nerve function (or the motor branch to triceps).[28] For elbow extension, Bertelli and Ghizoni[27] reported poor outcomes after C6 root to radial nerve grafting, because only 40% of patients achieved grade 3 motor strength (M3). Malungpaishrope and colleagues[28] reported their results for simultaneous third-fourth intercostal nerve transfer to the axillary nerve, combined with fifth-sixth intercostal nerve transfer to the triceps branch. Only 30% of patients achieved M3 elbow extension. It should be noted, however, that a delicate balance of reinnervation of elbow flexors and extensors is required. If the triceps becomes too powerful relative to the flexors, it may negate the function of elbow flexion, which is the priority.

Total Arm BPI

The outcomes of total plexus treatment are completely different in comparison to the encouraging results seen in upper arm treatment. Part of this problem is associated with the unfavorable results of hand function after reconstruction. Elbow flexion, the first priority in reconstruction, could be restored by reinnervation of the biceps muscle with the spinal accessory nerve (77% ≥M3)[19]; multiple intercostal nerves (81% ≥M3)[29]; and interposition nerve grafts from C5 root (90% ≥M3).[27] Shoulder reinnervation could be achieved by single nerve transfer.[25] Alternatively, the shoulder could be arthrodesed if donor nerves are inadequate.

Regain of elbow and shoulder function takes priority over hand function reconstruction because of more successful reinnervation of the proximal muscles compared to the distal muscles. However, treatment planning may depend on the primary method selected for hand reconstruction. Currently available methods include primary functioning free muscle transfers or nerve transfer[30–32] for the restoration of finger flexion. Our current treatment algorithm for total arm BPI is presented in **Fig. 7**. The methods selected for each patient depend on multiple factors including the following:

1. Time period after injury and the degree of muscle atrophy: a long time period after the injury worsens the outcomes of nerve transfer, especially for motor function. If patients present at approximately 6 months or later after injury, primary functioning free muscle transfers are preferred.
2. Associated vascular injury: this occurs approximately 10% of the time when total root avulsion is present. In cases of associated vascular injury, we prioritize and focus on the nerve transfer method regardless of the degree of vascular injury and previous treatment.

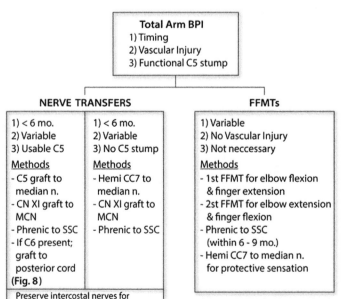

Total Arm BPI 1) Timing 2) Vascular Injury 3) Functional C5 stump		
NERVE TRANSFERS		**FFMTs**

1) < 6 mo.
2) Variable
3) Usable C5
 	
Methods
- C5 graft to
  median n.
- CN XI graft to
  MCN
- Phrenic to SSC
- If C6 present;
  graft to
  posterior cord
(Fig. 8)
	1) < 6 mo.
	2) Variable
	3) No C5 stump
	
	Methods
	- Hemi CC7 to
	  median n.
	- CN XI graft to
	  MCN
	- Phrenic to SSC
		1) Variable
		2) No Vascular Injury
		3) Not neccessary
		
		Methods
		- 1st FFMT for elbow flexion
		  & finger extension
		- 2st FFMT for elbow extension
		  & finger flexion
		- Phrenic to SSC
		  (within 6 - 9 mo.)
		- Hemi CC7 to median n.
		  for protective sensation

Preserve intercostal nerves for secondary FFMT if needed.		

Fig. 7. Treatment algorithm for total arm BPI. Factors that guide the decision-making process for treatment include timing, vascular injury, and the status of the C5 nerve stump. (1) With longer delays between injury and surgery, especially 6 months after injury, the results of nerve transfer become worse. (2) If vascular injury is present, despite vascular repair, the possibility of free muscle transfer failure is very high. (3) An intact C5 root stump can be transferred to the median nerve with the expectations of extrinsic finger flexion and protective sensation. FFMTs, functioning free muscle transfers; Hemi CC7, hemicontralateral C7 spinal nerve; CN XI, spinal accessory.

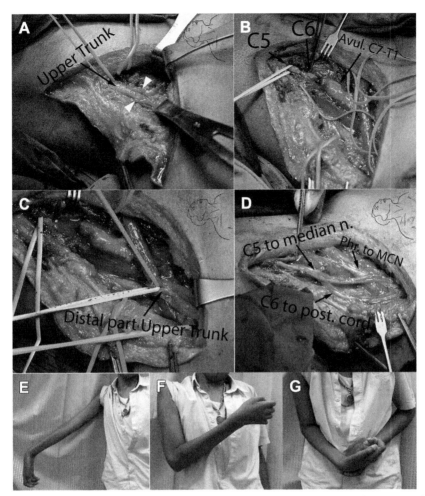

Fig. 8. (*A, B*) Rupture of the upper trunk (*arrowheads*) and avulsion of C7-T1 roots is demonstrated in a patient with total arm BPI. (*C*) The distal part of upper trunk was located distally posterior to the clavicle. (*D*) Treatment consists of (1) C5 grafting to the median nerve, (2) phrenic grafting to the musculocutaneous nerve (MCN), (3) spinal accessory transfer to the suprascapular nerve, and (4) C6 grafting to the posterior cord. (*E–G*) At 14 months after surgery, the patient had recovered shoulder abduction, elbow flexion, and extrinsic finger flexion.

3. The presence or absence of a functional C5 nerve root stump: electrical stimulation of the long thoracic or dorsal scapular nerves is used to gauge C5 nerve root function.[33] Nerve transfer of the C5 root to the median nerve with interposition nerve grafting is expected to lead to extrinsic finger flexion and protective sensation (**Fig. 8**).

SUMMARY

Traumatic adult brachial plexus treatment requires multiple well-planned primary and secondary reconstructive procedures. Intractable neuropathic pain threatens the quality of life despite motor and sensory nerve reconstruction. Realistic patient expectations should be set with the idea that no single procedure is capable of guaranteeing promising results or return to the preinjury status. It is not uncommon to perform secondary functioning free muscle transfers after unsuccessful nerve transfers, or even after failed primary functioning free muscle transfers.

REFERENCES

1. Yeoman P, Seddon H. Brachial plexus injuries: treatment of the flail arm. J Bone Joint Surg Br 1961;43: 493–500.
2. Leechavengvongs S, Witoonchart K, Uerpairojkit C, et al. Nerve transfer to deltoid muscle using the nerve to the long head of the triceps, part II: a report of 7 cases. J Hand Surg Am 2003;28(4):633–8.
3. Standring S. Gray's anatomy: the anatomical basis of clinical practice. Philadelphia: Elsevier Health Sciences; 2008.

4. Songcharoen P, Shin AY. Brachial plexus injury: acute diagnosis and treatment. In: Berger RA, Weiss AP, editors. Hand surgery. Philadelphia: Lippincott Williams & Wilkins; 2003. p. 1005–25.

5. Narakas AO. The treatment of brachial plexus injuries. Int Orthop 1985;9(1):29–36.

6. Chuang DC. Adult brachial plexus reconstruction with the level of injury: review and personal experience. Plast Reconstr Surg 2009;124(Suppl 6):e359–69.

7. Kline DG. Timing for brachial plexus injury: a personal experience. Neurosurg Clin N Am 2009; 20(1):24–6, v.

8. Seddon HJ. Three types of nerve injury. Brain 1943; 66(4):237–88.

9. Sunderland S. A classification of peripheral nerve injuries producing loss of function. Brain 1951;74(4): 491–516.

10. MacKinnon SE, Dellon AL. Surgery of the peripheral nerve. New York: Thieme Medical Pub; 1988.

11. Yeoman P. Cervical myelography in traction injuries of the brachial plexus. J Bone Joint Surg Br 1968; 50(253–260):32–3.

12. Nagano A, Ochiai N, Sugioka H, et al. Usefulness of myelography in brachial plexus injuries. J Hand Surg Br 1989;14(1):59–64.

13. Amrami KK, Port JD. Imaging the brachial plexus. Hand Clin 2005;21(1):25–37.

14. Doi K, Otsuka K, Okamoto Y, et al. Cervical nerve root avulsion in brachial plexus injuries: magnetic resonance imaging classification and comparison with myelography and computerized tomography myelography. J Neurosurg 2002;96(Suppl 3): 277–84.

15. Harper CM. Preoperative and intraoperative electrophysiologic assessment of brachial plexus injuries. Hand Clin 2005;21(1):39–46.

16. Robert EG, Happel LT, Kline DG. Intraoperative nerve action potential recordings. Neurosurgery 2009;65(Suppl 4):A97–104.

17. Kobayashi J, Mackinnon SE, Watanabe O, et al. The effect of duration of muscle denervation on functional recovery in the rat model. Muscle Nerve 1997;20(7):858–66.

18. Spinner RJ, Shin AY, Hébert-Blouin M, et al. Traumatic brachial plexus injury. In: Wolfe SW, Hotchkiss RN, Pederson WC, editors. Green's operative hand surgery. 6th edition. Philadelphia: Churchill Livingstone Elsevier; 2010. p. 1235–92.

19. Songcharoen P, Mahaisavariya B, Chotigavanich C. Spinal accessory neurotization for restoration of elbow flexion in avulsion injuries of the brachial plexus. J Hand Surg Am 1996;21(3):387–90.

20. Birch R. Brachial plexus injury: the London experience with supraclavicular traction lesions. Neurosurg Clin N Am 2009;20(1):15–23, v.

21. Coulet B, Boretto JG, Lazerges C, et al. A comparison of intercostal and partial ulnar nerve transfers in restoring elbow flexion following upper brachial plexus injury (C5-C6 ± C7). J Hand Surg Am 2010;35(8):1297–303.

22. Mackinnon SE, Novak CB, Myckatyn TM, et al. Results of reinnervation of the biceps and brachialis muscles with a double fascicular transfer for elbow flexion. J Hand Surg Am 2005;30(5): 978–85.

23. Liverneaux PA, Diaz LC, Beaulieu JY, et al. Preliminary results of double nerve transfer to restore elbow flexion in upper type brachial plexus palsies. Plast Reconstr Surg 2006;117(3):915–9.

24. Carlsen BT, Bishop AT, Spinner RJ, et al. Comparison of single and double nerve transfer for elbow flexion after brachial plexus injury: level 3 evidence. J Hand Surg Am 2009;34(Suppl 7):26–7.

25. Songcharoen P, Wongtrakul S, Spinner RJ. Brachial plexus injuries in the adult. nerve transfers: the Siriraj Hospital experience. Hand Clin 2005;21(1):83–9.

26. Chuang ML, Chuang DC, Lin IF, et al. Ventilation and exercise performance after phrenic nerve and multiple intercostal nerve transfers for avulsed brachial plexus injury. Chest 2005;128(5):3434–9.

27. Bertelli JA, Ghizoni MF. Reconstruction of complete palsies of the adult brachial plexus by root grafting using long grafts and nerve transfers to target nerves. J Hand Surg Am 2010;35(10):1640–6.

28. Malungpaishrope K, Leechavengvongs S, Witoonchart K, et al. Simultaneous intercostal nerve transfers to deltoid and triceps muscle through the posterior approach. J Hand Surg Am 2012;37(4): 677–82.

29. Nagano A, Tsuyama N, Ochiai N, et al. Direct nerve crossing with the intercostal nerve to treat avulsion injuries of the brachial plexus. J Hand Surg Am 1989;14(6):980–5.

30. Doi K. Management of total paralysis of the brachial plexus by the double free-muscle transfer technique. J Hand Surg Eur Vol 2008;33(3): 240–51.

31. Chuang DC. Nerve transfer with functioning free muscle transplantation. Hand Clin 2008;24(4): 377–88, vi.

32. Songcharoen P, Wongtrakul S, Mahaisavariya B, et al. Hemi-contralateral C7 transfer to median nerve in the treatment of root avulsion brachial plexus injury. J Hand Surg Am 2001;26(6):1058–64.

33. Flores LP. Functional assessment of C-5 ventral rootlets by intraoperative electrical stimulation of the supraclavicular segment of the long thoracic nerve during brachial plexus surgery. J Neurosurg 2008; 108(3):533–40.

34. Oberle J, Antoniadis G, Kast E, et al. Evaluation of traumatic cervical nerve root injuries by intraoperative evoked potentials. Neurosurgery 2002;51(5): 1182–8 [discussion: 1188–90].

35. Malessy MJ, van Duinen SG, Feirabend HK, et al. Correlation between histopathological findings in C-5 and C-6 nerve stumps and motor recovery following nerve grafting for repair of brachial plexus injury. J Neurosurg 1999;91(4):636–44.

36. Hattori Y, Doi K, Ohi R, et al. Clinical application of intraoperative measurement of choline acetyltransferase activity during functioning free muscle transfer. J Hand Surg Am 2001; 26(4):645–8.

Orthopedic Evaluation and Surgical Treatment of the Spastic Shoulder

Surena Namdari, MD, MSc[a],*,
Keith Baldwin, MD, MPH, MSPT[b], John G. Horneff, MD[b],
Mary Ann Keenan, MD[b]

KEYWORDS

• Spastic shoulder • Orthopedic evaluation • Surgical treatment • Brain injury

KEY POINTS

• Spastic shoulder deformity can cause substantial limitation in active and passive upper extremity function.
• When deformities and lack of function persist and neurologic recovery has plateaued, preoperative planning should be initiated.
• The key is to characterize the patient's motor control using a comprehensive physical examination, and when indicated, dynamic polyelectromyography and selective local anesthetic nerve blocks to identify the offending muscles.
• Treatment options include selective tendon releases, fractional tendon lengthenings, biceps suspension, arthrodesis, and arthroplasty, and must be determined after a careful review of the patient's specific clinical presentation.

INTRODUCTION

Disorders of acquired spasticity most commonly include traumatic brain injury and cerebrovascular accidents and cause disruption of upper motor neuron inhibitory pathways. The result is upper motor neuron syndrome, which can manifest in spasticity, dyssynergic muscle activation, muscle weakness, and contractures. Most commonly, the patient's shoulder assumes an adduction and internal rotation deformity, and this is the focus of this review. Patients can present with other patterns of deformity (eg, abduction, extension) depending on the pattern of muscle dyssynergy; however, these are beyond the scope of this review.

Patients with spastic shoulder deformity often describe substantial limitation in active and passive upper extremity function. When deformities and lack of function persist and neurologic recovery has plateaued, preoperative planning should be initiated to address residual spasticity and muscle contraction dyssynergy. The evaluation and surgical treatment of the spastic shoulder is uncommonly discussed. The determination of motor control necessitates a comprehensive physical examination and often includes dynamic polyelectromyography (poly-EMG) and selective local anesthetic nerve blocks to identify the offending muscles. Corresponding shoulder disease, including glenohumeral subluxation and arthrosis, must also be identified and treated. Treatment

Funding Sources/Conflicts of Interest: None.
[a] Thomas Jefferson University Hospital, Rothman Institute, 925 Chestnut Street, 5th Floor, Philadelphia, PA 19107, USA; [b] Department of Orthopedic Surgery, Hospital of the University of Pennsylvania, 2 Silverstein, 3400 Spruce Street, Philadelphia, PA 19104, USA
* Corresponding author.
E-mail address: surena.namdari@gmail.com

orthopedic.theclinics.com

options include selective tendon releases, fractional tendon lengthenings, biceps suspension, arthrodesis, and arthroplasty, and must be determined after a careful review of the patient's specific clinical presentation.

Upper Motor Neuron Syndrome

Upper motor neuron syndrome is defined as the change in motor control that occurs after an upper motor neuron injury, such as a cerebrovascular accident, spinal cord injury, traumatic brain injury, or other acquired central nervous system injury. Characteristics of upper motor neuron syndrome include the presence of spasticity and other forms of involuntary muscle overactivity, voluntary weakness, and a variety of motor control abnormalities that impair the regulation of voluntary movement. Patients with upper motor neuron lesions can present with highly variable combinations of impaired voluntary movement and involuntary muscle contractions. Of these 2 defects, it is the spastic and involuntary muscle contractions that may be painful and debilitating. Seventeen percent to 48% of patients who suffer a cerebrovascular accident are affected by spasticity,[1,2] and approximately one-third of patients with traumatic brain injury experience some level of limb spasticity.[3] With the annual number of stroke at 780,000 and a combined 1.7 million new spinal cord and traumatic brain injuries in the United States each year, the sequelae of upper motor syndrome are a source of substantial morbidity, which require skilled medical treatment.[4,5]

In the early stages of upper motor neuron syndrome, the imbalance of neurologic signals results in sustained muscle contraction found in the stretch reflex. In normal neuromuscular physiology, the stretching of a muscle body causes the muscle spindle Ia afferent neurons to excite motor neurons, which respond with contraction of agonist and relaxation of antagonist muscles.[6] The result of this balance is muscular tone, which allows the body to control itself within space and resist or influence forces within its environment. When an upper motor neuron injury occurs, the balance is shifted toward excitatory inputs, which result in motor neurons with lower threshold potentials and longer discharges. As a result, patients often experience unopposed muscle contraction or dyssynergic muscle activity.[6] In this clinical scenario, the normal stretch reflex that exists to protect the body from outside forces acts as a debilitating factor. Continued contractions lead to changes within the muscle tissue itself, as fibrous and adipose tissue begin to replace the normal contractile sarcomeres.[7] Remaining sarcomeres become shortened as a result of their constantly contracted state, and normal elastic tissue is lost. These sustained muscle contractions can lead to stereotypical postures of the various joints, namely the adduction and internal rotation deformity seen most commonly in the shoulder.[8,9]

Patients with spastic shoulders after upper motor neuron injury can either lack all motor control (hemiplegia) or have variable levels of preserved motor control (hemiparesis). This is a critical distinction in the evaluation of the spastic shoulder and one that is underscored throughout this review. Based on the degree of preserved motor control, the clinical picture often involves a combination of active and passive functional problems. Regardless of the specific patterns of spasticity and muscle overactivity, treatment should begin with nonoperative intervention aimed at preventing and treating the passive and dynamic components of spasticity.

Nonoperative Treatments

Medications

Nonoperative treatments for shoulder spasticity include oral medications, which have the benefit of being noninvasive. The most common targets of antispasmodic medications are the γ aminobutyric acid (GABA) system, the α_2 adrenergic system, and the sarcoplasmic reticulum calcium release system within muscle tissue. Baclofen and benzodiazepines act as agonists on GABA-B and GABA-A receptors, respectively, and are helpful in decreasing the release of excitatory neurotransmitters responsible for firing motor neuron signals.[8] These medications are not without side effects, because both can cause drowsiness, and baclofen can cause urinary incontinence, sexual dysfunction, and lower seizure threshold. Even more concerning is the potential for rebound spasticity seen within 48 hours of discontinued use of baclofen. Despite these concerns, baclofen remains the preferred drug treatment of spasticity and can be administered orally or intrathecally.[9]

Tizanidine is an ∞_2 receptor agonist that inhibits excitatory pathways in the spinal cord and brain by enhancing noradrenergic activity. One of the benefits of this drug is that it has enhanced tolerability compared with the GABA agonists.[8] Side effects include dry mouth and gastrointestinal irritation. Tizanidine should be avoided in patients with hypotension because it can exacerbate this condition. Its most concerning side effect is acute hepatitis, which must be accounted for with early liver enzyme monitoring.

Dantrolene is commonly known as a treatment in the acute setting of malignant hyperthermia caused by general anesthesia. It works by blocking the calcium release from the sarcoplasmic reticulum, which causes muscle cell contraction and interferes with the excitation-contraction coupling seen in muscle tissue. Unlike the medications mentioned earlier, dantrolene works directly on muscle tissue and is less likely to cause sedation and dizziness.[8] However, it does also require liver enzyme monitoring because of risk of acute hepatitis.

Physical therapy

Physical therapy can offer a gradual and long-term approach to maintaining range of motion. It is typically an integral adjunct of the nonoperative and surgical treatment of spastic patients throughout their lifetime. The key to the physical therapy treatment of a patient with upper motor neuron syndrome is to start as soon as possible and to continue as long as possible.[10] Passive stretching helps to decrease the excitatory threshold of the motor neurons and prevent the loss of elastic connective tissue. This treatment can be labor intensive for the patient and the therapist. Exercise machines can often take the place of a physical therapist. Posteraro and colleagues[11] reported on a regimen of active robot-assisted training, which avoids shoulder flexor patterns (active shoulder adduction and internal rotation movements) and which showed improved shoulder and elbow motor function in poststroke participants after 3 months of intervention. Overly aggressive passive range of motion can cause injury to soft tissue or bone, resulting in heterotopic bone formation.[12] Spastic patients often have concomitant disuse osteopenia of the involved extremity, and so, an internal rotation contracture makes a person vulnerable to a spiral fracture of the humerus with even gentle manipulation. As a result, it is important for the physical therapist to be aware of a patient's limitations and contour therapy regimens to their abilities without causing iatrogenic harm. Furthermore, it is important to recognize when gains in motion with physical therapy have plateaued and surgery is advisable rather than continued, or more aggressive, manipulation.

Chemodennervation

The 2 most common injection treatments for spasticity are botulinum toxin and phenol. Botulinum toxin is prepared from the *Clostridium botulinum* bacterium and works by binding to presynaptic nerve endings and blocking the release of acetylcholine. This treatment prevents the motor neuron signals from carrying out their excitatory inputs on muscle tissue. This paralytic toxin can target specific muscle groups through carefully placed injections. In a randomized, double-blind trial of 37 poststroke patients with shoulder spasticity, the injection of botulinum toxin was found to improve hygiene and Disability Assessment Scale scores compared with placebo injections of saline.[13] However, the same injections offered no improvement in pain scores for patients. Such results emphasize the importance of a multiple modality approach to nonoperative therapy. In addition, the effects of botulinum toxin injections disappear as new nerve endings grow and reinnervation of specific muscle groups occurs over a few months. Patients who undergo this treatment should be reassessed every 4 to 6 weeks and offered repeat injections if success is met with previous injections.[8]

Phenol is another injection available for the treatment of spasticity. It causes local destruction of peripheral neural tissue. Phenol blocks are especially effective for powerful muscle groups that cause limb deformity and are performed by physicians skilled in ultrasound guidance. A study of 13 hemiplegic patients with shoulder spasticity[14] showed that phenol injection of the subscapular nerves afforded patients immediate improvement in range of motion and pain relief. Similarly, phenol injections of the pectoralis major have been used with success in reducing shoulder spasticity.[15] However, injection of a mixed motor sensory nerve with caustic agents, such as phenol, can cause complex regional pain syndrome[16] or muscle fibrosis and are no longer commonly performed. Intramuscular injections of botulinum toxin do not cause this problem but have the disadvantage of being temporary.

Preoperative Evaluation of the Spastic Shoulder

Physical examination

The preoperative evaluation should begin with an understanding of the patient's level of cognitive impairment and social support system. Both of these variables are important in dictating a patient's ability to comply with postoperative instructions and rehabilitation. Cognitive impairment, learning ability, and short-term memory can often be evaluated by the appropriateness of a patient's response to questions, ability to follow commands, psychological testing, and by direct testing of learning ability in a rehabilitation setting.[17] Patients being considered for surgery have often failed physical therapy, and feedback from the physical therapist and caretakers can be helpful in understanding the patient's cognitive abilities. Aphasia is the loss of ability to communicate properly and can be expressive or receptive. Receptive aphasia is associated with a poor prognosis for rehabilitation, because the patient cannot understand instructions. However, a patient with expressive aphasia may be able to undergo rehabilitation because they are able to understand and follow instructions.[17] Presence of apraxia, an inability to perform a learned movement in the absence of motor impairment, is an important consideration when discussing expectations of surgery.[17] Patients with apraxia should be counseled that the prognosis for improvement in active motor function is poor. It is necessary to understand a patient's social support system, including family and caregivers, because these members can be important in clarifying a patient's active or passive goals of treatment; the social support system is important in the postoperative recovery process.

As noted earlier, patients with spastic shoulders after upper motor neuron injury can either lack all motor control (hemiplegia) or have variable levels of preserved motor control (hemiparesis). In evaluating the spastic shoulder, it becomes crucial to identify the clinical pattern of motor function, characterize the patient's ability to control their muscles, and the influence of stiffness and contractures on both exacerbating symptoms and masking intact motor control. A fixed limb deformity may be caused by severe spasticity or alternatively by soft tissue contracture of muscles, tendons, and ligaments. Differentiating between these 2 causes can be clinically challenging. Like all joints, the glenohumeral joint is traversed by agonist and antagonist muscles that can facilitate movement and stabilize the joint in patients with normally functioning anatomy or can result in patterns of dyssynergy and dysfunction in those with upper motor neuron injury. Through clinical evaluation, the physician can observe asymmetry in form or movement, palpate muscles for tone and spasticity, and assess muscle strength. Along with testing passive range of motion, the ability to actively initiate movement and maintain the arm in space is important to identify clinically. Contractures are common, and the shoulder is often held in an adducted and internally rotated posture. Triceps, biceps, and brachioradialis reflexes should be tested with a reflex hammer to confirm presence of spasticity. Spasticity can be measured by resistance to passive movement and graded by the Ashworth scale.[18,19] With this scale, 0 means no increase in tone (none); 1 means a slight increase in tone, giving a catch when the limb is moved in flexion or extension (mild); 2 means a more marked increase in tone but the limb is easily flexed (moderate); 3 means a considerable increase in muscle tone (passive movement is difficult) (severe); and 4 means the

limb is rigid in flexion or extension (very severe). In cases of inferior glenohumeral subluxation, a sulcus sign is often encountered, and leaving the arm unsupported may be painful for the patient. If a patient's symptoms are relieved by manual reduction of the subluxation, the pain is considered mechanical in nature and potentially amenable to surgical stabilization.

A thorough evaluation of the neurologic status of the limb is important, because patients present with various levels of impaired sensibility. Sensibility to light touch, as well as 2-point discrimination, is an important preoperative consideration. Patients with significant sensory impairments and a lack of protective sensation may be poor candidates for surgical intervention. Proprioception, a patient's understanding of the position of a limb in space, is also important to determine preoperatively. Proprioception can be determined by the up-or-down test at the distal interphalangeal joint.[20] Lack of proprioception does not represent a contraindication to surgery; however, like sensibility, it is not improved by neuro-orthopedic intervention and should be discussed with patients to generate realistic expectations regarding surgical outcomes.[21,22]

Imaging/advanced testing

Radiographs Evaluation of the spastic shoulder should always include plain radiographs (anterior-posterior view, scapular-Y view, and axillary view). Spasticity and contractures that create a rigid adduction deformity may prevent acquisition of an axillary view, and a Velpeau view[23] may be more appropriate. Radiographs are important to rule out subluxation of the humeral head, heterotopic ossification, or joint arthrosis, which can contribute to stiffness. Advanced imaging techniques, such as magnetic resonance imaging or computed tomography, are often unnecessary unless one of the diseases mentioned earlier is present.

Dynamic poly-EMG Historically, clinical examination has been the mainstay of evaluation and decision making for patients who have spastic limb deformities. Clinical assessment, supplemented by instrumented laboratory analysis with dynamic poly-EMG, has helped characterize movement disorders and has been shown to improve the outcomes of treatment.[17,24] In our practice, dynamic poly-EMG is used in cases in which there is preserved motor control and the surgical preference is for selective tendon lengthening rather than tendon/muscle releases.[22] As noted earlier, in patients who show volitional control in the limb, the major clinical question is whether the limited shoulder motion is a result of absent or weak muscle activity or the result of inappropriate activity (dyssynergy or cocontraction) of the antagonist muscles.[22] For example, an inability to actively externally rotate the shoulder may be a result of weakness in the shoulder external rotators or a problem with dyssynergic activity of the internal rotators during attempted external rotation. In this situation, dynamic poly-EMG may reveal a normally active posterior deltoid during attempted external rotation but dyssynergic activity of the pectoralis major and latissimus dorsi (**Fig. 1**). As a result, a hypothesis can be generated that lengthening, or effectively weakening, the pectoralis major and latissimus dorsi could improve active external rotation.

During dynamic poly-EMG testing, sensors are placed on multiple muscles, and information is recorded while the person is moving. EMG recordings and movement tracings are often obtained from specific muscles, including the lateral head of the triceps, pectoralis major, teres major, and latissimus dorsi during passive motion by the examiner and attempted active motion by the patient. Poly-EMG data can interpret whether effort-related initiation, modulation, and termination of voluntary activity are present in a given muscle.[25] Poly-EMG can also identify dyssynergy or cocontraction, defined as inappropriate muscle firing during antagonist motion. If a patient has preserved motor control in agonist muscle groups, weakening antagonist muscles that are dyssynergic by fractional lengthening can result in improved active function.

Selective neurologic blockade Selective neurologic blocks can be used as an adjunct to the diagnostic evaluation and preoperative planning of patients with spastic shoulder disease. When cocontraction is present in a muscle with appropriate agonist activity, it is thought that removing the dyssynergic activity results in improved volitional motion. However, if contractures are too rigid, fractional lengthening may be ineffective in sufficiently tempering the effects of the antagonist muscle and a tendon release may be necessary. Although EMG may show motor function in the posterior deltoid and dyssynergic activity in the internal rotators during attempted external rotation, fractional lengthening may not yield a substantial gain in external rotation if severe contractures of the musculotendinous units of the pectoralis major and latissimus dorsi are present. In cases in which there is a question regarding whether contractures are too rigid to result in substantial recovery of active motor function with fractional lengthening, selective bupivacaine blocks of dyssynergic muscles can be used to temporarily relieve spasticity and to show improvement in motion. Deformity caused by spasticity improves after a nerve block, but deformity caused by a fixed contracture does not change after administration of local anesthetic.[17]

Surgical Treatment of the Spastic Shoulder

Shoulder tenotomies

Shoulder tenotomies are appropriate to consider in patients with upper motor neuron disease without voluntary control of their limb (hemiplegia) (**Fig. 2**). These contractures can cause pain and interfere with axillary hygiene and activities of daily living. Although the limb may be functionless, improving the position of the arm may improve the function of the patient by making self-care and caregiver-assisted care, such as dressing and axillary hygiene, easier. For example, making a shoulder passively flexible can result in a hemiplegic patient becoming independent in upper

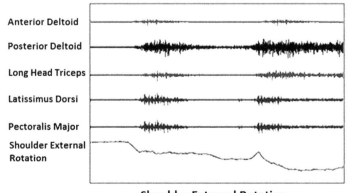

Shoulder External Rotation

Fig. 1. Normally active posterior deltoid during attempted external rotation but dyssynergic activity of the pectoralis major, latissimus dorsi, and to a lesser extent, the long head of the triceps.

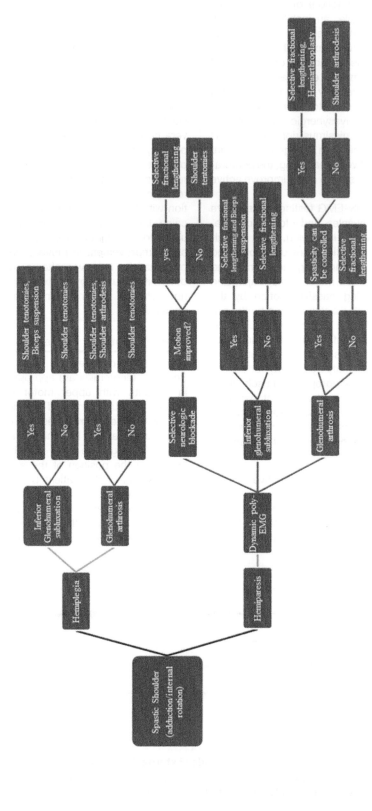

Fig. 2. Algorithm for surgical decision making and treatment of the spastic shoulder.

body dressing. Previous EMG studies have shown that the adduction and internal rotation deformity is caused by spasticity and myostatic contracture of the pectoralis major, latissimus dorsi, teres major, and subscapularis muscles.[25] Unless there is a question regarding the presence or absence of active motor control on preoperative physical examination, we do not routinely obtain dynamic poly-EMGs of patients without preserved motor control. In the nonfunctional extremity, all 4 involved muscles should be released.[21]

This technique has been previously described.[21] The patient is positioned supine on a hand table with a bolster under the scapula, or in a modified (30°–45°) beach chair position. A full beach chair is avoided because of commonly encountered medical comorbidities in these patients and concern for adequate cerebral perfusion. A 7-cm incision is made in the anterior portion of the shoulder approximating the deltopectoral interval.[21,25] The cephalic vein is identified and retracted laterally with the deltoid. In the distal portion of the interval, the sternal and clavicular heads of the pectoralis major are identified along the lateral border of the intertubercular groove of the humerus and released. The subscapularis tendon is then identified and carefully tenotomized from the lesser tuberosity, taking care to avoid violating the underlying glenohumeral joint capsule. Dissection is then carried deep and medial. The brachial plexus and axillary artery are retracted carefully. The tendon insertion of the latissimus dorsi is identified just distal to the muscular portion of the subscapularis and medial to the intertubercular groove and is also released from the humerus. The arm can be further externally rotated, and the teres major tendon can be identified deep to the latissimus dorsi insertion and also released. A drain is placed in the deep wound before closure to minimize postoperative hematoma.

Postoperative rehabilitation is critical to maintain correction and decrease the possibility of recurrence. The limb should be placed in slight abduction and external rotation. This position can often be simply achieved by patients with several pillows placed at the side. Self-assisted passive range-of-motion exercises are started immediately on the first postoperative day, including supine forward elevation, external rotation, and horizontal abduction. In some cases, the skin may be too frail to begin immediate range of motion. In these cases, the patient is immobilized in a favorable position (slight abduction and external rotation) and range of motion is started after 2 to 3 weeks.

We studied 36 hemiplegic patients who underwent releases of the pectoralis major, subscapularis, latissimus dorsi, and teres major for adduction and internal rotation contractures after upper motor neuron injury.[21] Preoperative indications for surgery were pain, and difficulty with dressing, skin care, or hygiene. Average follow-up was 14.3 months. Although 53% of patients reported preoperative pain, all noted improved pain relief, with 95% being pain free at final follow-up. Patients showed significant improvements in passive range of motion in extension (20°–34°), flexion (49°–125°), abduction (43°–105°), and external rotation (1°–45°). All patients noted improvement in hygiene, skin care, and caregiver-assisted dressing, and 97% were satisfied with the outcome of surgery. There were 2 hematomas that resolved without intervention, and no postoperative infections or neurovascular injuries.

Shoulder fractional lengthenings

Hemiparetic patients with selective motor control (hemiparesis) have the potential to achieve a greater degree of function, because some level of active motion is preserved. These patients often show a flexion synergy pattern, in which the spastic flexors and internal rotators are mass activated when the patient attempts to perform a functional task. In this population, functional limitations can be a result of either contracted muscles or abnormal patterns of activation and spasticity. The clinical question is often whether the lack of function observed is a result of weakness of agonist muscles or inappropriate activation of antagonist muscles. As noted earlier, dyssynergy or cocontraction in antagonist muscle groups may be inhibiting functional agonist muscle activity. In theory, if antagonist muscle groups are creating a mass activation pattern that results in loss of function, selectively lengthening these muscles should produce functional improvement. In this subset of patients, we routinely obtain dynamic poly-EMG studies to clarify the clinical picture and to generate a plan for selective tendon fractional lengthening.[22] The most commonly involved muscles are the pectoralis major, latissimus dorsi, teres major, and long head of the triceps, which act in cocontraction with activation of the shoulder flexors during attempted flexion.

This technique has been previously described.[22] The patient may be positioned as described in the shoulder tenotomy technique. Again, a standard deltopectoral incision is made. The goal of fractional lengthening is to cut the tendon at the musculotendinous junction as it overlaps the muscle. When performed in this manner, the tendon lengthens based on the amount of spasticity in the limb. The undersurface of the pectoralis major must be exposed, because the tendinous portion is found on the undersurface of the muscle.

Enough proximal exposure must be available to identify the musculotendinous portions of the latissimus dorsi, teres major, and long head of the triceps in the deep portion of the wound near the medial humerus. The triceps tendon may be found deep to and superior to the tendinous portions of the latissimus dorsi and teres major. The brachial plexus must be retracted medially. Meticulous hemostasis must be obtained, followed by placement of a drain.

No immobilization is generally required. When the patient is resting, a pillow is recommended at the side to allow the tendon to heal in a lengthened position and to prevent recurrence. Active and active-assistive range of motion exercises are initiated on the first postoperative day. Resistive exercises and passive stretching are avoided for 3 to 4 weeks to avoid rupture of the lengthened muscles.

We reported our experience with 34 hemiparetic patients who underwent selective fractional lengthening for spastic shoulder contractures after upper motor neuron injury.[22] All patients had difficulty with activities of daily living, including skin care, hygiene, and dressing. All patients underwent lengthening of the pectoralis major, latissimus dorsi, and teres major. In addition, 4 patients underwent lengthening of the long head of the triceps based on findings on dynamic poly-EMG. At mean 1 year of follow-up, there were significant improvements in active flexion (59°–116°), abduction (51°–95°), and external rotation (6°–45°). Of patients who had pain preoperatively, 88% were pain free and 92% were satisfied with the outcome of surgery. One patient who did not comply with postoperative instructions experienced a recurrence and did not have pain relief.

Inferior glenohumeral subluxation

After an injury involving a hemisphere of the brain, there is flaccid paralysis contralateral to the involved side. During this period of flaccid paralysis, a subluxation of the glenohumeral joint often occurs. This subluxation is most commonly self-limiting and asymptomatic. During the flaccid paralysis stage and before the onset of spasticity, a sling to support the arm[26] or functional electrical stimulation[27–29] to maintain the glenohumeral joint in a reduced position can be an important means of prophylaxis against persistent subluxation as spasticity develops. In some patients, painful subluxation of the glenohumeral joint and corresponding spasticity persist.[30] If the pain is relieved by manual reduction of the glenohumeral joint, and alleviated by support of the limb in a sling, surgical correction of the subluxation may be considered. The biceps suspension procedure is

our technique of choice for this condition. Dynamic poly-EMG is performed if other sequelae of upper motor neuron disease with preserved motor control are being treated concomitantly. If the biceps suspension procedure is unsuccessful, a shoulder arthrodesis is also a possible surgical treatment option.

The biceps suspension technique has been previously described.[30,31] The patient is positioned supine with the arm resting on a hand table. In general, supine positioning reduces the glenohumeral joint without the need for any proximally directed force. A standard deltopectoral approach is used. Lengthenings or releases of the adductor/internal rotator muscles are performed as dictated by the preoperative plan. The tendon of the long head of the biceps is identified in the intertubercular groove. The biceps tendon is dissected from the groove, but the rotator interval is not violated. The biceps is then cut at its musculotendinous junction, and all muscle fibers are sharply removed from the tendon. A Krackow stitch using a stout suture such as number 2 Fiberwire (Arthrex, Naples, FL) is placed at the distal end of the biceps tendon, tubularizing it. The intertubercular groove is then subperiosteally exposed, and 2 5-mm drill holes, 1 proximal and 1 distal in the groove, are made (approximately 2 cm apart). A curved curette is used to connect the 2 holes, with care not to break the bone bridge between the drill holes. A suture passer or free needle is used to pass the tendon through the drill holes from proximal to distal. Traction is placed on the tendon to reduce the subluxation. The biceps is then sewn to itself with a number 2 Fiberwire. Meticulous hemostasis is obtained, and a deep drain is placed. The repair is protected in a sling for 3 months. Gentle self-assisted passive range of motion can be started on the first postoperative day, but the arm should be supported at all times to prevent strain on the repair.

Our experiences with this procedure have been described in a series of 11 patients at minimum 2-year clinical follow-up.[30] Nine patients had complete reduction of the subluxation on postoperative radiographs; 1 had a partial reduction; and 1 had recurrent subluxation. Nine patients were satisfied with the outcome of surgery. All patients noted a decrease in pain, and 10 patients reported an improvement in the appearance of their shoulder.

Shoulder arthrosis/arthroplasty

The combination of increased tone in the shoulder musculature, contractures, and glenohumeral arthrosis can be a challenging clinical problem. A major clinical question remains whether the patient has preserved motor control. If the patient is hemiplegic and lacks motor control, a shoulder arthrodesis is often the most reliable treatment option for pain relief and repositioning of the limb in space. During fusion, contracture releases can allow for positioning of the limb in an appropriate position for fusion. In general, we place the shoulder in 20° of flexion, 30° of abduction, and 40° of internal rotation. It is critical to provide sufficient abduction to allow for axillary hygiene. No study has specifically evaluated the outcomes of shoulder fusion in patients with upper motor neuron injury. Thin skin and muscle atrophy can lead to postoperative wound complications from prominent hardware, because plates often rest below the skin surface. Skin may require Z-plasty during closure, hardware should be minimized when possible, and local muscle flaps should be considered for particular complex cases.

If the patient is hemiparetic and has some level of preserved motor control, the secondary clinical question is whether spasticity can be controlled sufficiently to allow for stability of a shoulder arthroplasty. The pain of the surgery can often produce increased muscle tone in the acute postoperative setting, thus creating a cycle of pain and spasticity that can put the arthroplasty at risk for instability. As a result, we generally avoid placement of a glenoid implant because of theoretic concern of early loosening and wear from eccentric loading resulting from shoulder spasticity. Hattrup and colleagues[32] described 3 cases of total shoulder arthroplasty in patients with upper motor neuron injury and glenohumeral arthrosis. Although arthroplasty was effective in relieving pain in all 3 patients, 2 patients experienced postoperative subluxation. In their small series, the 1 patient without postoperative subluxation of the glenohumeral joint underwent botulinum toxin injections in muscles selectively chosen after assessment of the patient's dystonic pattern on physical examination. In our experience, patients with preserved active motor control and glenohumeral joint arthrosis can benefit from shoulder hemiarthroplasty, if combined with appropriate treatment of shoulder spasticity.[33] The surgeon should not allow the presence of arthrosis to distract from the standard workup of spasticity. In cases of preserved motor control, a dynamic poly-EMG should be obtained; and if necessary, selective neurogenic blockade can be helpful in fully delineating patterns of spasticity. At the time of arthroplasty, appropriate muscle fractional lengthenings and botulinum injections (ie, deltoid) for muscle groups that cannot be lengthened are important to control postoperative spasticity and joint stability. When inferior glenohumeral joint subluxation is also present, a biceps suspension procedure can be similarly added to the treatment plan of hemiarthroplasty and selective fraction lengthenings.[33]

SUMMARY

The spastic shoulder presents unique diagnostic and treatment challenges to the orthopedic surgeon. The ability to distinguish between hemiplegia and hemiparesis represents the first step in identifying the clinical pattern of motor function. Dynamic poly-EMG and selective nerve blocks can be helpful in tailoring the treatment plan in patients with preserved motor control. When the appropriate treatment strategy is selected, the spastic shoulder can be successfully treated with selective tendon releases, fractional tendon lengthenings, biceps suspension, arthrodesis, or arthroplasty.

REFERENCES

1. Anson CA, Shepherd C. Incidence of secondary complications in spinal cord injury. Int J Rehabil Res 1996;19(1):55–66.
2. Esquenazi A, Albanese A, Chancellor MB, et al. Evidence-based review and assessment of botulinum neurotoxin for the treatment of adult spasticity in the upper motor neuron syndrome. Toxicon 2013;67:115–28.
3. Wedekind C, Lippert-Gruner M. Long-term outcome in severe traumatic brain injury is significantly influenced by brainstem involvement. Brain Inj 2005; 19(9):681–4.
4. Stroke. In Centers for Disease Control and Prevention. Edited, 2012. Available at: http://www.cdc.gov/stroke. Accessed February 11, 2013.
5. Injury prevention & control: Traumatic brain injury. In Centers for Disease Control and Prevention. Edited, 2012. Available at: http://www.cdc.gov/Traumatic BrainInjury. Accessed February 11, 2013.
6. Nielsen JB, Crone C, Hultborn H. The spinal pathophysiology of spasticity–from a basic science point of view. Acta Physiol (Oxf) 2007;189(2):171–80.
7. Gracies JM. Pathophysiology of spastic paresis. I: paresis and soft tissue changes. Muscle Nerve 2005;31(5):535–51.
8. Kheder A, Nair KP. Spasticity: pathophysiology, evaluation and management. Pract Neurol 2012; 12(5):289–98.
9. Tafti MA, Cramer SC, Gupta R. Orthopaedic management of the upper extremity of stroke patients. J Am Acad Orthop Surg 2008;16(8):462–70.
10. Logan LR. Rehabilitation techniques to maximize spasticity management. Top Stroke Rehabil 2011; 18(3):203–11.

11. Posteraro F, Mazzoleni S, Aliboni S, et al. Upper limb spasticity reduction following active training: a robot-mediated study in patients with chronic hemiparesis. J Rehabil Med 2010;42(3):279–81.

12. Cipriano CA, Pill SG, Keenan MA. Heterotopic ossification following traumatic brain injury and spinal cord injury. J Am Acad Orthop Surg 2009;17(11):689–97.

13. Marciniak CM, Harvey RL, Gagnon CM, et al. Does botulinum toxin type A decrease pain and lessen disability in hemiplegic survivors of stroke with shoulder pain and spasticity?: a randomized, double-blind, placebo-controlled trial. Am J Phys Med Rehabil 2012;91(12):1007–19.

14. Hecht JS. Subscapular nerve block in the painful hemiplegic shoulder. Arch Phys Med Rehabil 1992;73(11):1036–9.

15. Botte MJ, Keenan MA. Percutaneous phenol blocks of the pectoralis major muscle to treat spastic deformities. J Hand Surg Am 1988;13(1):147–9.

16. Mailis A, Furlan A. Sympathectomy for neuropathic pain. Cochrane Database Syst Rev 2003;(2):CD002918.

17. Braun RM, Botte MJ. Treatment of shoulder deformity in acquired spasticity. Clin Orthop Relat Res 1999;(368):54–65.

18. Ashworth B. Preliminary trial of carisoprodol in multiple sclerosis. Practitioner 1964;192:540–2.

19. Brashear A, Zafonte R, Corcoran M, et al. Inter- and intrarater reliability of the Ashworth Scale and the Disability Assessment Scale in patients with upper-limb poststroke spasticity. Arch Phys Med Rehabil 2002;83(10):1349–54.

20. Epstein O. Clinical examination. Philadelphia: Mosby/Elsevier; 2008. p. 439.

21. Namdari S, Alosh H, Baldwin K, et al. Shoulder tenotomies to improve passive motion and relieve pain in patients with spastic hemiplegia after upper motor neuron injury. J Shoulder Elbow Surg 2011;20(5):802–6.

22. Namdari S, Alosh H, Baldwin K, et al. Outcomes of tendon fractional lengthenings to improve shoulder function in patients with spastic hemiparesis. J Shoulder Elbow Surg 2012;21(5):691–8.

23. Bloom MH, Obata WG. Diagnosis of posterior dislocation of the shoulder with use of Velpeau axillary and angle-up roentgenographic views. J Bone Joint Surg Am 1967;49(5):943–9.

24. Bhakta BB, Cozens JA, Bamford JM, et al. Use of botulinum toxin in stroke patients with severe upper limb spasticity. J Neurol Neurosurg Psychiatr 1996;61(1):30–5.

25. Pill SG, Keenan MA. Neuro-orthopaedic management of extremity dysfunction in patients with spasticity from upper motor neuron syndromes. In: Brashear A, Mayer NH, editors. Spasticity and other forms of muscle overactivity in the upper motor neuron syndrome: etiology, evaluation, management, and the role of botulinum toxin. New York: WE MOVE; 2008. p. 119–42.

26. Williams R, Taffs L, Minuk T. Evaluation of two support methods for the subluxated shoulder of hemiplegic patients. Phys Ther 1988;68(8):1209–14.

27. Chantraine A, Baribeault A, Uebelhart D, et al. Shoulder pain and dysfunction in hemiplegia: effects of functional electrical stimulation. Arch Phys Med Rehabil 1999;80(3):328–31.

28. Faghri PD, Rodgers MM, Glaser RM, et al. The effects of functional electrical stimulation on shoulder subluxation, arm function recovery, and shoulder pain in hemiplegic stroke patients. Arch Phys Med Rehabil 1994;75(1):73–9.

29. Kobayashi H, Onishi H, Ihashi K, et al. Reduction in subluxation and improved muscle function of the hemiplegic shoulder joint after therapeutic electrical stimulation. J Electromyogr Kinesiol 1999;9(5):327–36.

30. Namdari S, Keenan MA. Outcomes of the biceps suspension procedure for painful inferior glenohumeral subluxation in hemiplegic patients. J Bone Joint Surg Am 2010;92(15):2589–97.

31. Namdari S, Keenan MA. Biceps suspension procedure for treatment of painful inferior glenohumeral subluxation in hemiparetic patients. JBJS Essential Surgical Techniques 2011;01(02):1–10.

32. Hattrup SJ, Cofield RH, Evidente VH, et al. Total shoulder arthroplasty for patients with cerebral palsy. J Shoulder Elbow Surg 2007;16(5):e5–9.

33. Namdari S, Keenan MA. Treatment of glenohumeral arthrosis and inferior shoulder subluxation in an adult with cerebral palsy: a case report. J Bone Joint Surg Am 2011;93(23):e1401–5.

Lateral Epicondylitis
Review of Injection Therapies

Christopher H. Judson, MD, Jennifer Moriatis Wolf, MD*

KEYWORDS

- Lateral epicondylitis • Injection therapies • Placebo

KEY POINTS

- There are several described injection therapies for lateral epicondylitis, but no 1 treatment has been agreed upon. There is a scarcity of large, blinded, uniformly designed randomized trials.
- Botulinum toxin, autologous blood, platelet-rich plasma, hyaluronic acid, and prolotherapy injections have all demonstrated benefit over placebo in studies of varied size and quality.
- Glucocorticoid injections are effective at reducing pain in the short-term; however, they are no different than placebo beyond 8 weeks.
- Polidocanol and glycosaminoglycan injections have not shown any superiority over placebo.

INTRODUCTION

Lateral elbow epicondylitis, also known as tennis elbow, is a common musculoskeletal condition affecting 1% to 3% of the adult population.[1,2] Men and women are equally affected, and presentation most often occurs between the ages of 35 and 50 years.[3] Patients report pain in the lateral elbow and weakened grip, especially with wrist extension. Symptoms can be present, on average, between 6 months and 2 years.[2,4]

Although originally thought to be an inflammatory condition, lateral epicondylitis is perhaps better characterized as a tendinopathy, as there are no inflammatory cells in pathologic specimens.[3,5,6] Alfredson and colleagues[6] found normal levels of PGE-2, an inflammatory marker, in tissue specimens from surgery on patients with lateral epicondylitis. The pathologic findings have instead been described as angiofibroblastic tendinosis, which typically occurs at the origin of the extensor carpi radialis brevis, or less commonly the extensor

digitorum communis.[5] It is hypothesized that the extensor muscle origin at the lateral humeral epicondyle is susceptible to microtrauma from overuse and eccentric loading, and potentially an inadequate vascular supply. Studies have described 2 relatively hypovascular zones in the common extensor origin, at the origin of the lateral epicondyle, and 2 to 3 cm distal along the tendinous insertion.[7] Additionally, Smith and colleagues[8] described a disparity in the vasodilator and vasoconstrictor innervation of the blood vessels in the extensor origin.

TREATMENT

There have been numerous described methods for therapy. Unfortunately, there has been no single agreed-upon treatment for lateral epicondylitis. The most conservative treatment is observational, or a wait-and-see approach. Most patients will report improvement of symptoms by 1 year after initial onset.[9] Activity modification and nonsteroidal

Disclosures: Salary from Journal of Hand Surgery, Elsevier Inc (J.M. Wolf).
Department of Orthopaedic Surgery, University of Connecticut Health Center, 263 Farmington Avenue, Farmington, CT 06030, USA
* Corresponding author.
E-mail address: JMWolf@uchc.edu

orthopedic.theclinics.com

anti-inflammatory drugs (NSAIDs) have been described for symptomatic pain relief. Other conservative treatments include various types of physiotherapy, including exercises, bracing, and ultrasound.

For those patients who do not respond to these treatment modalities, injections have been utilized prior to any surgical treatment. Historical injections included lidocaine, alcohol, and carbolic acid.[3] Currently, the combination of corticosteroids with a local anesthetic is most widely used. However, in recent literature there have been an increasing number of alternate injectable substances described in randomized controlled trials (RCTs). These include botulinum toxin, autologous blood, platelet-rich plasma, hyaluronic acid, polidocanol, glycosaminoglycan, and prolotherapy.

Beyond injections, operative interventions are available for refractory cases. It is estimated that only 4% to 11% of patients will eventually progress to surgical intervention.[4] These include open, percutaneous, or arthroscopic release of the extensor origin, debridement of the extensor origin, denervation of the lateral epicondyle, and anconeus rotation.[4] This article reviews the different types of injection therapies for lateral epicondylitis described in the literature.

TYPES OF INJECTIONS
Glucocorticoids

Glucocorticoid injections have a long history in the treatment of lateral epicondylitis, with descriptions of their use as early as the 1950s.[10] Originally, when lateral epicondylitis was believed to be an inflammatory process, steroid injections were thought to act as a local anti-inflammatory modality. However, as the understanding of the pathology of lateral epicondylitis has evolved, so have the explanations for the beneficial effects of steroid injections. Although there are few inflammatory cells present in the affected tissue, studies have shown an increase in the levels of substance P, or neurokinin-1, receptors in patients suffering from lateral epicondylitis.[11] This demonstrates a possible neurogenic cause for pain in lateral epicondylitis. Corticosteroids have been shown to reduce substance P levels in other parts of the body, suggesting that steroid injections may provide relief for pain of a neurogenic origin in lateral epicondylitis.[4,12]

Many different steroids have been utilized as injection therapies for lateral epicondylitis. Price and colleagues[13] compared hydrocortisone with 2 different doses of triamcinolone and found both 10 mg and 20 mg doses of triamcinolone to be

superior to hydrocortisone in the first 8 weeks, with no differences beyond this time point.

There have been numerous randomized trials comparing steroid injections with local anesthetic or saline injections, as well as with NSAIDs, physiotherapy, and a wait-and-see protocol. Overall, most studies have shown that in the acute follow-up time period, patients receiving steroid injections have improved Visual Analog Scale (VAS) pain scores and functional scores during the first 2 to 6 weeks after injection.[9,14] Other studies, however, found no significant difference even in the short term between steroid injections and placebo injections.[15,16] Lindenhovius and colleagues[15] performed a double-blind RCT of 64 patients treated with steroid or lidocaine and found no significant difference in disabilities of the arm, shoulder, and hand (DASH) or pain scores at 1 or 6 months follow-up. In another double-blind RCT comparing steroid with bupivacaine in 39 subjects, Newcomer and colleagues[16] found no significant differences in outcomes from 8 weeks to 6 months.

In the longer term, steroid injections may even be harmful in the treatment of lateral epicondylitis. Smidt and colleagues[9] performed an RCT with long-term follow-up at 1 year of 185 patients, comparing corticosteroid injections with physiotherapy (PT) and a wait-and-see strategy. They defined success as patients rating themselves as completely recovered or much improved. Although corticosteroids performed better than PT and the wait-and-see groups at 6 weeks (92% vs 47% and 32% success, respectively), these patients were worse at 52 weeks (69% vs 91% and 83% success, respectively).[9] The authors hypothesize that steroid injections worsen long-term results by either weakening the tendon or by allowing patients to further aggravate their tendinosis initially by relieving pain in the short term.

Steroid injections are not without risks. In Gaujoux-Viala's meta-analysis of 744 patients receiving injections for shoulder or elbow tendonitis, 10.7% of patients had transient pain after injection, and 4.0% of patients had skin atrophy or depigmentation.[17] No tendon ruptures or infections were reported in this large study group, indicating that although these have been reported in the literature after Achilles tendon injections, their occurrence is exceedingly rare.[17-19]

Overall, steroid injections have a long track record in the treatment of lateral epicondylitis and have been shown to have a beneficial effect on pain in the short term, averaging 6 weeks for many patients. However, there is no evidence that patients do any better with corticosteroid injections than with no treatment beyond 6 to 8 weeks, and in some studies, patients receiving steroid injections have inferior long-term outcomes compared with controls.

Botulinum Toxin

Botulinum toxin A is a presynaptic acetylcholine blocker that has the ability to cause a palsy of skeletal muscle.[4] Botulinum toxin is theorized to help healing in lateral epicondylitis by causing a reversible partial paralysis of the wrist extensors that can last 2 to 4 months.[20] This in turn avoids microtrauma to the tendon and allows the pathologic tissue to heal.[4,21] Botulinum toxin A was first described in the treatment of lateral epicondylitis in 1997 by Morre and colleagues.[22] Since then, several RCTs have shown promising results for botulinum toxin for tennis elbow.

Wong and colleagues[20] (2005) evaluated 60 patients who received a blinded injection of botulinum toxin or placebo. Patients in the botulinum toxin group had significantly lower VAS pain scores at 4 and 12 weeks ($P = .006$). Espandar and colleagues[23] in 2010 saw similar reductions in pain from 4 to 16 weeks, with 100% follow-up. This study used anatomic measurement to guide injection placement. In the largest RCT evaluating botulinum toxin, Placzek and colleagues[21] (2007) compared botulinum toxin and placebo in 130 patients in a multicenter double-blind RCT. Patients in the treatment group showed significantly improved VAS and clinical pain scores at 6, 12, and 18 weeks after injection compared with controls ($P = .001$). There were no significant differences in grip strength.

However, not all trials have shown positive results for botulinum toxin. In 2005, Hayton and colleagues[24] stratified 40 patients into botulinum toxin and placebo groups. They found no difference between the groups at 3 months with regard to pain, grip strength, or quality of life. Lin and colleagues[25] (2010) compared botulinum toxin with corticosteroid injection at 4, 8, and 12 weeks in a small double-blinded RCT of 19 elbows. They found significantly decreased pain scores in the steroid group at 4 weeks compared with botulinum toxin, but no difference in VAS pain scores at 8 and 12 weeks. Grip strength was consistently higher in the corticosteroid-treated group.

The major adverse effect seen with botulinum toxin injection is finger and wrist extensor weakness. Wong and colleagues[20] found a 13% incidence of mild paresis in the fingers at 4 weeks after injection. Placzek and colleagues[21] showed no difference in grip strength, but significantly decreased strength in third finger extension, lasting from 2 to 14 weeks ($P = .001–.007$). Espandar and colleagues[23] observed similar weakness of third and fourth finger extension in almost all patients. Wong and Hayton reported that this weakness was not tolerated by a small percentage of patients whose work required intricate hand movements.[20,24]

Randomized trials of botulinum toxin injection for tennis elbow have shown promising results in relieving pain, at the expense of weakness in the finger extensors. However, these results have not been shared by all studies, and no RCTs have evaluated patients beyond 4 months, so longer-term follow-up is needed.

Autologous Blood

Autologous blood injection for the treatment of lateral epicondylitis was first described by Edwards and Calandruccio.[26] The authors noted that techniques such as forceful closed manipulation, traumatic injection, and percutaneous release resulted in improved outcomes for patients, and theorized that this was due to bleeding at the extensor origin following the trauma. This bleeding would then stimulate an inflammatory cascade to begin a healing response for the tendinopathy. They proposed that autologous blood injection, specifically composed of 2 to 3 mL of autologous blood combined with lidocaine, would deliver the cellular and humoral mediators to the elbow for a similar healing process.

In their case series of 28 patients with lateral epicondylitis symptoms present for 6 or more months who had failed conservative therapy, Edwards and Calandruccio found that after receiving 1 to 3 autologous blood injections, pain scores and Nirschl stages decreased at an average follow-up of 9.5 months.[26] Overall, they found 79% relief of pain following autologous blood injections.

There have been several RCTs evaluating autologous blood injections for lateral epicondylitis, although only 1 study with comparison to a placebo injection. Wolf and colleagues[27] performed an RCT of 28 patients comparing autologous blood, corticosteroid, and a saline injection. The study was double-blinded, and patients were evaluated at 2 weeks, 2 months, and 6 months after injection with VAS, DASH, and the patient-related forearm evaluation. Although all of these outcomes demonstrated improvement from baseline in each group, there were no significant differences in any of the groups.

In 2010, Ozturan compared autologous blood injection to both corticosteroid injection and extracorporeal shock wave therapy in a 3-armed randomized trial of 60 patients.[28] Although corticosteroid treatment showed the best outcomes at 4 weeks, success rates at 1 year were greatest for the autologous blood (83%) and extracorporeal shock wave therapy (90%) groups, compared with only 50% for the corticosteroid group. Kazemi directly compared autologous blood with corticosteroid injections in a short-term RCT of 60 patients.[29] At 8 weeks, autologous blood was significantly more effective at decreasing pain scores and increasing quick DASH scores.

There have been few adverse effects demonstrated from autologous blood injections. Most commonly, authors have cited the pain after injection as the most difficult for patients. Ozturan described 89% of patients having no more pain after 2 days, and the remaining 11% of patients had pain from 4 to 6 days.[28] Additionally, 21% of patients had elbow erythema; 16% had swelling, and 21% had nausea. Wolf and colleagues[27] and Kazemi and colleagues[29] described no adverse effects.

Autologous blood injections offer numerous factors to stimulate a healing cascade in the degenerative tendinous origin, and studies have shown beneficial effects for patients receiving these injections in the short and long term, especially compared with steroid injections. Although the literature has not definitively shown any benefit compared with placebo in small studies, this may warrant further investigation.

Platelet-rich Plasma

Autologous platelet-rich plasma (PRP) is a concentrated source of platelets and platelet-derived growth factors that has been used in numerous medical fields. PRP is theorized to enhance the healing of wounds, bone, and tendons through release of specific growth factors upon platelet activation.[30] For lateral epicondylitis, the reasoning for use is similar to that of autologous blood injections, but proponents of PRP laud the increased concentration of platelets and therefore platelet-derived growth factors.[30] PRP has been used for various musculoskeletal diagnoses, and Mishra and Pavelko[31] were the first to study its efficacy in lateral epicondylitis treatment.

PRP is prepared by drawing up 30 to 60 cc of blood from the patient and using a US Food and Drug Administration (FDA)-approved blood separation device to centrifuge the blood for 15 minutes to isolate PRP.[30] This produces 3 to 6 mL of PRP, which can be combined with 1 to 2 mL of local anesthetic for injection.

Mishra and Pavelko[31] treated 20 patients with chronic lateral epicondylitis with PRP in an unblinded prospective study. They found that patients who received PRP injections had significantly

better VAS scores at 8 weeks than placebo. At final follow-up of 1 to 3 years, 93% of patients had reduction in VAS pain scores.

There have been few RCTs evaluating PRP in the treatment of tennis elbow. Peerbooms and colleagues[32] evaluated 100 patients in a double-blind randomized trial comparing PRP with corticosteroid injection.[32,33] The authors defined successful treatment as greater than 25% reduction in VAS score with no reintervention. They found that although the corticosteroid group showed slightly more improvement at 4 weeks, VAS and DASH scores were significantly better for the PRP group at 26 and 52 weeks ($P<.001$ and $P = .005$). Overall, 73% of the PRP group versus 49% the corticosteroid group had successful outcomes. In a 2-year follow-up study, the authors found that 81% of PRP patients met their definition of success as opposed to 40% of the corticosteroid group.[33]

Krogh and colleagues[34] compared PRP with corticosteroid and placebo injections in 60 patients in a randomized, double-blind trial. Corticosteroids showed improved pain relief at 1 month compared with PRP and placebo. However, at 3 months follow-up, there were no significant differences between the groups.

Creaney and colleagues[35] and Thanasas and colleagues[36] both compared PRP with autologous blood injections in RCTs of 28 and 150 patients, respectively, who had failed first-line therapy for lateral epicondylitis. Creaney and colleagues[35] defined success as a 25-point reduction in the patient-related tennis elbow evaluation. They found 66% success for the PRP group and 72% success for the autologous blood group, which was not significantly different. They found that twice as many patients in the autologous blood group (20% vs 10%) sought eventual surgery. Thanasas and colleagues[36] found their PRP group to have significantly better pain improvement than autologous blood at 6 weeks ($P<.05$), but that the differences were not significant beyond this time point.

Regarding the safety of PRP, similar to autologous blood, there are no concerns for immunogenic reactions. Several patients have reported postinjection pain that can last up to 3 to 4 weeks.[32] Thanasas and colleagues[36] found that patients who received PRP had more postinjection pain as compared to autologous blood injections.

PRP has certainly shown benefits in a difficult cohort of patients with chronic lateral epicondylitis who have failed other therapies. Although it has not shown superiority compared with corticosteroids or placebo at 3 months, its superiority to corticosteroids in long-term follow-up was demonstrated in 1 large double-blinded RCT with

2 years follow-up.[33] On the other hand, PRP has not been shown to have a clinical advantage to autologous blood injection thus far in the literature. Therefore, with the current body of evidence, it is difficult to justify the additional expense of preparing PRP compared with autologous blood injections for lateral epicondylitis.

OTHER INJECTIONS
Hyaluronic Acid

Hyaluronic acid is a high-molecular weight glycosaminoglycan found in diverse tissues throughout the body, including within connective tissue. It has been noted to function as an induction agent for early inflammation, as well as an inflammatory mediator.[37,38] Hyaluronic acid has been utilized as an intra-articular viscosupplementation agent for osteoarthritis, and has been proven to be relatively safe in this application. Its use was expanded to include soft tissues when Petrella and colleagues[37] demonstrated its safety and success in the treatment of acute ankle sprains.

Petrella and colleagues[38] performed an RCT comparing hyaluronic acid injections with placebo in 331 racquet sport athletes with tennis elbow. The study was blinded to patients but not to the physicians or those collecting data. Two injections of 1.2 mL of 1% sodium hyaluronic acid and placebo were given 1 week apart, and outcomes were measured at 1 and 2 weeks, as well as at 1, 3, and 12 months. Patients treated with hyaluronic acid had a significantly lower VAS pain score and global assessment of elbow injury. Patients' grip strength and satisfaction were significantly improved versus the control from 1 month to 1 year after injection ($P<.01$ and $P<.05$). Eighty-nine percent of these athletes were able to return to pain-free sport in the hyaluronic acid group at an average of 18 days; however, no one in the control group was able to perform this feat.

Adverse events were rare in this study with an equivalent number of patients reporting pain after receiving hyaluronic acid as those receiving saline.[38] No other adverse events were reported.

Overall, hyaluronic acid has been shown to be safe and effective in 1 large, RCT for use in lateral epicondylitis versus placebo in the time frame of 1 to 12 months. The reason for its effectiveness has yet to be determined; 1 hypothesis would be that it induces an inflammatory healing response. The expense of this treatment must be considered in the analysis and cost evaluation of its use. Additional RCTs would be helpful in determining if consistent results can be obtained for determining a more definitive role in lateral epicondylitis injection therapy.

Polidocanol

Polidocanol is a local anesthetic, as well as a sclerosant, that has also been used in the treatment of varicose veins.[39] Its use in lateral epicondylitis therapy was first studied by Zeisig and colleagues[39] with the hypothesis that areas of increased blood flow in the extensor origin seen on ultrasound and color Doppler might be a source of pain. Based on this theory, the authors proposed injecting a sclerosing agent into these increased blood flow areas to decrease pain.

Zeisig and colleagues[39] completed a prospective, randomized double-blind trial comparing injections of polidocanol and lidocaine with epinephrine in 34 patients. All injections were given with ultrasound and color Doppler guidance. At 3 months and 12 months, there were no significant differences in satisfaction, pain, or grip strength between the groups, although all patients had improved pain and grip strength compared with baseline. A crossover analysis was performed allowing those not satisfied at 3 months to receive a polidocanol injection. The study reported no adverse events in either group.

Glycosaminoglycan

Glycosaminoglycans are polysaccharides found throughout the human body. They have been reported to inhibit clotting factor formation as well as catabolic enzymes in connective tissues.[40] With these properties, beneficial effects for the chronic degenerative angiofibromatosis seen in lateral epicondylitis have been proposed. Glycosaminoglycans have been used for other tendinopathies such as Achilles and patellar tendonitis with some benefit.[41]

Akermark and colleagues[40] performed a double-blind trial of 60 patients comparing glycosaminoglycan injections with placebo. Patients in the treatment group demonstrated significantly better reduction of pain scores from 3 to 12 weeks, but no significant difference beyond this point. Treatment failures, although slightly lower for the glycosaminoglycan group, were not significantly different. The incidence of painful injections was almost 3 times higher for glycosaminoglycan injections compared with placebo, and 6% of patients had local hematomas.

Prolotherapy

Prolotherapy, named because of hypothesized proliferative effects on tissue, has been utilized in the treatment of chronic musculoskeletal pain for over a century.[42] There is no standard solution used for all prolotherapy injections, as this is reported to vary based on practitioner and the condition being treated. The basic principle is to give multiple injections of a small amount of irritant or sclerosing solution over the course of many weeks. The most commonly used irritants are hypertonic dextrose, phenol-gylcerine-glucose, and sodium morrhuate.[42] The mechanism of action has not been confirmed for these irritants; however, it is hypothesized that hypertonic dextrose causes nearby cells to rupture from osmosis, while sodium morrhuate can attract inflammatory mediators.[43] A Cochrane review of randomized trials evaluating prolotherapy for lower back pain concluded these therapies were not effective by themselves, but may be effective as adjuvant therapies for low back pain.[44]

One RCT has compared prolotherapy with placebo in the treatment of lateral epicondylitis. Scarpone and colleagues[45] compared prolotherapy with hypertonic dextrose and sodium morrhuate to a saline injection in a prospective, randomized, double-blind trial including 24 patients. Subjects received 3 injections over 8 weeks and were found to have significantly improved pain scores and isometric strength at 16 weeks compared with placebo ($P<.001$). No objective or validated outcomes were measured at 52 weeks, but fewer subjects in the prolotherapy arm (0/10) sought additional treatment as compared with the control arm (4/10). Adverse effects were minimal, with all subjects in the treatment and placebo arms reporting self-limited postinjection pain.[45] Seventeen percent of subjects receiving prolotherapy had local erythema and discomfort at the injection site 1 day after injection, but this resolved with acetaminophen and codeine.

In a randomized double-blind controlled trial by Carayannopoulos and colleagues,[46] 24 patients received either prolotherapy or corticosteroid injections. Both groups showed improvement in VAS and DASH scores by 3 and 6 months; however, there were no differences between the groups.

INJECTION TECHNIQUE

Injection of the lateral epicondyle can be performed in a number of different ways, and no 1 method is agreed upon in the literature. Nonetheless, basic guidelines can be followed. Informed consent should be obtained prior to any injection. Risks of the injection should include risks specific to the injected substance, as well as pain and infection. Sterile technique should be practiced. The location and exact technique for injection may vary between practitioners.

The injection location has been described most commonly at the point of maximum tenderness;

however, studies have used injection points anywhere from just over the bony prominence of the lateral epicondyle to a point one-third of the distance down the forearm in line with the posterior interosseous nerve.[23] Most clinicians will attempt to introduce the needle into the tendon of the pathologic extensor carpi radialis brevis (ECRB), the location of which can be seen in **Fig. 1**.

Different methods have been described for the injection, including a single-shot technique and a peppering technique, where the injection is placed into multiple areas without withdrawing it from the skin. Proponents for the latter technique hypothesize that it may stimulate bleeding and create openings in the degenerative hypovascular tissue, allowing an improved healing response.[47] Okcu and colleagues[47] performed a randomized study using a single corticosteroid injection with either immediate withdrawal of the needle or the attempted creation of a hematoma with 30 to 40 redirections and reinsertions into the bone without removing the needle from the skin. The authors had a high loss to follow-up, but in the 62% of patients followed an average of 21 months, the group that received the peppering technique had significantly better DASH scores ($P = .017$).

Dogramaci and colleagues[48] divided 75 patients into 3 groups in a randomized trial comparing a single-shot steroid injection, lidocaine injection with a peppering technique, and steroid injection with a peppering technique. They found that although all groups showed improvement at 3 weeks and 6 months, the corticosteroid group injected with peppering technique had superior outcomes at 6 months.

In a randomized trial of 120 patients injected via the peppering technique, Altay and colleagues[49] found no difference at 1 year between those injected with local anesthetic versus corticosteroid. However, it is unknown whether corticosteroid

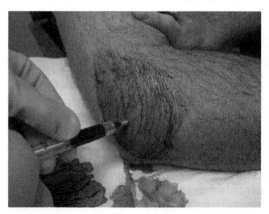

Fig. 1. Patient undergoing autologous blood injection.

would provide a long-term benefit at 1 year, regardless of what injection technique was utilized. In another small randomized trial, Bellapianta and colleagues[50] compared peppered and single injection technique in 19 patients and found no significant differences between the groups.

Zeisig and colleagues[39] also described a technique of ultrasound guidance in order to deposit the injected substance in the area of the tendinous origin with the most degenerative changes. However, there have been no trials comparing ultrasound guidance with blind injections for lateral epicondylitis.

In summary, multiple injection techniques and locations have been described, with little consistent evidence that any 1 technique is better than another. Randomized trials have demonstrated results in favor of and against the peppering technique, although these trials have usually used corticosteroid injections. It may be that a peppering technique is more valuable when injecting a substance such as autologous blood, PRP, or botulinum toxin, in which a larger area of dispersal of growth factors or a wider area of paralysis could be expected. Future trials evaluating injection technique with these substances will be needed.

SUMMARY

Lateral epicondylitis is a common musculoskeletal ailment affecting adults, and there is no definitively agreed upon therapy with consistent results. It is thought to be self-limited, but it often takes extended time to resolve. As with the majority of orthopedic conditions, the first line in the treatment algorithm includes conservative therapies, comprised of activity modification and physiotherapy with braces, exercise, and ultrasound. However, a prolonged symptomatic course is not uncommon with conservative management, and many patients will seek additional treatment.

Injection therapies represent a crucial minimally invasive modality on the spectrum between conservative therapies and surgery. Injections are a reasonable option for patients who fail conservative measures or for those who desire more than conservative treatment and are informed of the risks of injection. The choice of what injection or injections to offer patients, however, is not clearly defined.

Comparing the results of RCTs remains difficult in the lateral epicondylitis literature. Inclusion criteria are often different, with some trials including patients who have had and failed different conservative therapies and even injections. The average disease duration prior to injection can vary highly between trials. Outcome measures are variable, with pain being reported during activity or at rest in different studies. With regards to specific trials addressing injections, different injection techniques and even numbers of injections result in an inconsistency that makes direct comparison difficult.

Krogh and colleagues[51] performed a systematic review and meta-analysis of 17 trials with 1381 patients comparing injection therapies in lateral epicondylitis. Unfortunately, only 3 of these studies had a low risk of bias. They found that glucocorticoid injections were no different than placebo beyond 8 weeks. Botulinum toxin showed a small benefit. Autologous blood and PRP were shown to be superior to placebo, as were prolotherapy and hyaluronic acid. Polidocanol and glycosaminoglycan were comparable to placebo. The largest effect size was seen with hyaluronic acid, followed by prolotherapy, autologous blood, PRP, and botulinum toxin.

Lateral epicondylitis continues to be a difficult problem to treat, with no well-defined treatment. As the understanding of the pathology of lateral epicondylitis has evolved, so have the possible injection therapies. Currently there are a number of new injection therapies with encouraging results. Certainly, large randomized trials with consistent outcome measures and long-term follow-up will aid in the comparison of these injections. At this time, evidence is most supportive for autologous blood, PRP, and botulinum toxin. Glucocorticoids, although historically the mainstay of injection therapy, appear to be effective in the short term only. Cost analysis will be important given the high prices of many of these therapies.

REFERENCES

1. Allander E. Prevalence, incidence, and remission rates of some common rheumatic diseases or syndromes. Scand J Rheumatol 1974;3(3):145–53.
2. Verhaar JA. Tennis elbow. Anatomical, epidemiological and therapeutic aspects. Int Orthop 1994; 18(5):263–7.
3. Faro F, Wolf JM. Lateral epicondylitis: review and current concepts. J Hand Surg Am 2007;32(8): 1271–9.
4. Calfee RP, DaSilva MF, Patel A, et al. Management of lateral epicondylitis: current concepts. J Am Acad Orthop Surg 2008;16(1):19–29.
5. Nirschl RP, Ashman ES. Elbow tendinopathy: tennis elbow. Clin Sports Med 2003;22(4):813–36.
6. Alfredson H, Ljung BO, Thorsen K, et al. In vivo investigation of ECRB tendons with microdialysis technique–no signs of inflammation but high amounts of glutamate in tennis elbow. Acta Orthop Scand 2000;71(5):475–9.

7. Bales CP, Placzek JD, Malone KJ, et al. Microvascular supply of the lateral epicondyle and common extensor origin. J Shoulder Elbow Surg 2007;16(4): 497–501.

8. Smith RW, Papadopolous E, Mani R, et al. Abnormal microvascular responses in a lateral epicondylitis. Br J Rheumatol 1994;33(12):1166–8.

9. Smidt N, van der Windt DA, Assendelft WJ, et al. Corticosteroid injections, physiotherapy, or a wait-and-see policy for lateral epicondylitis: a randomised controlled trial. Lancet 2002;359(9307): 657–62.

10. Baily RA, Brock BH. Hydrocortisone in tennis elbow; a controlled series. Proc R Soc Med 1957; 50(6):389–90.

11. Ljung BO, Alfredson H, Forsgren S. Neurokinin 1-receptors and sensory neuropeptides in tendon insertions at the medial and lateral epicondyles of the humerus. Studies on tennis elbow and medial epicondylalgia. J Orthop Res 2004;22(2):321–7.

12. Callebaut I, Vandewalle E, Hox V, et al. Nasal corticosteroid treatment reduces substance P levels in tear fluid in allergic rhinoconjunctivitis. Ann Allergy Asthma Immunol 2012;109(2):141–6.

13. Price R, Sinclair H, Heinrich I, et al. Local injection treatment of tennis elbow–hydrocortisone, triamcinolone and lignocaine compared. Br J Rheumatol 1991;30(1):39–44.

14. Hay EM, Paterson SM, Lewis M, et al. Pragmatic randomised controlled trial of local corticosteroid injection and naproxen for treatment of lateral epicondylitis of elbow in primary care. BMJ 1999; 319(7215):964–8.

15. Lindenhovius A, Henket M, Gilligan BP, et al. Injection of dexamethasone versus placebo for lateral elbow pain: a prospective, double-blind, randomized clinical trial. J Hand Surg Am 2008;33(6): 909–19.

16. Newcomer KL, Laskowski ER, Idank DM, et al. Corticosteroid injection in early treatment of lateral epicondylitis. Clin J Sport Med 2001;11(4):214–22.

17. Gaujoux-Viala C, Dougados M, Gossec L. Efficacy and safety of steroid injections for shoulder and elbow tendonitis: a meta-analysis of randomised controlled trials. Ann Rheum Dis 2009;68(12): 1843–9.

18. Bedi SS, Ellis W. Spontaneous rupture of the calcaneal tendon in rheumatoid arthritis after local steroid injection. Ann Rheum Dis 1970;29(5): 494–5.

19. Cowan MA, Alexander S. Simultaneous bilateral rupture of Achilles tendons due to triamcinolone. Br Med J 1961;1(5240):1658.

20. Wong SM, Hui AC, Tong PY, et al. Treatment of lateral epicondylitis with botulinum toxin: a randomized, double-blind, placebo-controlled trial. Ann Intern Med 2005;143(11):793–7.

21. Placzek R, Drescher W, Deuretzbacher G, et al. Treatment of chronic radial epicondylitis with botulinum toxin A. A double-blind, placebo-controlled, randomized multicenter study. J Bone Joint Surg Am 2007;89(2):255–60.

22. Morre HH, Keizer SB, van Os JJ. Treatment of chronic tennis elbow with botulinum toxin. Lancet 1997;349(9067):1746.

23. Espandar R, Heidari P, Rasouli MR, et al. Use of anatomic measurement to guide injection of botulinum toxin for the management of chronic lateral epicondylitis: a randomized controlled trial. CMAJ 2010;182(8):768–73.

24. Hayton MJ, Santini AJ, Hughes PJ, et al. Botulinum toxin injection in the treatment of tennis elbow. A double-blind, randomized, controlled, pilot study. J Bone Joint Surg Am 2005;87(3):503–7.

25. Lin YC, Tu YK, Chen SS, et al. Comparison between botulinum toxin and corticosteroid injection in the treatment of acute and subacute tennis elbow: a prospective, randomized, double-blind, active drug-controlled pilot study. Am J Phys Med Rehabil 2010;89(8):653–9.

26. Edwards SG, Calandruccio JH. Autologous blood injections for refractory lateral epicondylitis. J Hand Surg Am 2003;28(2):272–8.

27. Wolf JM, Ozer K, Scott F, et al. Comparison of autologous blood, corticosteroid, and saline injection in the treatment of lateral epicondylitis: a prospective, randomized, controlled multicenter study. J Hand Surg Am 2011;36(8):1269–72.

28. Ozturan KE, Yucel I, Cakici H, et al. Autologous blood and corticosteroid injection and extracorporeal shock wave therapy in the treatment of lateral epicondylitis. Orthopedics 2010;33(2):84–91.

29. Kazemi M, Azma K, Tavana B, et al. Autologous blood versus corticosteroid local injection in the short-term treatment of lateral elbow tendinopathy: a randomized clinical trial of efficacy. Am J Phys Med Rehabil 2010;89(8):660–7.

30. Sampson S, Gerhardt M, Mandelbaum B. Platelet rich plasma injection grafts for musculoskeletal injuries: a review. Curr Rev Musculoskelet Med 2008;1(3–4):165–74.

31. Mishra A, Pavelko T. Treatment of chronic elbow tendinosis with buffered platelet-rich plasma. Am J Sports Med 2006;34(11):1774–8.

32. Peerbooms JC, Sluimer J, Bruijn DJ, et al. Positive effect of an autologous platelet concentrate in lateral epicondylitis in a double-blind randomized controlled trial: platelet-rich plasma versus corticosteroid injection with a 1-year follow-up. Am J Sports Med 2010;38(2):255–62.

33. Gosens T, Peerbooms JC, van Laar W, et al. Ongoing positive effect of platelet-rich plasma versus corticosteroid injection in lateral epicondylitis: a double-blind randomized controlled trial with

2-year follow-up. Am J Sports Med 2011;39(6): 1200–8.

34. Krogh TP, Fredberg U, Stengaard-Pedersen K, et al. Treatment of lateral epicondylitis with platelet-rich plasma, glucocorticoid, or saline: a randomized, double-blind, placebo-controlled trial. Am J Sports Med 2013;41(3):625–35.

35. Creaney L, Wallace A, Curtis M, et al. Growth factor-based therapies provide additional benefit beyond physical therapy in resistant elbow tendinopathy: a prospective, single-blind, randomised trial of autologous blood injections versus platelet-rich plasma injections. Br J Sports Med 2011;45(12):966–71.

36. Thanasas C, Papadimitriou G, Charalambidis C, et al. Platelet-rich plasma versus autologous whole blood for the treatment of chronic lateral elbow epicondylitis: a randomized controlled clinical trial. Am J Sports Med 2011;39(10):2130–4.

37. Petrella RJ, Petrella MJ, Cogliano A. Periarticular hyaluronic acid in acute ankle sprain. Clin J Sport Med 2007;17(4):251–7.

38. Petrella RJ, Cogliano A, Decaria J, et al. Management of tennis elbow with sodium hyaluronate periarticular injections. Sports Med Arthrosc Rehabil Ther Technol 2010;2:4.

39. Zeisig E, Fahlström M, Ohberg L, et al. Pain relief after intratendinous injections in patients with tennis elbow: results of a randomised study. Br J Sports Med 2008;42(4):267–71.

40. Akermark C, Crone H, Elsasser U, et al. Glycosaminoglycan polysulfate injections in lateral humeral epicondylalgia: a placebo-controlled double-blind trial. Int J Sports Med 1995;16(3):196–200.

41. Sundqvist H, Forsskahl B, Kvist M. A promising novel therapy for Achilles peritendinitis: double-blind comparison of glycosaminoglycan polysulfate and high-dose indomethacin. Int J Sports Med 1987;8(4):298–303.

42. Rabago D, Slattengren A, Zgierska A. Prolotherapy in primary care practice. Prim Care 2010;37(1): 65–80.

43. Rabago D, Best TM, Zgierska AE, et al. A systematic review of four injection therapies for lateral epicondylosis: prolotherapy, polidocanol, whole blood and platelet-rich plasma. Br J Sports Med 2009;43(7):471–81.

44. Dagenais S, Yelland MJ, Del Mar C, et al. Prolotherapy injections for chronic low-back pain. Cochrane Database Syst Rev 2007;(2):CD004059.

45. Scarpone M, Rabago DP, Zgierska A, et al. The efficacy of prolotherapy for lateral epicondylosis: a pilot study. Clin J Sport Med 2008;18(3):248–54.

46. Carayannopoulos A, Borg-Stein J, Sokolof J, et al. Prolotherapy versus corticosteroid injections for the treatment of lateral epicondylosis: a randomized controlled trial. PM R 2011;3(8):706–15.

47. Okçu G, Erkan S, Sentürk M, et al. Evaluation of injection techniques in the treatment of lateral epicondylitis: a prospective randomized clinical trial. Acta Orthop Traumatol Turc 2012;46(1):26–9.

48. Dogramaci Y, Kalaci A, Savaş N, et al. Treatment of lateral epicondilitis using three different local injection modalities: a randomized prospective clinical trial. Arch Orthop Trauma Surg 2009;129(10): 1409–14.

49. Altay T, Gunal I, Ozturk H. Local injection treatment for lateral epicondylitis. Clin Orthop Relat Res 2002;(398):127–30.

50. Bellapianta J, Schwartz F, Lisella J, et al. Randomized prospective evaluation of injection techniques for the treatment of lateral epicondylitis. Orthopedics 2011;34(11):e708–12.

51. Krogh TP, Bartels EM, Ellingsen T, et al. Comparative effectiveness of injection therapies in lateral epicondylitis: a systematic review and network meta-analysis of randomized controlled trials. Am J Sports Med 2012;41(6):1435–46.

Hand Infections

Orrin I. Franko, MD[a], Reid A. Abrams, MD[b],*

KEYWORDS

• Hand infections • Paronychia • Tenosynovitis • Animal bites

KEY POINTS

- Acute hand infections are most commonly caused by *Staphylococcus* spp and *Streptococcus* spp, with an increasing prevalence of methicillin-resistant *Staphylococcus aureus* (MRSA).
- Empiric antibiotic coverage should be withheld until cultures have been obtained. Then it should begin with broad-spectrum treatment directed by the injury environment and mechanism, including strong consideration for coverage of MRSA.
- The cornerstone of surgical treatment includes incision, drainage, debridement, and irrigation followed by daily dressing changes.
- Herpetic whitlow is a viral infection that may mimic acute bacterial infections and typically resolves spontaneously without treatment.
- Flexor tenosynovitis can be diagnosed by the classic signs of fusiform swelling, flexed resting posture, flexor sheath tenderness, and pain with passive extension.
- Septic arthritis of the wrist is typically diagnosed by a joint aspirate white blood cell count greater than 50,000 with 75% polymorphonuclear lymphocytes. It should be treated as soon as possible.
- Bite injuries should always be explored for involvement of an underlying joint or tendon, especially human bite clenched fist injuries over the metacarpal head.
- Necrotizing fasciitis is a life-threatening condition with a mortality rate of 33% that requires emergent surgical debridement.

INTRODUCTION

Infections of the hand are present in all communities, but prevalence is dependent on patient factors such as immunodeficiency (HIV, diabetes, malnutrition) and exposure (occupation, intravenous drug use). The epidemiology of cultured organisms has demonstrated a trend toward increasing rates of methicillin-resistant *Staphylococcus aureus* (MRSA) species, although many infections are polymicrobial or culture-negative.[1] Rapid treatment of these infections with appropriate surgical decompression, debridement, and antibiotics, followed by wound care and hand therapy is required to minimize or prevent lasting sequelae.

MICROBIOLOGY

The most common hand pathogens are *S aureus*, *Streptococcus* spp, and gram-negative species. *Staphylococcus* is the primary organism in 50% to 80% of infections.[2] MRSA species are becoming more prevalent both in community and hospital settings with current rates as high as 78%.[3–7] Industrial and home-acquired infections routinely involve a single gram-positive organism, whereas infections from intravenous drug use, bites, mutilating farm injuries, and those associated with diabetes mellitus are generally polymicrobial with gram-positive, gram-negative, and anaerobic species.[2,8–12] Some of the most

Funding Sources: None.
Conflict of Interest: None.
[a] University of California, San Diego School of Medicine, San Diego, CA, USA; [b] Division of Hand and Microvascular Surgery, Department of Orthopedic Surgery, University of California, San Diego School of Medicine, 200 West Arbor Street 8894, San Diego, CA 92103, USA
* Corresponding author.
E-mail address: raabrams@ucsd.edu

Orthop Clin N Am 44 (2013) 625–634
http://dx.doi.org/10.1016/j.ocl.2013.06.014
0030-5898/13/$ – see front matter © 2013 Elsevier Inc. All rights reserved.

common risk factors for various bacteria include the following:

- MRSA infections are more common in patients with diabetes mellitus, immunocompromised patients, intravenous drug abusers, prisoners, and homeless individuals[5–7]
- Alpha-hemolytic streptococcus and *S aureus* are the most common pathogens in human bite infections[2,9,10]
- *Eikenella corrodens* is isolated in approximately one-third of human bite wounds[2,9]
- *Pasteurella multocida* commonly infects animal bite and scratch wounds[13]
- Necrotizing fasciitis can be caused by group A streptococcus alone or infections can be polymicrobial, involving alpha-hemolytic and beta-hemolytic streptococci, *Staphylococcus* spp, and anaerobes[14]
- Fungi and atypical mycobacterium cause chronic indolent infections.

ANTIBIOTICS

Empiric antibiotics should be administered after performing cultures and Gram stain. Initial antibiotics should be aimed only at suspected organisms because overly broad coverage can select for resistant organisms, is costly, and needlessly exposes patients to side effects. However, increasing rates of MRSA suggest that empiric treatment to cover methicillin-resistant organisms is routinely advised, particularly in urban regions.[1] **Box 1** serves as a guide for the selection of appropriate antibiotic treatment.

Box 1
Antibiotic selection guide

- Cefazolin and penicillin G: intravenous antibiotic coverage for aerobic and anaerobic pathogens in serious infections requiring incision and drainage and hospitalization[15]
- Gentamicin (gram-negative coverage): if intravenous drug abuse is involved or the patient is diabetic[11,15]
- Vancomycin: the drug of choice for cases of methicillin resistant MRSA. Occasionally MRSA is sensitive to Septra, quinolones, tetracyclines, or rifampin; however, rifampin should never be used as a single agent
- Penicillin G (parenteral) or first-generation cephalosporin: empiric coverage for human bites; however, some investigators also recommend aminoglycoside coverage[2,10]

- Piperacillin-tazobactam or ampicillin-sulbactam: good initial coverage for human and animal bites
- High doses penicillin G and aminoglycoside: empiric coverage for necrotizing faciitis[14]
- Clindamycin: used for both anaerobic coverage and, in the case of hemolytic streptococcal infection, to stop toxin production

---

PATIENT FACTORS

Immunosuppressive drugs, acquired AIDS, and diabetes mellitus predispose patients to hand infections. In diabetic hand infection, treatment is often delayed, resolution slowed, repeated debridement is often necessary, and amputations are frequent (20%–63%) to control infection or because of poor function.[11,16] Hand infections in AIDS patients are typically from routine pathogens with atypical presentations and unusually virulent courses. Herpetic lesions are unusually dire and often require antiviral treatment.[17] Diabetes, alcohol, and intravenous drug abuse are risk factors for necrotizing fasciitis.[14]

INCISION AND WOUND MANAGEMENT

Successful management of hand infections predates antibiotics. Incision and drainage remains the basis of treatment. Straight incisions are preferred to avoid flap necrosis. Placement over tendons or neurovascular structures is discouraged. Highly contaminated wounds should be left open and dressed with moist gauze and a splint, immobilizing digits in the intrinsic-plus posture and maintaining the breadth of the first web space. Sometimes repeated debridement is necessary until the wound is clean enough for delayed closure or healing by secondary intention. Wound closure over irrigation or suction drainage is sometimes feasible. Vacuum-assisted closure therapy (also known as negative pressure wound therapy) has transformed the management of large open wounds arising from extensive debridement, such as in necrotizing fasciitis.[18,19] Wounds should be reexamined at 24 to 48 hours. Dressings are changed daily thereafter. Incorporating whirlpools or soaks can help encourage continued drainage. Hand therapy is initiated after inflammation and swelling have begun to resolve, usually before the wound has healed.

MANAGEMENT OF INFECTIONS UNIQUE TO THE HAND
Paronychia

An acute paronychia is an abscess beneath the eponychial fold.[20] It can remain superficial to the nail plate, localized to the radial or ulnar side, or the infection can spread transversely around the entire nail fold. The abscess can track proximally around and deep to the nail plate between the nail and matrix.[20] Manicures, artificial nails, nail biting, or hangnails are common causes. Eponychial swelling, tenderness, erythema, and drainage are characteristic. S aureus is the most common pathogen, followed by Streptococcus pyogenes, Pseudomonas pyocyanea, and Proteus vulgaris.[21]

Although early infections can be treated with oral antibiotics alone, the safest approach is drainage whenever an abscess is present under a digital block. When possible, the nail should be elevated and retained; however, if necessary, it should be removed fully or partially to achieve adequate decompression. An incision across the eponychial fold should be avoided to prevent late nail fold deformity. Soaks can be started immediately and antibiotics should be administered for at least 5 to 7 days, or until resolution of the infection.[22]

If an abscess is not present, nonoperative treatment with antibiotics is performed in conjunction with warm soaks 3 to 4 times per day.[21,23,24] One study examined the use of topical antibiotics in a retrospective fashion and concluded that gentamicin antibiotic alone was superior to a combined steroid-antibiotic ointment.[24] When oral antibiotics are selected, options include amoxicillin with clavulanic acid (Augmentin); however, in areas with high rates of MRSA infections, clindamycin or trimethoprim-sulfamethoxazole (Bactrim, Septra) may be first-line agents.[25–27]

Chronic paronychias can result from excessive exposure to moisture; they are characterized by intermittent periods of inflammation around the eponychium. Eventually there is separation of the nail fold from the underlying nail plate. A cheese-like drainage may exude from beneath the eponychium. Candida albicans, atypical mycobacteria, and gram-negative bacteria have all been implicated.[2,20] Treatment is challenging. The most successful interventions are marsupialization or total nail removal.[20] Adjunctive topical steroid-antifungal ointment (3% Vioform in Mycolog) or oral antifungal medications have been recommended (itraconazole, fluconazole).[20]

Felon

Felons are painful abscesses in the digital pulp, typically following a puncture wound. Tense distension can compromise soft tissue and distal phalanx vascularity. The most common organism is S aureus.[20] Expeditious drainage is necessary to prevent digital pad necrosis, distal phalanx osteomyelitis, or flexor tenosynovitis. Fish-mouth incisions should be avoided because they can compromise pulp vascularity.[20] The point of maximal tenderness guides incision placement with high lateral (made just below the fingernail) and midvolar configurations preferred.[20] Proximal probing can inoculate the flexor sheath and should be avoided. The wound should be dressed with loose gauze packing, which is removed in 24 to 48 hours, followed by warm daily soaks and gauze dressing changes until healing by secondary intention.

Herpetic Whitlow

Herpetic whitlow is a viral infection of the digital tip caused by herpes simplex virus (HSV), resulting from exposure to genital (HSV-2) or oral (HSV-1) lesions. A painful cytolytic infection occurs 2 to 14 days after contact, usually maturing in 14 days. Viral shedding, and the risk of infecting others, persists until lesion epithelialization is complete.[28] As the infection subsides, the virus becomes latent, retreating to the sensory ganglia, avoiding immune clearance.[28] The natural history of the infection results in complete resolution without treatment, usually in 3 weeks.[29] The diagnosis of herpetic whitlow is made based on history and clinical examination. Patients may present with flu-like prodromal symptoms before the lesion appears. The lesion is often preceded with throbbing pain, tingling, or numbness at the lesion site. A single vesicle and/or additional vesicles may coalesce as a single larger bulla with clear vesicular fluids that can be often mistaken for a pustule. Unlike a felon, herpetic whitlow vesicles do not appear on the pulp of the digit. Nonoperative treatment is the best option because, typically, the vesicles unroof, form ulcers, crust, and flake off over 2 to 3 weeks.

The disease demonstrates a bimodal age distribution that usually effects children less than 10 years of age (HSV-1) or young adults between 20 and 30 years (HSV-1 or 2).[30] Although diagnosis is typically by history and physical examination, it can be confirmed with cultures of the vesicular fluid, Tzanck smear, direct fluorescent antibody testing, or a rise in serum antibody titers. Superinfections can follow unnecessary incision and drainage and, for this reason, it is important not to mistake the clear vesicular fluid for pus. Acyclovir, famciclovir, or valacyclovir may benefit patients troubled by frequent recurrences, to abort recurrent infections in patients who have a prodrome, decrease the clinical course in particularly protracted cases, and they are usually necessary to induce remission in patients with AIDS.[28,31]

Flexor Tenosynovitis

Pyogenic flexor tenosynovitis results when a puncture wound inoculates the flexor sheath. The sheath is a mesothelium-lined closed space, extending from the proximal end of the A1 pulley to the distal interphalangeal joint. The thumb sheath is contiguous with the radial bursa and the small finger sheath is contiguous with the ulnar bursa. The radial and ulna bursae extend proximal to the carpal tunnel. In 50% to 80% of individuals, the radial and ulnar bursae communicate (**Fig. 1**).[2] S aureus, Streptococcus spp, and gram-negative organisms are the most common pathogens. Less often, chronic indolent infections, characterized by abundant tenosynovitis, can be caused by fungi and atypical mycobacterium.[32] The classic clinical symptoms of a septic or pyogenic flexor tenosynovitis was described by

Kanavel[33] and includes fusiform swelling, sheath tenderness, flexed resting posture, and pain on passive extension of the involved digit. Typically, patients with a pyogenic flexor tenosynovitis will have most, but not necessarily all, of these signs (**Box 2**).

Box 2
Kanavel signs

- Flexed resting posture of the involved digit
- Flexor sheath tenderness
- Digital fusiform swelling
- Pain on passive digital extension[2]

Treatment should be instituted expeditiously because a delay can result in tendon vascular compromise and necrosis, adhesions, or extension into adjoining deep spaces (**Box 3**).

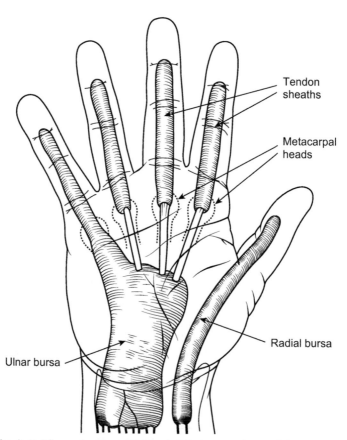

Tendon sheaths

Metacarpal heads

Radial bursa

Ulnar bursa

Fig. 1. Anatomy of the digital flexor sheaths, radial, and ulnar bursae. The small finger sheath is contiguous with the ulnar bursa and the thumb flexor sheath is contiguous with the radial bursa. The proximal extents of the radial and ulnar bursae are the carpal tunnel and Parona space and, in 5% to 80% of persons, the two bursae communicate.

Box 3
Deep space infection sources

- Horseshoe abscess: infection of the thumb flexor sheath can spread through communication of the radial and ulnar bursae extending into the small finger sheath
- Parona space: extensive proximal spread from any digit can lead to involvement of Parona space
- Thenar space: proximal spread from the index finger flexor sheath can cause infection of the thenar space
- Midpalmar space: proximal extension from the long or ring finger sheaths

---

Early infections (within 24 hours) can be treated with observation, elevation, splinting, and intravenous antibiotics.[2,34] Surgical drainage is prudent if there is no improvement within 24 hours or if initial presentation is delayed 24 hours or more beyond the onset of symptoms. A popular treatment method is limited incisions at the proximal and distal ends of the flexor sheath, catheter insertion into one end, and either continuous or intermittent through-and-through irrigation. Extravasation is common with this technique probably due to sheath erosions or inaccurate catheter placement resulting in digital swelling and stiffness. This can be avoided by adding a midlateral incision, which facilitates catheter placement and better drainage, especially when the infection consists of viscous purulent material. In digits compromised by infection, zigzag Bruner incisions should be avoided to prevent flap tip necrosis and poor tendon coverage.

Recommended treatment includes a proximal incision made just proximal to the A1 pulley, near the distal palmar crease. For the midlateral approach, an incision is made from the metacarpophalangeal joint flexion crease to the distal

interphalangeal joint flexion crease. An angiocatheter or No. 5 pediatric feeding tube is placed in the sheath for irrigation. After thorough irrigation, the catheter can be removed, or left for continuous irrigation. After 48 hours, the wet dressing and catheter are removed and digital motion is started. Wounds are left open and they typically heal rapidly by secondary intention.

Deep Space Infections

The deep spaces (**Fig. 2**) of the hand include the thenar, midpalmar, Parona, and the interdigital web spaces.[35] Deep space infections arise from penetrating inoculation or contiguous spread and, rarely, hematogenous seeding. *S aureus,* streptococci and coliforms are the common pathogens.[2]

Thenar space infections can result from contiguous proximal spread from index finger flexor tenosynovitis. Infection can spread around the distal edge of the adductor pollicis and first dorsal interosseous muscles to involve the dorsal first web (or in the interval between the adductor pollicis and first dorsal interosseous) causing a pantaloon-shaped abscess.[36] The first web becomes markedly swollen and the thumb rests in palmar abduction because thenar space volume is largest in this thumb position. Dorsal, palmar, combined dorsal and palmar, and transcommissural[36] incisions have been described, with many surgeons preferring the two-incision approach.[2,32] Incisions paralleling the first web commissure are discouraged to avoid web contracture.

Direct penetration or contiguous spread from the flexor sheaths of the middle two fingers may cause infection of the deep palmar space.[36] The palm becomes markedly tender and swelling obscures the normal concavity. Dorsal hand swelling may be so impressive that the palmar process may be mistaken for a dorsal infection.

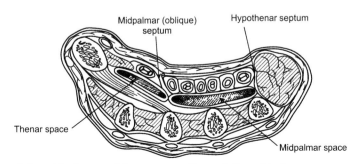

Fig. 2. Cross section of the midpalmar and thenar spaces through the midpalm.

Passive motion of the middle two fingers elicits pain. Transverse or oblique palmar incisions have been routinely used for drainage.

Parona space is bordered by the pronator quadratus, digital flexors, flexor pollicis longus, and flexor carpi ulnaris. Involvement of this space usually results from contiguous spread from the radial or ulnar bursae.[32] Symptoms may include acute carpal tunnel syndrome and pain with finger flexor motion. Management is similar to the other deep space infections, emphasizing wide exposure and thorough drainage, avoiding placement of incisions directly over the flexor tendons and median nerve to avoid desiccation.

Old-fashioned collar buttons were dumb-bell shaped, securing the collar closure by passing each end through overlapping buttonholes. Collar button abscess describes a web space infection that spreads palmarly and dorsally through a narrow fascial hole in the middle. It usually results from contiguous spread of an infected palmar blister, skin fissure, or puncture. Due to adherence of the palmar skin and underlying fascia, instead of spreading peripherally, the infection is forced to expand dorsally through a perforation in the palmar fascia (distal to the bifurcation of the neurovascular bundle) to involve the subcutaneous tissue of the dorsal web.[2,36] The involved web is swollen and the adjacent digits are abducted. A palmar incision can be used with excision of the palmar fascia in the interdigital space, which allows drainage of the palmar and dorsal extension of the infection, or palmar and dorsal incisions can be used.[36] Transverse incisions should be avoided to prevent a web contracture.

After adequate debridement of deep space abscesses, wounds can be loosely approximated over an irrigating catheter. If there is any doubt regarding the adequacy of the drainage or tissue viability, the wound should be left open for daily wet loose gauze packing dressing changes and possibly repeat trips to the operating room.

Septic Arthritis

Hand joint infections are typically caused by penetrating injuries, extension from contiguous infections, or from hematogenous spread. Bacterial toxins, proteolytic enzymes, bactericidal enzymes of synovial and reticuloendothelial origin, and proteoglycanolytic enzymes of cartilaginous origin are released and mediate cartilage destruction.[37] Increased intraarticular pressure impedes synovial perfusion and can

result in cartilage damage, capsular and bony erosion, sinus formation, and osteomyelitis.[37]

The most common bacteria for septic arthritis in the hand include S aureus and beta-hemolytic streptococcus.[2,37] Hemophilus influenza should be considered in unvaccinated young children. Neisseria gonorrhoeae should be considered in sexually active patients with atraumatic septic arthritis.[2,37] S aureus, gram negative rods, anaerobes, polymicrobial infections, positive blood cultures, and osteomyelitis portend a poor outcome.[37]

Examination reveals a painful, swollen, and erythematous joint that assumes the posture that accommodates maximal joint volume. Motion, active or passive, and axial loading is painful. A puncture wound may be identified. Hematogenous spread is suspected in patients with systemic symptoms. Crystalline arthropathies may present similarly. It has been demonstrated that serum white blood cell count, erythrocyte sedimentation rate, and C-reactive protein are not particularly useful for diagnosing a septic joint.[38] If possible, the involved joint should be aspirated and sent for culture, Gram stain, cell count, and crystal analysis (Box 4).

Box 4
Characteristic fluid for joint sepsis

- A friable mucin clot

- A white blood cell count of more than 50,000 of which more than 75% are polymorphonuclear lymphocytes

- A glucose 40 mg less than the fasting blood glucose[2,37]

- Gram stain may not show organisms[37]

Of note, the threshold white blood cell count of 50,000 has been examined more closely in recent years with newer studies suggesting that sensitivity for detecting septic arthritis of the wrist is as low as 47% to 61% and that a value of 17,500 cells may increase sensitivity to 83% with a specificity of 67%.[39,40] Treating joint sepsis with serial aspirations is unreliable in the hand.[37] Definitive incision and drainage evacuates the offending exudate, allows removal of pannus and necrotic debris, and diminishes intraarticular pressure. Studies have demonstrated that septic wrists drained more than 16 hours after presentation had worse results compared with those surgically treated within 10 hours (Box 5).[41]

Postoperatively, the wound can be loosely closed over an irrigation catheter or left open and closed later. The hand is splinted for 24 to 48 hours in a functional position, after which drains and splints are removed and motion is encouraged. Parenteral antibiotics are continued until resolution of local and systemic signs. Thereafter, parenteral or oral antibiotics are given for the duration of 2 to 4 weeks after the initial debridement.[37]

Bites from Humans and Other Animals

A true human bite wound is rare compared with the more typical clenched fist injury, which usually presents with a wound over the metacarpal head. When the metacarpophalangeal joint is examined in extension, the wound may appear innocuous due to retraction of lacerations in the extensor mechanism and joint capsule proximal to the skin laceration. Radiographs may show a fracture, foreign body (eg, a tooth) or osteomyelitis.

Group A streptococcus, S aureus, and E corrodens are the most common strains isolated from human bite wounds.[9] E corrodens is associated with 7% to 29% of human bite infections and is variably susceptible to cephalosporins and not susceptible to penicillinase-resistant penicillins.[9] Bacteroides spp have been the most commonly isolated anaerobes, usually associated with mixed cultures.

Animal bites are most frequently inflicted by dogs, cats, and rodents, often involving the hand.[42] Dog bites account for 80% to 90% of domestic animal bites. Only 2% require hospitalization and they rarely become infected, whereas up to 50% of cat bites may become infected with up to 37% requiring admission.[43–47] P multocida,

Staphylococcus spp, Streptococcus spp, and some anaerobes are the usual pathogens.[42,43] A hallmark of P multocida infection is rapid onset and intense cellulitis, with symptoms occurring sometimes within hours. Empiric antibiotics typically include amoxicillin-clavulanate or penicillin V. Patients who are allergic to penicillin can be treated with alternative antibiotics, including doxycycline, tetracycline, or ciprofloxacin.[48,49]

Acute uninfected bite wounds should be extended, explored and debrided. Of note, cat bites tend to be caused by longer, slender teeth causing puncture wounds that seal off and form abscesses quickly, thus necessitating open debridement. Dog bites, on the other hand, are more likely to cause lacerations that stay open by themselves.[44] If a joint is entered, splinting, elevation, and hospitalization with parenteral antibiotics have been recommended for 48 hours.[10] In the setting of an uninfected wound in which no tendon or joint was injured, debridement and antibiotics did better than debridement alone with no significant difference in outcome if the antibiotics were given intravenously or orally.[50]

Infected bites require hospitalization, debridement, and intravenous antibiotics. Often, repeat debridement at 48 hours is prudent. Warm soaks or whirlpools and wet gauze dressing changes are started 24 to 48 hours after debridement.[10] Generally, tendon repairs are best delayed and wounds are left open to heal by secondary intention.[32]

Necrotizing Fasciitis

Necrotizing fasciitis is a life-threatening and limb-threatening soft tissue infection involving the fascial layer. It occurs primarily, but not exclusively, in the indigent and in abusers of drugs and alcohol.[14] The extremities are the most frequently involved areas of the body. In one study, 63% of cases arose out of intravenous drug abuse.[14] In about half of cases, one organism was isolated and, most frequently, it was group A streptococcus.[14] Otherwise, infections were polymicrobial, involving alpha-hemolytic and beta-hemolytic streptococci, S aureus, and anaerobes.[14,51]

Necrotizing fasciitis presents with a spectrum of clinical findings that includes painful and rapidly advancing cellulitis with tensely swollen and shiny skin. Radiographs may demonstrate gas in the tissue.[52] Bullae and ecchymoses appear within days. Systemic signs may initially be lacking, although a leukocytosis is consistently present.[14] Azotemia in the absence of shock or hypotension is an early tipoff to streptococcal toxic shock syndrome, which frequently accompanies necrotizing fasciitis due to the hemolytic streptococci.

With disease progression, hemodynamic instability in the face of an otherwise trivial-appearing cellulitis should increase suspicion for necrotizing fasciitis. The definitive diagnosis is made at surgery when fibrinous necrotic fascia is found accompanied by liquefaction of the subcutaneous fat and a characteristic foul-smelling thin fluid referred to as dishwater pus (**Fig. 3**). There is usually thrombosis of subcutaneous vessels and, depending on the stage of the disease, the skin may or may not appear viable. The muscle is usually spared. Wide debridement of the involved fascia and necrotic skin is the definitive treatment. Due to the tendency for rapid advancement of the infection, the authors' strategy is to first identify the proximal extent of the involved fascia through exploratory incisions and to start debridement at this level and progress distally. Cultures and Gram stain are taken at the first opportunity and antibiotics are started emergently. Skilled supportive medical care is imperative, often requiring ICU management. Empiric antibiotic treatment should be started early with vancomycin and clindamycin. The addition of clindamycin is important for suppression of the toxins produced by strep and staph species.[52,53]

Mortality has ranged from 8.7% to 33%. The single-most important factor influencing morbidity and mortality is early and adequate debridement.[14] Negative prognostic factors include age more than 50 years, underlying chronic illness, diabetes mellitus, and involvement of the trunk.

Mycobacterial Infections

Seventy-five percent of atypical mycobacterial infections involve the hand.[2,54] *Mycobacteria marinum* is the common organism, usually caused by wounds associated with contaminated swimming pools, fish tanks, piers, boats, fish bites or injuries from fish fins or spines.[54] Infections can be cutaneous (verrucal), subcutaneous (granulomatous), or deep (involving tendon, joint or bursal synovium or bone).[54] Tenosynovial infection is the most frequent deep manifestation. Variation from a typical rheumatoid pattern should alert the clinician. Misdiagnosis often delays appropriate treatment.[54] Skin tests and smears for acid-fast organisms are unreliable.[2,54] When smears are negative, fungal infections, though rare, should be ruled out. Typically, systemic symptoms are absent and white blood cell count and sedimentation rate are normal.[54] Granulomas are noted on histology. Cultures must be incubated in Lowenstein-Jensen media at 30°C for up to 6 to 8 weeks.[54] Superficial infections are usually self-limited unless the lesions are picked at or biopsied without antibiotic coverage, in which case subcutaneous lesions can ensue.[54] A subcutaneous lesion requires debridement and 2 to 6 months of antibiotics and deep lesions require tenosynovectomy, synovectomy, or debridement of the involved bone or joint, with antibiotic duration from 4 to 24 months.[54] In cases of digital flexor tenosynovitis, the tenosynovium is completely removed, preserving the annular pulleys. Wrist dorsal tenosynovial infection is excised through a longitudinal incision and retinacular flaps. An extensile carpal tunnel approach is used to excise involved the flexor tenosynovium at the wrist.[32] Minocycline is the antibiotic of choice. Ethambutol and rifampin are alternatives in case of allergy or organism insensitivity.[2,54]

Fungal Infections

Fungal infections of the upper extremities can be cutaneous, subcutaneous, deep, or systemic.[53] Cutaneous lesions often involve the skin or nails. Keratinophilic fungi colonize glabrous skin (tinea corporis), the interdigital areas and palms (tinea manuum), or nails (onychomycosis), causing a pruritic scaling of the skin or nail deformity. Diagnosis can be made with potassium hydroxide preparations and fungal cultures. Skin infections are treatable with topical agents such as tolnaftate

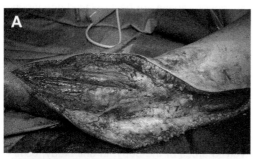
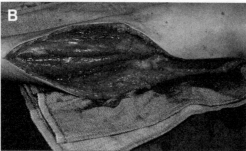

Fig. 3. Intraoperative photos of a patient with necrotizing fasciitis before (*A*) and after (*B*) the involved fascia was excised. The classic and telltale finding is the layer of purulent, thickened, and friable fascia ordinarily not present between the subcutaneous layer and muscle. Note the lack of muscle involvement.

and miconazole. Onychomycosis typically occurs in hands exposed to constant moisture and begins as a minor paronychial infection, progressing to whole nail involvement characterized by thickening, softening, discoloration, and cracking. Psoriatic nail deformities can mimic onychomycosis. Onychomycosis is notoriously resistant to treatment. Nail removal and application of topical agents is less successful than systemic griseofulvin, ketoconizole,[53] fluconazole, or itraconazole. The cure rate ranges from 57% to 80%.[53]

Rare subcutaneous and deep fungal infections are often overlooked in the differential diagnosis of hand infections. Sporotrichosis is a common subcutaneous fungal lesion occurring predominantly in the upper extremities.[53] Subcutaneous implantation is the typical mode of transmission usually by plant handling (rose thorns, cacti, sphagnum moss). Ulceration occurs at the initial puncture site with eventual nodules forming along lymphatics that in turn can ulcerate. Cultures secure the diagnosis because standard stains are rarely helpful. Oral potassium iodide is the treatment of choice.

Deep fungal infections of the hand involve tenosynovium, joints, or bone. They may be caused by pathogenic fungi (histoplasmosis, blastomycosis, coccidioidomycosis) or opportunists (mucormycosis, aspergillosis, Candida). Infections usually enter through the pulmonary route with musculoskeletal infections occurring via hematogenous spread. Treatment requires debridement and antifungals.

ACKNOWLEDGMENTS

To Mia Savoie, MD, quintessential infectious disease clinician, colleague, and teacher. I am grateful for previous and ongoing collaboration in the care of patients with hand infections, and for her assistance with this review article.

REFERENCES

1. Fowler JR, Ilyas AM. Epidemiology of adult acute hand infections at an urban medical center. J Hand Surg Am 2013;38(6):1189–93.
2. Hausman MR, Lisser SP. Hand infections. Orthop Clin North Am 1992;23:171–85.
3. Bach HG, Steffin B, Chhadia AM, et al. Community-associated methicillin-resistant Staphylococcus aureus hand infections in an urban setting. J Hand Surg Am 2007;32(3):380–3.
4. LeBlanc DM, Reece EM, Horton JB, et al. Increasing incidence of methicillin-resistant Staphylococcus aureus in hand infections: a 3-year county hospital experience. Plast Reconstr Surg 2007;119(3):935–40.
5. O'Malley M, Fowler J, Ilyas AM. Community-acquired methicillin-resistant Staphylococcus aureus infections of the hand: prevalence and timeliness of treatment. J Hand Surg Am 2009;34(3):504–8.
6. Salgado CD, Farr BM, Calfee DP. Community-acquired methicillin-resistant Staphylococcus aureus: a meta-analysis of prevalence and risk factors. Clin Infect Dis 2003;36(2):131–9.
7. Wilson PC, Rinker B. The incidence of methicillin-resistant Staphylococcus aureus in community-acquired hand infections. Ann Plast Surg 2009; 62(5):513–6.
8. Fitzgerald RH, Cooney WP, Washington JA, et al. Bacterial colonization of mutilating hand injuries and its treatment. J Hand Surg 1977;2A:85–9.
9. Goldstein EJ, Citron DM, Wield B, et al. Bacteriology of human and animal bite wounds. J Clin Microbiol 1978;8:667–72.
10. Mann RJ, Hoffeld TA, Farmer CB. Human bites of the hand. J Hand Surg Am 1977;2:97–104.
11. Mann RJ, Peacock JM. Hand infections with diabetes mellitus. J Trauma 1977;17:376–80.
12. Reyes FA. Infections secondary to intravenous drug abuse. Hand Clin 1989;5:629–33.
13. Arons MS, Fernando L, Polayesw IM. Pasteurella multocida—the major cause of hand infections following domestic animal bites. J Hand Surg Am 1982;7:47–52.
14. Schecter A, Meyer A, Schecter G, et al. Necrotizing fasciitis of the upper extremity. J Hand Surg Am 1982;7:15–20.
15. Speigel JD, Szabo RM. A protocol for the treatment of severe infections of the hand. J Hand Surg Am 1988;13:254–9.
16. Glass KD. Factors related to the resolution of treated hand infections. J Hand Surg Am 1982;7:338–94.
17. Glickel SZ. Hand infections in patients with acquired immunodeficiency syndrome. J Hand Surg Am 1988;13:770–5.
18. Phelps JR, Fagan R, Pirela-Cruz MA. A case study of negative pressure wound therapy to manage acute necrotizing fasciitis. Ostomy Wound Manage 2006;52(3):54–9.
19. Pirela-Cruz MA, Machen MS, Esquivel D. Management of large soft-tissue wounds with negative pressure therapy-lessons learned from the war zone. J Hand Ther 2008;21(2):196–202 [quiz: 203].
20. Canales FL, Newmeyer WL, Kilgore ES. The treatment of felons and paronychias. Hand Clin 1989; 5:515–23.
21. Rockwell PG. Acute and chronic paronychia. Am Fam Physician 2001;63(6):1113–6.
22. Ritting AW, O'Malley MP, Rodner CM. Acute paronychia. J Hand Surg Am 2012;37(5):1068–70 [quiz page: 1070].

23. Jebson PJ. Infections of the fingertip. Paronychias and felons. Hand Clin 1998;14(4):547–55, viii.

24. Wollina U. Acute paronychia: comparative treatment with topical antibiotic alone or in combination with corticosteroid. J Eur Acad Dermatol Venereol 2001;15(1):82–4.

25. Brook I. Aerobic and anaerobic microbiology of paronychia. Ann Emerg Med 1990;19(9):994–6.

26. Brook I. Paronychia: a mixed infection. Microbiology and management. J Hand Surg Br 1993; 18(3):358–9.

27. Tosti R, Ilyas AM. Empiric antibiotics for acute infections of the hand. J Hand Surg Am 2010; 35(1):125–8.

28. Fowler JR. Viral infections. Hand Clin 1989;5: 613–27.

29. Rubright JH, Shafritz AB. The herpetic whitlow. J Hand Surg Am 2011;36(2):340–2.

30. Gill MJ, Arlette J, Buchan KA. Herpes simplex virus infection of the hand. J Am Acad Dermatol 1990; 22(1):111–6.

31. Laskin OL. Acyclovir and suppression of frequently recurring herpetic whitlow. Ann Intern Med 1985; 102(4):494–5.

32. Siegel DB, Gelberman RH. Infections of the hand. Orthop Clin North Am 1988;19:779–89.

33. Kanavel AB. Infections of the hand, edition 7, Philadelphia: Lea & Febiger; 1943. p. 241–2.

34. Henry M. Septic flexor tenosynovitis. J Hand Surg Am 2011;36(2):322–3.

35. McDonald LS, Bavaro MF, Hofmeister EP, et al. Hand infections. J Hand Surg Am 2011;36(8): 1403–12.

36. Burkhalter WE. Deep space infections. Hand Clin 1989;5:53–9.

37. Freeland AE, Senter BS. Septic arthritis and osteomyelitis. Hand Clin 1989;5:533–52.

38. Margaretten ME, Kohlwes J, Moore D, et al. Does this adult patient have septic arthritis? JAMA 2007;297(13):1478–88.

39. Coutlakis PJ, Roberts WN, Wise CM. Another look at synovial fluid leukocytosis and infection. J Clin Rheumatol 2002;8(2):67–71.

40. Li SF, Cassidy C, Chang C, et al. Diagnostic utility of laboratory tests in septic arthritis. Emerg Med J 2007;24(2):75–7.

41. Rashkoff ES, Burkhalter WE, Mann RJ. Septic arthritis of the wrist. J Bone Joint Surg Am 1983; 65(6):824–8.

42. Jaffe AC. Animal bites. Pediatr Clin North Am 1983; 30:405–13.

43. Aghababian RV, Conte JE. Mammalian bite wounds. Ann Emerg Med 1980;9:79–83.

44. Benson LS, Edwards SL, Schiff AP, et al. Dog and cat bites to the hand: treatment and cost assessment. J Hand Surg Am 2006;31(3):468–73.

45. Goldstein EJ. Bite wounds and infection. Clin Infect Dis 1992;14(3):633–8.

46. Griego RD, Rosen T, Orengo IF, et al. Dog, cat, and human bites: a review. J Am Acad Dermatol 1995; 33(6):1019–29.

47. Kizer KW. Epidemiologic and clinical aspects of animal bite injuries. JACEP 1979;8(4):134–41.

48. Freshwater A. Why your housecat's trite little bite could cause you quite a fright: a study of domestic felines on the occurrence and antibiotic susceptibility of *Pasteurella multocida*. Zoonoses Public Health 2008;55(8–10):507–13.

49. Kwo S, Agarwal JP, Meletiou S. Current treatment of cat bites to the hand and wrist. J Hand Surg Am 2011;36(1):152–3.

50. Zubowica VN, Gravier M. Management of early bites of the hand: a prospective randomized study. Plast Reconstr Surg 1991;88:111–4.

51. Wilkerson R, Paull W, Coville FV. Necrotizing fasciitis. Review of the literature and case report. Clin Orthop Relat Res 1987;216:187–92.

52. Stevens DL, Bisno AL, Chambers HF, et al. Practice guidelines for the diagnosis and management of skin and soft-tissue infections. Clin Infect Dis 2005;41(10):1373–406.

53. Hitchcock TF, Amadio PC. Fungal infections. Hand Clin 1989;5:599–611.

54. Hurst LC, Amadio PC, Badalamente MA, et al. *Mycobacterial marinum* infections of the hand. J Hand Surg Am 1987;12:428–35.

Os Acromiale
A Review and an Introduction of a New Surgical Technique for Management

Peter S. Johnston, MD[a,*], E. Scott Paxton, MD[b],
Victoria Gordon, BA[b], Matthew J. Kraeutler, BS[b],
Joseph A. Abboud, MD[b], Gerald R. Williams, MD[b]

KEYWORDS

- Os acromiale • Acromion • Ossification center • Synchondrosis • Shoulder • Arthroscopy

KEY POINTS

- An os acromiale can be found at the basi-acromion, meta-acromion, meso-acromion, or pre-acromion level, with a meso-acromion as the most common. The os is named for the most anterior portion on the unstable fragment.
- The prevalence of os acromiale is 1% to 30%, with 42% to 61% being bilateral and a higher prevalence in the male and African American population.
- Most patients with an os acromiale can be treated nonoperatively, but multiple surgical procedures have been reported in the treatment of a symptomatic os acromiale, including open or arthroscopic excision of the os fragment, open reduction and internal fixation (ORIF) with or without bone grafting, arthroscopic subacromial decompression with acromioplasty, and arthroscopically assisted reduction-internal fixation.
- Open fragment excision has limited indications and is recommended for symptomatic pre-acromion with a relatively small fragment or as a salvage procedure after a failed ORIF. In the latter scenario, arthroscopic excision is probably a better option, as it has the possible benefit of less periosteal and deltoid attachment injury, possibly lending to better results than open excision.
- ORIF techniques and approaches associated with the most success include those with rigid fixation and preservation of the vascularity of the os acromiale (likely the acromiale branch of the thoracoacromial artery). Even in cases of successful union, patients still may have hardware discomfort requiring hardware removal; however, there are minimal complications that arise from most ORIF cases.
- Resection of the synchondrosis without excision of the entire os acromiale has shown promising results in a small number of patients with short-term follow-up and presents a novel approach to patients with a symptomatic os acromiale.

INTRODUCTION

Os acromiale is a developmental defect that arises from the lack of an osseous union between the ossification centers of the acromion, resulting in a fibrocartilaginous tissue connection. This anatomic abnormality occurs more frequently in the male and black demographic than in the white and female population.[1] It is common that os acromiale is diagnosed through incidental radiographic findings and has been noted that traumatic events can cause the onset of symptoms from a previously asymptomatic os acromiale.[1-5] Surgical treatment is typically recommended only after nonsurgical management

[a] Southern Maryland Orthopaedic and Sports Medicine, 23000 South Moakley Street, Suite 102, Leonardtown, MD 20650, USA; [b] Rothman Institute, Thomas Jefferson University, 925 Chestnut Street, Philadelphia, PA, 19107, USA
* Corresponding author.
E-mail address: pjohnston4@hotmail.com

Orthop Clin N Am 44 (2013) 635–644
http://dx.doi.org/10.1016/j.ocl.2013.06.015
0030-5898/13/$ – see front matter © 2013 Elsevier Inc. All rights reserved.

has failed to relieve symptoms. Procedures commonly used include open or arthroscopic excision of the os fragment,[5,6] open reduction and internal fixation (ORIF) with or without bone grafting,[3,7–12] arthroscopic subacromial decompression with acromioplasty,[9,13–16] and arthroscopically assisted reduction-internal fixation.[17] After reviewing the literature, we report on a case series of 6 patients with a symptomatic meso os acromiale treated with a new technique involving arthroscopic acromioplasty in conjunction with the excision of the acromial nonunion site with creation of a 5-mm to 7-mm gap between the anterior and posterior fragments. We have demonstrated it to be a safe and effective technique in this case series. This arthroscopic partial resection of an os acromiale is considered as an alternative option for treating a symptomatic meso os acromiale.

ANATOMY

There are 4 centers of ossification of the acromion: the basi-acromion, the meta-acromion, the meso-acromion, and the pre-acromion (**Fig. 1**). The basi-acromion typically fuses with the scapular spine by age 12, and all 4 centers should unite by ages 15 to 18. However, some do not have complete ossification until as late as age 25 years.[18] Diagnosis of os acromiale should not be finalized until after this time point.

One of the main functions of the acromion is to provide the origin of the deltoid muscle. The meta-acromion provides the origin of the posterior deltoid muscle, the meso-acromion anchors the middle portion of the deltoid, and the pre-acromion supports the anterior deltoid fibers along with the coracoacromial (CA) ligament.

An os acromiale is named by the most anterior ossification center that did not fuse. A meso-acromion involves the failure of the anterior acromial apophysis (including the pre-acromion and meso-acromion) to unite with the posterior portion of the acromion (including the meta-acromion and the basi-acromion). By definition, a pre-acromion exists when the synchondrosis is anterior to the acromio-clavicular joint, a meso-acromion exists when the sychondrosis extends into the acromio-clavicular joint, a meta-acromion has the synchondrosis posterior to the acromioclavicular joint, and a basi-acromion occurs in the junction of the acromion and spine of the scapula.

PREVALENCE

The first instance of os acromiale was defined by Gruber[19] in 1863, when 3 of 100 cadavers presented with os acromiale involving a distinct synovial joint. Prevalence of os acromiale has been reported in 1% to 30% of the general population, with 41% to 62% of cases presenting with bilateral involvement.[5,20–22] Genetic causes may attribute to the relatively high 30% rate found in the excavated remains of a Philadelphia congregation from the nineteenth century.[23] Sammarco[1] examined 2367 scapulas from the Hamann-Todd Osteological Collection at the Cleveland Museum of Natural History and discovered more prevalence of os acromiale in the black and male population with 13.2% in black individuals compared with 5.8% in white individuals and 8.5% in males compared with 4.9% in females; 8.0% of the skeletons had os acromiale, of which 33.3% were bilateral.[1] No study has yet to determine if os acromiale occurs more frequently in symptomatic patients with shoulder pain than in the general population.[1]

PATHOPHYSIOLOGY

Many os acromiale diagnoses are made incidentally with radiographic imaging. The primary source of shoulder pain is often unrelated to the os acromiale. In symptomatic cases of os acromiale, there are 2 likely etiologies of pain: motion at the nonunion site or an impingement syndrome. Patients often experience localized pain and tenderness at the nonunion site on movement of the unstable fragment if a painful synchondrosis is present. Many times an asymptomatic os becomes symptomatic after a traumatic episode

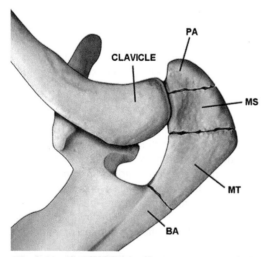

Fig. 1. Diagram of the ossification centers of the acromion. BA, basi-acromion; MS, meso-acromion; MT, meta-acromion; PA, pre-acromion. (*Reprinted from* Frizziero A, Benedetti MG, Creta D, et al. Painful os acromiale: conservative management in a young swimmer athlete. J Sports Sci Med 2012;11:352–6; with permission.)

disrupting the fibrous union. Magnetic resonance imaging (MRI) or bone scan may illustrate the inflammatory response at the nonunion site.[12,13,24,25] Alternatively, the subacromial space maybe reduced due to flexion of the anterior fragment with deltoid contraction and elevation of the arm. Symptoms of external impingement are produced as a result of this decrease in the subacromial space with this dynamic process. The presence of a meso-acromion has been associated with rotator cuff pathology, ranging from tendonitis to full-thickness tears of the rotator cuff.[5,6,18,20–22,26–31]

NONSURGICAL MANAGEMENT

Nonsurgical treatment for a patient who first presents with an isolated symptomatic os acromiale is generally recommended as the initial approach. Physical therapy, in conjunction with nonsteroidal anti-inflammatory drugs, is prescribed similar to a typical impingement treatment protocol. Subacromial corticosteroid injections are also widely used to relieve symptoms and may delay or eliminate the need for surgical intervention. Full-thickness rotator cuff tears have been reported to be associated with an os acromiale as often as 50% of the time; therefore, surgery may be recommended earlier for these patients than our typical patients with external impingement without an os acromiale.[12]

SURGICAL MANAGEMENT

Surgical treatment typically occurs once all nonsurgical means have been exhausted. Multiple surgical procedures have been reported in the treatment of an os acromiale, including open or arthroscopic excision of the os fragment, ORIF with or without bone grafting, arthroscopic subacromial decompression with acromioplasty, and arthroscopically assisted reduction-internal fixation. Depending on the case, certain techniques may be more effective than others; however, each has its benefits and disadvantages. In general, management techniques that address the os acromiale itself (fragment excision or ORIF) are used only when the nonunion site is tender and specifically a cause of pain. Otherwise, attention is focused only on managing the concomitant pathology (impingement or rotator cuff tear) and the os acromiale is ignored.

Fragment Excision

Open fragment excision has had mixed results due to deltoid weakness and dysfunction postoperatively. Mudge and colleagues[6] had 8 patients with rotator cuff tears associated with an os acromiale. Six underwent fragment excision and rotator cuff repair, including suturing of the deltoid to the acromion. Four had excellent results, but the other 2 had poor results.

Armengol and colleagues[32] had a case series of 41 patients with an os acromiale in conjunction with rotator cuff tears. Five patients had an open fragment excision, but all 5 had poor results. Warner and colleagues[12] had 3 patients who underwent fragment excision and only 1 had satisfactory results. The other 2 patients with poor results had meso-acromion fragment excision with lingering weakness and pain. The successful case involved resection of a pre-acromion.

Open fragment excision has limited indications and is recommended for symptomatic pre-acromion with a relatively small fragment or as a salvage procedure after a failed ORIF. In the latter scenario, arthroscopic excision is probably a better option.

In a recent case series reporting on deltoid function after arthroscopic excision of either pre-acromion or meso-acromion, Campbell and colleagues[33] demonstrated no decrease in deltoid function or strength compared with the contralateral arm and found no difference in results when the excision was performed with or without a rotator cuff repair. Additionally, Wright and colleagues[15] reported on 13 patients after an arthroscopic excision of a meso-acromion and had no decrease in anterior deltoid strength and no occurrence of deltoid detachment. Arthroscopic excision has the possible benefit of less periosteal and deltoid attachment injury, possibly lending to better results than open excision.

ORIF

Because complications arise from the fragment excision, many surgeons advocate internal fixation of the unfused os acromiale with bone grafting. Techniques to provide stability include the use of tension-band wires, sutures, or cannulated screws with or without the use of bone graft.[34]

Peckett and colleagues[3] reviewed 26 patients presenting with symptomatic meso os acromiale that were treated with either K-wires or screws and a tension band. Twenty-four had a satisfactory result with 96% union. Average time to union was 4 months. Eight cases had persistent pain postoperatively that was relieved by wire and screw removal. Seventeen of the 26 patients had a concomitant rotator cuff tear, and only 11 of these were repairable. They concluded that ORIF with bone grafting should be used for patients with symptomatic meso os acromiale, but a substantial number of patients require hardware removal.[3]

Warner and colleagues[12] reported on 11 patients who underwent ORIF with iliac crest bone grafting comparing 2 fixation techniques. Each technique incorporated debridement of the nonunion site with incorporation of iliac crest autograft spanning the debrided nonunion site. Four patients (5 shoulders) underwent ORIF with a tension-band procedure including the use of pins and wires. Four of 5 of these procedures resulted in persistent nonunion. The other 7 patients had an ORIF using cannulated screws, and an 18-guage wire passed through the screws in a figure of 8 fashion. Six of 7 were successful unions. Mean time for satisfactory radiographic and clinical union was approximately 9 weeks. Nine of the 12 patients required hardware removal to alleviate postoperative pain. The investigators advocated that stabilization and bone grafting should be performed in conjunction with figure of 8 wires through cannulated screws because there was a higher rate of union.

Hertel and colleagues[8] reported on 15 shoulders in 12 patients who underwent ORIF for unstable os acromiale fragments using tension band wiring without the use of bone grafting. Two surgical approaches were used. An anterior deltoid-off approach was used on 7, whereas the other 8 shoulders were approached trans-acromially to preserve the deltoid origin. Union occurred in 3 of 7 cases approached anteriorly and in 7 of 8 shoulders repaired without detachment of the deltoid. The investigators concluded that fusion was more successful when the vascularity of the acromial epiphysis was maintained, likely through the acromiale branch of the thoracoacromial artery.[8]

Atoun and colleagues[17] reported on arthroscopically assisted internal fixation of the symptomatic unstable os acromiale with absorbable screws. In their series, 8 patients presented with symptomatic meso os acromiale and had satisfactory results 3 to 6 months postoperatively. Two patients experienced hardware irritation that was treated with trimming of the prominent subcutaneous screw. Full union was achieved in 6 patients, partial union in 1 patient, and failed union in 1 patient. The fusion results were all verified by radiographs. This arthroscopic technique was the first of its kind to aid in the fixation of os acromiale.[17]

Techniques and approaches associated with the most success include those with rigid fixation and preservation of the vascularity of the os acromiale.[8] Even in cases of successful union, patients still may have hardware discomfort requiring hardware removal; however, there are minimal complications that arise from most ORIF cases.

Arthroscopic Subacromial Decompression with Acromioplasty

Arthroscopic subacromial decompression is primarily used when impingement with or without a rotator cuff tear is present and the nonunion site is nontender and considered to be incidental. Potential advantages compared with open procedures include more rapid rehabilitation, better range of motion, and shorter surgical times.[15,35–38] As with other treatment options presented for this problem, the results are variable.

Jerosch and colleagues[39] analyzed 12 patients with an os acromiale of 122 patients who were all treated with arthroscopic subacromial decompression. At follow-up visits, the patients presenting with os acromiale had slightly better outcomes. Therefore, the arthroscopic subacromial decompression procedure was a recommended alternative to other more invasive and complicated procedures.

Hutchinson and Veenstra[14] had 3 asymptomatic os acromiale patients who underwent arthroscopic decompression for impingement syndrome associated with an unstable os acromiale. All 3 patients were initially satisfied with results postoperatively, but at 1-year follow-up, they all had symptoms return. Two patients even required more surgery. The arthroscopic decompression ultimately failed for all 3 patients. The investigators came to the conclusion that arthroscopic subacromial decompression should not be recommended for impingement secondary to an unstable os acromiale.

Armengol and colleagues[32] reported the results of 42 cases of os acromiale (including 33 patients with meso os acromiale) that were associated with partial or full-thickness rotator cuff tears. The patients were treated in 1 of 3 ways: resection for 5 patients, ORIF for 14 patients, and modified acromioplasty for 22 patients. Their acromioplasty technique involved removal of the acromial spur with preservation of the superior cortex and deltoid fascia. Only half of the patients who had an ORIF had satisfactory outcomes, with 86% needing revision surgery for hardware issues, whereas the modified acromioplasty yielded 86% satisfactory results.

Abboud and colleagues[28] treated 19 patients who had os acromiale associated with rotator cuff tears. Eleven (53%) of the patients had satisfactory results, including 4 who were treated with open acromioplasty and 3 treated with arthroscopic acromioplasty. The remaining 3 patients were treated with ORIF. The 7 patients treated with acromioplasty achieved improved outcome scores in all categories but external rotation. It is important to note that all 3 patients who had workers' compensation claims did not have satisfactory results with the acromioplasty procedure.[28]

CASE SERIES

Here we present a new technique for managing symptomatic meso os acromiale and present our results. The clinical outcome of this series of 6 patients with a symptomatic meso os acromiale who underwent this new technique have demonstrated favorable outcomes thus far.

We retrospectively identified 6 patients who underwent partial resection of a meso os acromiale by the senior author between March 2008 and March 2011. The study group consisted of 4 men and 2 women, with a mean age of 53 years (range, 36–65 years) at the time of surgery. The dominant shoulder was symptomatic in 3 (50%) of the patients. No patients were involved in a workers' compensation program. Patients had a mean follow-up of 25 months (range 5–36 months, median 22 months). All patients had the insidious onset of pain with no identifiable traumatic event.

All patients had pain over the anterolateral and superior aspect of the shoulder that was exacerbated with overhead activities. In addition, all patients exhibited localized point tenderness over the dorsal aspect of the acromion at the nonunion site. Anteroposterior, scapular Y, and axillary radiographs of the shoulder along with an MRI were obtained in all patients preoperatively. The diagnosis of meso os acromiale was confirmed preoperatively by use of radiographs and MRI, demonstrating a failure of fusion at the level of the mid to posterior margin of the acromioclavicular joint. Impingement and rotator cuff pathology were diagnosed based on physical examination and confirmed with MRI.

The decision for surgery was based on history, physical examination, and MRI. All patients failed a course of nonoperative treatment, including nonsteroidal anti-inflammatories, activity modification, and physical therapy. Surgical management was directed by the underlying pathoanatomy in addition to addressing the os acromiale. Rotator cuff tears were diagnosed in 4 of the 6 patients in our series: 1 with a high-grade partial supraspinatus tear, 2 with full-thickness supraspinatus tears, and 1 with full-thickness tears of the supraspinatus and infraspinatus. These patients underwent double-row repair with acromioplasty and partial os resection. Patients without high-grade partial or full-thickness rotator cuff tears were treated with acromioplasty and partial os resection alone.

SURGICAL METHOD

After standard diagnostic arthroscopy, the scope is placed in the subacromial space from a standard posterior portal, and after a subtotal bursectomy and release of the CA ligament, the integrity of the rotator cuff is evaluated. A lateral portal is established approximately at the level of the os acromiale. Optimal portal placement can be facilitated through the use of a spinal needle. In the absence of a rotator cuff tear, acromioplasty and partial resection of the os acromiale is performed. With the arthroscope in the anterolateral portal, a burr is introduced posteriorly and a cutting block technique is used for the acromioplasty as described by Caspari and Thal (**Fig. 2**).[40] The arthroscope is then moved back to the posterior portal and an arthroscopic shaver is introduced through the lateral portal (**Fig. 3**). Resection of the os acromiale is started with the shaver to better define the anterior and posterior fragments and to create a space for the arthroscopic burr. Next, the burr is placed in the anterolateral portal and approximately 5 mm of the anterior and posterior fragments are resected. Resection is evenly divided between the anterior and posterior

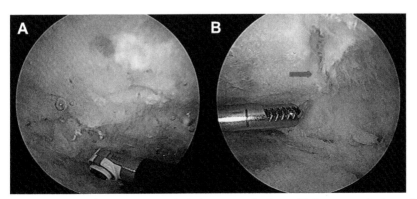

Fig. 2. View from lateral portal (*A*) os acromiale before acromioplasty. (*B*) Post acromioplasty. Red Arrow = nonunion site.

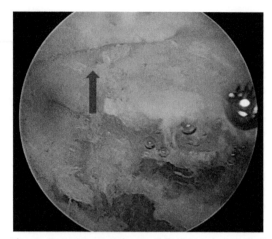

Fig. 3. Posterior portal view of os acromiale. Red arrow = nonunion site.

fragments. Care is taken to preserve the acromial attachment site of the posterior acromioclavicular joint capsular ligaments. This attachment includes portions on both the anterior and posterior acromial fragments and both should be preserved. The arthroscope is then moved back to the lateral portal to confirm that bone has been resected symmetrically from superior to inferior. In addition, percutaneously placed spinal needles can be used to confirm the amount of bone resection (**Fig. 4**). Any bony debris is suctioned from the subacromial space. Any rotator cuff tear can be addressed before or after the acromioplasty and partial os resection.

POSTOPERATIVE REHABILITATION

Postoperative protocol was determined by additional procedures in 4 of the 6 cases. In those that did not have additional pathology (2 cases), the rehabilitation was as follows. Patients were placed in a sling postoperatively until their return visit 1 to 2 weeks postoperatively. At this visit, they were encouraged to discard the sling and use the extremity within the limits of pain for daily activities. Formal range of motion exercises were added if passive motion was not full at the first postoperative visit. Strengthening exercises are introduced after 4 weeks and return to full activity is expected at 3 to 4 months. The details of rehabilitation when a rotator cuff tear is also performed are beyond the scope of this article. However, in general, if a rotator cuff repair was also performed, active use of the shoulder is restricted for 6 weeks postoperatively and unrestricted return to activity is expected at 9 to 12 months depending on the tear size.

Outcomes were assessed at the initial interaction and at the latest follow-up with the validated University of Pennsylvania Shoulder Score (Penn Shoulder Score).[41,42] Additionally, patients were assessed postoperatively with a Single Assessment Numeric Evaluation (SANE) and QuickDASH (Disabilities of the Arm, Shoulder, and Hand) questionnaires. Patients were also examined for tenderness at the os acromiale site at final follow-up and the presence of any complications was noted.

RESULTS

All patients were available for follow-up. Overall, Penn Shoulder Scores increased from 50.6 (range 28–76, median 45) preoperatively to 78.5 (range 32–97, median 86.5) at the time of follow-up ($P = .12$) (**Table 1**). Breakdown of the pain portion of the Penn score demonstrated that the average pain significantly decreased from 5.6 preoperatively to 1.3 at the time of follow-up ($P = .027$). Active forward flexion, which increased from 143° (range 90–160°, median 158) preoperatively to 163° (range 135–180°, median 160) at the time of follow-up ($P = .23$), showed no statistical significance. Average SANE and QuickDASH scores at follow-up were 79.2 (range 70–90, median 77.5) and 15.9 (range 4.5–61.4, median 5.7), respectively. All patients had resolution of the localized

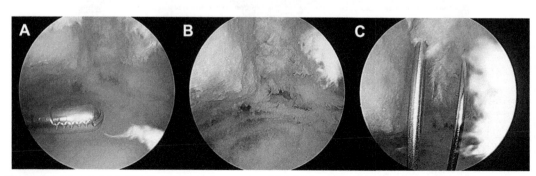

Fig. 4. Lateral portal. (*A, B*) Post resection of nonunion. (*C*) Spinal needles being used to verify width of resection (5–7 mm).

Table 1
Preoperative and postoperative outcome measures with associated _P_-value

Outcome	Preoperative	Postoperative	_P_ Value
Penn Shoulder Score	50.6	78.5	.12
Penn pain score	5.6	1.3	.027*
Active forward flexion	143	163	.23
SANE	—	79.2	—
QuickDASH	—	15.9	—

Statistically significant improvement in Penn pain scores.
* indicates statistical significance.
Abbreviations: DASH, Disabilities of the Arm, Shoulder, and Hand; Penn, University of Pennsylvania; SANE, Single Assessment Numeric Evaluation.

tenderness over the nonunion site and no patient required additional surgery for treatment of the os acromiale. In addition, no patient developed painful instability of the anterior os fragment or of the acromioclavicular joint.

The effect of rotator cuff pathology on outcome was not statistically significant, probably because of the small number of patients (**Table 2**). Four of 6 patients underwent rotator cuff repair for full-thickness or high-grade partial-thickness rotator cuff tears. The 2 patients with an isolated symptomatic meso os acromiale without full-thickness rotator cuff tears had better postoperative outcomes in all measures, although these differences were not significant: Penn, 90.5 versus 72.5

(_P_ = .30); SANE, 80 versus 78.75 (_P_ = .92); Quick-DASH: 5.7 versus 21.0 (_P_ = .34).

DISCUSSION

Symptomatic meso os acromiale is a challenging problem. After failure of nonoperative treatment, the previously described surgical approaches have yielded inconsistent outcomes. Concomitant pathology, including rotator cuff tendonitis and full-thickness tears, impingement secondary to instability of the os fragment or degenerative spurs, and acromioclavicular arthritis, can affect diagnosis and surgical outcome. The best surgical option for meso os acromiale remains controversial. Arthroscopic excision of the entire anterior fragment has had promising results and the senior author, before adopting the current technique of partial excision, performed it many times. Despite a lack of reported complications associated with complete arthroscopic excision and no reported deltoid strength deficits, the potential for deltoid detachment exists and reattachment is difficult.[33] One theory as to why an os acromiale becomes symptomatic is that repetitive stresses or destabilizing trauma across the nonunion site leads to local inflammation. As has been previously described, we have also recognized degenerative changes at the site of the nonunion, including cyst formation, hypertrophy, and sclerosis (**Fig. 5**).[43] These findings are also present in acromioclavicular joint arthropathy, which responds well to limited excision. The similarity of findings to acromioclavicular arthropathy is what first suggested the possibility of treating it with partial excision, similar to the resection performed for acromioclavicular arthropathy.

Table 2
Postoperative outcome measures for each individual patient and the associated operative diagnosis

Patient	Operative Diagnosis	Penn Shoulder Score	Penn Pain Score	SANE	Quick DASH
1	Os acromiale, impingement syndrome	97	0.25	90	6.82
2	Os acromiale, impingement syndrome	84	1.25	70	4.50
3	Os acromiale, rotator cuff tear	89	0.75	90	4.55
4	Os acromiale, rotator cuff tear	78	0	70	13.64
5	Os acromiale, rotator cuff tear, glenohumeral joint arthritis	91	1.0	85	4.55
6 (outlier)	Os acromiale, rotator cuff tear, glenohumeral joint arthritis	32	4.25	70	61.36

Abbreviations: DASH, Disabilities of the Arm, Shoulder, and Hand; Penn, University of Pennsylvania; SANE, Single Assessment Numeric Evaluation.

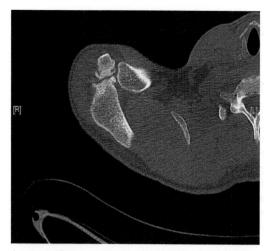

Fig. 5. Axillary computed tomography scan demonstrating os acromiale and associated cystic changes.

In theory, arthroscopic partial resection of the acromial nonunion site minimizes any abutment of the 2 fragments, which is believed to be a source of pain (**Fig. 6**). Combining this with an acromioplasty addresses impingement of the os fragment on the rotator cuff. All patients had resolution of the os acromiale tenderness and none developed any complications, including painful instability of either the anterior os fragment or the acromioclavicular joint. This latter finding is likely secondary to preservation of the posterior capsular ligaments. Moreover, if any patient had complained of residual pain at the nonunion site, any of the other described treatment options, including ORIF, would still be possible.

Although the preoperative and postoperative differences in outcome measures were not statistically significant, our sample size is likely too small

to have demonstrated a difference, even if one existed. Moreover, 1 patient in our series with an associated 2-tendon retracted rotator cuff tear also had glenohumeral arthritis that adversely affected the overall outcome and statistical significance.

Postoperative SANE and QuickDASH scores were 79.2 and 15.9, respectively. All patients had increased active forward flexion. An 11-point visual analog scale for pain was calculated by averaging the 4 pain questions in the Penn Shoulder Score, as described previously.[28] Using this scale and paralleling previous reports, the average pain significantly decreased from 5.6 preoperatively to 1.3 at the time of follow-up ($P = .027$).

Also notable was the prevalence of full-thickness rotator cuff tears in our cohort (4 of 6 patients). The impact of an associated rotator cuff repair on the outcome of surgical treatment of a symptomatic os acromiale has been previously reported by Abboud and colleagues.[28] The investigators demonstrated no difference in outcome of surgical treatment of os acromiale in the presence of rotator cuff repair. Although our sample size was small and differences were not statistically significant, we demonstrated better outcomes in patients undergoing acromioplasty and os resection without rotator cuff repair. One difference in the study by Abboud and colleagues[28] is that nearly 50% of patients were involved in workers' compensation claims compared with 0% in our cohort.

We are aware that this is a small group of patients and that further work is necessary to confirm these reasonable preliminary results. However, this technique offers a potential advantage over previously described procedures in that pain was predictably eliminated, especially at the nonunion site, complications were not identified (especially painful instability and need for any associated

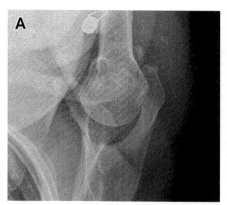

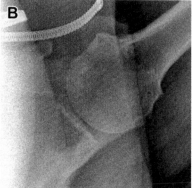

Fig. 6. Preoperative and postoperative radiographs of a 66-year-old woman with a symptomatic meso-acromion and a tear of the supraspinatus and upper one-third of the infraspinatus. (*A*) Preoperative axillary view demonstrating os acromiale at the level of the AC joint. (*B*) Postoperative axillary radiograph demonstrating the resection of the nonunion.

hardware removal), and other potential treatment options (ie, ORIF) were not compromised.

In conclusion, arthroscopic partial resection of os acromiale is another potential option for treating a symptomatic meso os acromiale without the complications of previous approaches. We have demonstrated it to be a safe and effective technique in this small series.

REFERENCES

1. Sammarco VJ. Os acromiale: frequency, anatomy, and clinical implications. J Bone Joint Surg Am 2000;82(3):394–400.
2. Burkhart SS. Os acromiale in a professional tennis player. Am J Sports Med 1992;20(4):483–4.
3. Peckett WR, Gunther SB, Harper GD, et al. Internal fixation of symptomatic os acromiale: a series of twenty-six cases. J Shoulder Elbow Surg 2004; 13(4):381–5.
4. Swain RA, Wilson FD, Harsha DM. The os acromiale: another cause of impingement. Med Sci Sports Exerc 1996;28(12):1459–62.
5. Edelson JG, Zuckerman J, Hershkovitz I. Os acromiale: anatomy and surgical implications. J Bone Joint Surg Br 1993;75(4):551–5.
6. Mudge MK, Wod VE, Frykman GK. Rotator cuff tears associated with os acromiale. J Bone Joint Surg Am 1984;66:427–9.
7. Demetracopoulos CA, Kapadia NS, Herickhoff PK, et al. Surgical stabilization of os acromiale in a fast-pitch softball pitcher. Am J Sports Med 2006; 34(11):1855–9.
8. Hertel R, Windisch W, Schuster A, et al. Transacromial approach to obtain fusion of unstable os acromiale. J Shoulder Elbow Surg 1998;7(6):606–9.
9. Sahajpal D, Strauss EJ, Ishak C, et al. Surgical management of os acromiale: a case report and review of the literature. Bull NYU Hosp Jt Dis 2007;65(4): 312–6.
10. Kurtz CA, Humble BJ, Rodosky MW, et al. Symptomatic os acromiale. J Am Acad Orthop Surg 2006;14: 12–9.
11. Ryu RK, Fan RS, Dunbar WH 5th. The treatment of symptomatic os acromiale. Orthopedics 1999; 22(3):325–8.
12. Warner JJ, Beim GM, Higgins L. The treatment of symptomatic os acromiale. J Bone Joint Surg Am 1998;80(9):1320–6.
13. Jerosch J, Hepp R, Castro WH. An unfused acromial epiphysis. A reason for chronic shoulder pain. Acta Orthop Belg 1991;57(3):309–12.
14. Hutchinson MR, Veenstra MA. Arthroscopic decompression of shoulder impingement secondary to os acromiale. Arthroscopy 1993;9(1):28–32.
15. Wright RW, Heller MA, Quick DC, et al. Arthroscopic decompression for impingement syndrome secondary to an unstable os acromiale. Arthroscopy 2000;16(6):595–9.
16. Harris JD, Griesser MJ, Jones GL. Systematic review of the surgical treatment for symptomatic os acromiale. Int J Shoulder Surg 2011;5(1):9–16.
17. Atoun E, van Tongel A, Narvani A, et al. Arthroscopically assisted internal fixation of the symptomatic unstable os acromiale with absorbable screws. J Shoulder Elbow Surg 2012;21(12):1740–5.
18. McClure JG, Raney RB. Anomalies of the scapula. Clin Orthop Relat Res 1975;110:22–31.
19. Gruber W. ÜberdieArten der Acromialknochen und accidentellen Acromialgelenke. Arch Anat Physiol Und wissensch Med 1863;24:373–8.
20. Grant JC. 6th edition. An atlas of anatomy, vol. 26. Baltimore (MD): Williams & Wilkins; 1972. p. 40.
21. Liberson F. Os acromiale: a contested anomaly. J Bone Joint Surg 1937;19:683–9.
22. Nicholson GP, Goodman DA, Flatlow EL, et al. The acromion: morphologic condition and age related changes. A study of 420 scapulas. J Shoulder Elbow Surg 1996;5:1–11.
23. Angel JL, Kelly JO, Parrington M, et al. Life stresses of the free black community as represented by the First African Baptist Church, Philadelphia, 1823-1841. Am J Phys Anthropol 1987;74:213–29.
24. Uri DS, Kneeland JB, Herzog R. Os acromiale: evaluation of markers for identification on sagittal and coronal oblique MR images. Skeletal Radiol 1997;26:31–4.
25. Satterlee CC. Successful osteosynthesis of an unstable mesoacromion in 6 shoulders: a new technique. J Shoulder Elbow Surg 1999;8:125–9.
26. Neer CS. Rotator cuff tears associated with os acromiale. J Bone Joint Surg Am 1984;66:1320–1.
27. Norris TR, Fischer J, Bigliani L, et al. The unfused acromial epiphysis and its relationship to impingement syndrome. Orthop Trans 1983;7:505–6.
28. Abboud JA, Silverberg D, Pepe M, et al. Surgical treatment of os acromiale with and without associated rotator cuff tears. J Shoulder Elbow Surg 2006;15(3):265–70.
29. Boehm TD, Matzer M, Brazda D, et al. Os acromiale associated with tear of the rotator cuff treated operatively. Review of 33 patients. J Bone Joint Surg Br 2003;85(4):545–9.
30. Boehm TD, Rolf O, Martetschlaeger F, et al. Rotator cuff tears associated with os acromiale. Acta Orthop 2005;76(2):241–4.
31. Burbank KM, Lemos MJ, Bell G, et al. Incidence of os acromiale in patients with shoulder pain. Am J Orthop (Belle Mead NJ) 2007;36(3):153–5.
32. Armengol J, Brittis DA, Pollock RG, et al. The association of unfused acromial epiphysis with tears of the rotator cuff: a review of 42 cases. J Shoulder Elbow Surg 1994;3:S14.
33. Campbell PT, Nizlan NM, Skirving AP. Arthroscopic excision of os acromiale: effects on deltoid

function and strength. Orthopedics 2012;35(11): e1601–5.

34. Ortiguera CJ, Buss DD. Surgical management of the symptomatic os acromiale. J Shoulder Elbow Surg 2002;11:521–8.

35. Altchek DW, Warren RF, Wickiewicz TL, et al. Arthroscopic acromioplasty. Technique and results. J Bone Joint Surg Am 1990;72:1198–207.

36. Ellman H. Arthroscopic subacromial decompression for chronic impingement. Two to five year results. J Bone Joint Surg Br 1991;73:395–8.

37. Esch J, Ozerkis LR, Helgager JA, et al. Arthroscopic subacromial depression. Results to the degree of rotator cuff repair. Arthroscopy 1988;4:241–9.

38. Norlin R. Arthroscopic subacromial decompression versus open acromioplasty. Arthroscopy 1989;5:1–11.

39. Jerosch J, Steinbeck J, Strauss JM, et al. Arthroskpische subakromiale decompression. Indikationbeim Os acromiale? Unfallchirurg 1994;97:69–73.

40. Caspari RB, Thal R. A technique for arthroscopic subacromial decompression. Arthroscopy 1992; 8(1):23–30.

41. Leggin BG, Michener LA, Shaffer MA, et al. The Penn shoulder score: reliability and validity. J Orthop Sports Phys Ther 2006;36(3):138–51.

42. Richman N, Curtis A, Hayman M. Acromion-splitting approach through an os acromiale for repair of a massive rotator cuff tear. Arthroscopy 1997;13(5): 652–5.

43. Pagnani MJ, Mathis CE, Solman CG. Painful os acromiale (or unfused acromial apophysis) in athletes. J Shoulder Elbow Surg 2006;15(4): 432–5.

MUSCULOSKELETAL ONCOLOGY

Preface

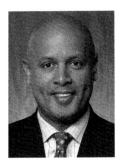

Felasfa M. Wodajo, MD
Editor

In the oncology section of this issue of *Orthopedic Clinics of North America*, we conclude our two-part series on soft tissue tumors in children. In "Malignant Soft Tissue Tumors in Children," Dr Thacker provides brief synopses of the most common pediatric soft tissue malignancies, such as rhabdomyosarcoma and synovial sarcomas, as well as reviewing the basics of biopsy and musculoskeletal imaging for soft tissue tumors. As readers are aware, soft tissue sarcomas are more common in adults than children. However, as orthopedic surgeons are often the first specialists consulted for masses in children, knowing the characteristics of the more common malignancies should help in planning appropriate workup and reducing unnecessary anxiety for parents.

Computer-aided navigation has already been shown to improve surgical technique in joint replacement surgery but may turn out to be even more important in orthopedic oncology, especially in challenging anatomical locations such as the pelvis. In "How Intraoperative Navigation Is Changing Musculoskeletal Tumor Surgery," Robert L. Satcher Jr, MD, PhD reviews the types of navigation equipment available, their usage in the operating room and surveys the available literature on the use of navigation in tumor surgery. Dr Satcher is currently Assistant Professor of Orthopaedic Oncology at The University of Texas MD Anderson Cancer Center in Houston. Between 2004 and 2011, he was also a Mission Specialist with NASA and was the first orthopedic surgeon to orbit the Earth, flying with the Space Shuttle in 2009. His research focuses on the development and prevention of bone metastases in carcinoma.

Felasfa M. Wodajo, MD
Musculoskeletal Tumor Surgery
Virginia Hospital Center
Arlington, VA 22205, USA

E-mail address:
wodajo@tumors.md

http://dx.doi.org/10.1016/j.ocl.2013.08.001
0030-5898/13/$ – see front matter

How Intraoperative Navigation is Changing Musculoskeletal Tumor Surgery

Robert L. Satcher Jr, MD, PhD

KEYWORDS

- Navigation • Computer • Tumor • Surgery • Sarcoma • Cancer • Musculoskeletal

KEY POINTS

- CAOS was implemented in musculoskeletal tumor surgery to enhance surgical precision.
- More study is needed to evaluate clinical outcomes in patients where CAOS is used to resect bone tumors.
- Future applications for CAOS include resection of soft tissue tumors.

INTRODUCTION

Computer-assisted orthopedic surgery (CAOS) was introduced in musculoskeletal tumor surgery recently to enhance surgical precision in resecting malignant and benign tumors. The origins of computer-assisted surgery were in other subspecialties; it has been used for more than 2 decades in maxillofacial surgery, and in neurosurgery for cranial biopsies and tumor resections. More recently, it has been used in orthopedic surgery for trauma, spine surgery for pedicle screw insertion, cup placement in hip arthroplasty, total knee replacement, and reconstructive surgery.

The initial use of intraoperative computer assistance for musculoskeletal tumor surgery was prompted by the difficulty in treating malignant pelvic and sacral tumors. A simulation by Cartiaux and colleagues[1–3] quantified this well-known difficulty, showing that the probability of experienced surgeons achieving negative surgical margins on plastic pelvic models was only 52%. A subsequent model showed that introducing CAOS improved cutting accuracy, and therefore the precision, of tumor resection.[1]

The first nontumor computed tomography (CT)–based computer-assisted osteotomy of the bony pelvis was performed in 1995 in patients with acetabular dysplasia, with the goal of improving the precision of required cuts for corrective periacetabular osteotomies.[4] Hufner and colleagues,[5] were the first to use computer-navigated instruments (chisels) to perform osteotomies in patients with sacral tumors. They demonstrated the advantage of visualizing the relationship between the chisel and the tumor for more accurate tumor resection. This technique was subsequently improved and expanded by various groups. Krettek and colleagues[6] added K-wires to visualize the preoperatively planned osteotomy levels for resecting pelvic tumors. Wong and colleagues[7,8] attached navigation trackers to conventional instruments (diathermy handle) to visualize the tumor in real time on the virtual CT images displayed on the navigation monitor. This visualization enabled clear identification of where cuts should be made for negative surgical margins through marking the bone surfaces with the diathermy needle.

The pace of development of CAOS has increased in the last 5 to 7 years as computer technology has become more sophisticated and intraoperative imaging systems have improved. The potential for enhanced surgical precision has

Department of Orthopaedic Oncology, MD Anderson Cancer Center, 1400 Pressler Street, Unit 1448, Houston, TX 77030, USA

E-mail address: rlsatcher@mdanderson.org

Orthop Clin N Am 44 (2013) 645–656

http://dx.doi.org/10.1016/j.ocl.2013.07.001

remained the impetus for increased interest by musculoskeletal oncologic surgeons. Current developments in CAOS for benign and malignant tumor resection are reviewed elsewhere in this issue. This article describes the technique, examines the limitations of navigation systems, and reviews recent clinical progress.

CAOS PRINCIPLES AND METHODS

Computer-assisted navigation provides a real-time, interactive, 3-dimensional (3D) digital map of a patient's anatomy, and helps track surgical instruments during the procedure. CAOS methods increase spatial accuracy during dissection, surgical resection, instrumentation, or other actions. The principles of CAOS are straightforward and similar to real-time interactive maps that use GPS (global positioning system) technology. Namely, a virtual or digital 3D patient is created from imaging studies, which is used to guide

surgical instruments that are tracked and mapped to this simulation. The essential steps for using CAOS are as follows:

1. Creation of a digital patient image, most commonly using magnetic resonance imaging (MRI) or CT scan of the anatomic region of interest, which will be used as a template. For oncology, the tumor is included in the image, and can be highlighted and distinguished from normal tissue to aid in visualization.
2. Preoperative planning of the surgical resection planes (ie, cuts in the bone and soft tissue) on the virtual patient image.
3. Viewing of the digital patient image intraoperatively by the surgeon on a video monitor.
4. Intraoperative matching of the patient anatomy with the digital patient image using a navigated device to localize anatomic landmarks on the patient—a process called *registration*. The surgeon validates the registration to ensure that an

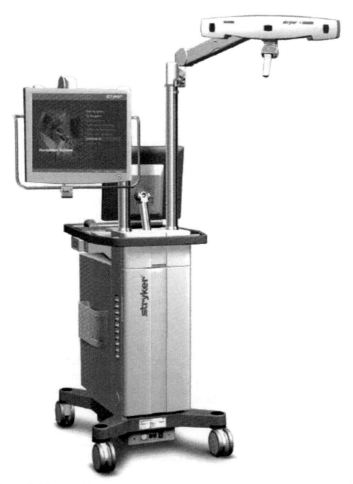

Fig. 1. Commercially available portable navigation system for computer-assisted orthopedic tumor surgery. The system includes an optical tracker, video monitor, and computer.

accurate matching has occurred between actual and virtual patient anatomy.

5. Use of navigated instruments whose positions are transferred into the digital patient image in real time to carry out the preoperative plan.

The source of errors in using CAOS systems are primarily caused by mismatch between the preoperatively acquired image and the real-time intraoperative patient anatomy. Consequently, the most recent process optimization strategies have focused on acquiring patient imaging intraoperatively via CT or MRI. Even without the intraoperative imaging, navigated accuracy errors of less than 0.5 mm are routinely reported.

Image-free navigation systems (eg. where no preoperative imaging is performed) are also available, but for tumor resections, only image-based systems have been used, because patient-specific surgical planning is required.[9] Typical components of a navigation system include a stereoscopic optical tracking system, positioning

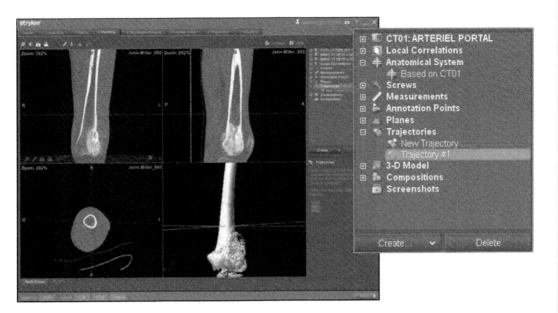

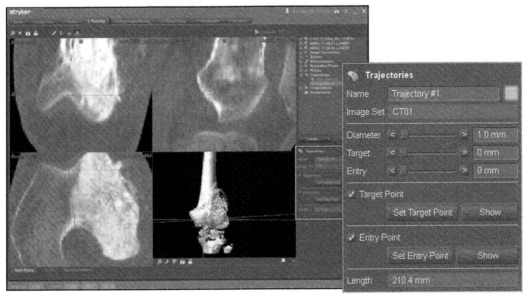

Fig. 2. Image of distal femur for preoperative planning that includes highlighting the tumor, selecting reference markers for registration, and planning and placing directional planes of reference for osteotomies. Annotations can be added to the images that will aid subsequent intraoperative execution of the plan.

sensors placed on the patient, tracked instruments, a video monitor to display virtual information, and a computer (**Fig. 1**). The centerpiece of a navigation system is the tracking system.[4,10]

Tracking can be performed optically or electromagnetically. The most common systems are optical, and use either passive infrared light–reflecting spheres, or active infrared light–emitting diodes in the surgical field. Electromagnetic tracking systems have fallen into disfavor for CAOS because of their inferior accuracy and the risk of malfunction from ferromagnetic and electromagnetic fields from other instruments commonly present in operating rooms. The primary disadvantage of optical systems is the need for an uninterrupted line-of-sight between the sensors and tracked devices/instruments.[4,10] Before surgery, the computer-navigated instruments must be calibrated for their geometry and shape to be incorporated in the virtual image of the patient. Current navigation systems are capable of tracking common surgical instruments, including osteotomes, diathermy handles, and drills.

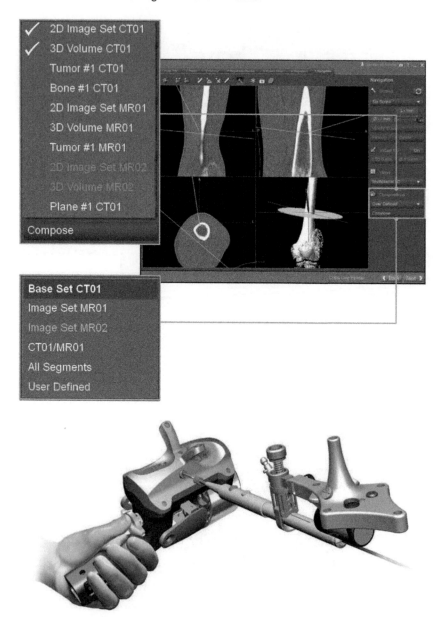

Fig. 3. Calibration of a diathermy for tracking during navigated surgery. Calibration can also be performed with pointers, patient trackers, and intraoperative imaging devices to define the projection of these objects within the virtual coordinate system in real time, and therefore execute the intended surgical plan.

PREOPERATIVE PLANNING

Preoperative planning has been emphasized to achieve the intended surgical goal.[8] Current systems allow the surgeon to view the patient images in 3D, and therefore accurately identify the tumor's spatial relationship to vital structures (eg, nerves, blood vessels). Recent recommendations also include using a large high-definition video monitor to minimize errors while viewing patient images.

During preoperative planning, the appropriate patient images (most commonly CT and MRI scans) are selected and can be combined or overlapped. The MRI adds soft tissue information to a CT scan, whereas other modalities, such as positron emission tomography (PET), can add physiologic information. The major steps in planning include highlighting the tumor, selecting reference markers for registration, and planning and placing directional planes of reference for osteotomies (**Fig. 2**). Annotations can be added to the images that will aid subsequent intraoperative execution of the plan. Finally, sites can be selected for the placement of patient tracking devices.

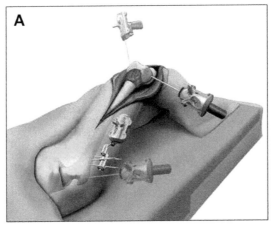

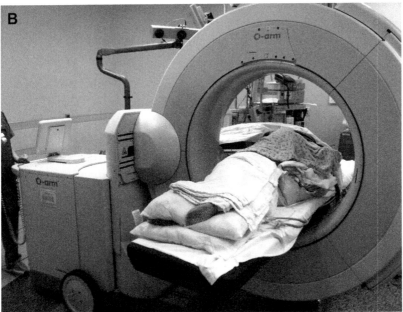

Fig. 4. (*A*) Registration of patient intraoperatively with surface matching to improve accuracy. The pointer is used to identify multiple points (at least 20) on several surfaces. The computer matches these surfaces to the virtual image of the femur from preoperative scanning, thereby improving the accuracy of navigation. (*B*) An alternative to patient registration is intraoperative scanning of the patient after application of the reference frame to the same bone or another nearby immobile structure. Note camera above patient. (Medtronic O-Arm and StealthStation Navigation, Medtronic Inc, MN, USA.)

REGISTRATION OF PATIENT TO IMAGE

Intraoperative registration of the patient to the patient images is the key step in the navigation process. Numerous registration concepts have been applied successfully for CAOS, using associated algorithms and hardware.[11] The goal of registration is to provide a one-to-one correspondence between the anatomic region of the patient and the virtual 3D model that was constructed from patient images. To compensate for intraoperative real-time patient movement, a tracking mechanism is also established, which creates a local coordinate system (dynamic reference frame) that moves with the patient. Calibration is subsequently performed with pointers, tracked surgical instruments, patient trackers, and intraoperative imaging devices to define the projection of these objects within the virtual coordinate system in real time, and therefore execute the intended surgical plan (**Fig. 3**).

Three-dimensional intraoperative registration is typically performed through identifying anatomic features that are clearly represented in the virtual patient image. Two methods are most often used:

1. Paired point matching (PPM): this is an invasive method that uses fixed markers implanted preoperatively in a separate procedure. These markers are radiopaque, and therefore identifiable on both the patient and the patient

A   B

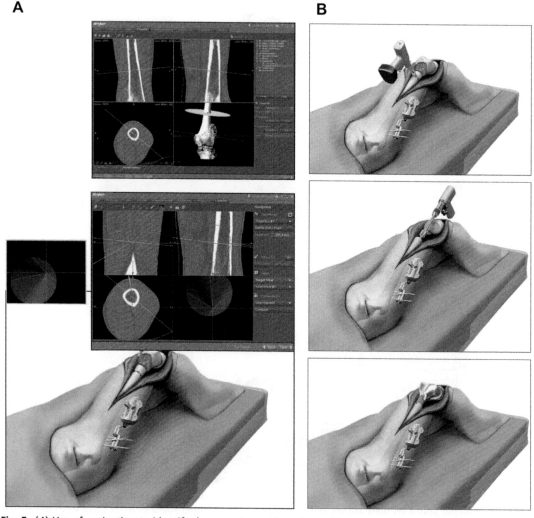

Fig. 5. (*A*) Use of navigation to identify the correct resection plane. After successful patient registration and instrument calibration, the patient anatomy and movements of calibrated instruments in the region of interest are navigated in real time using a video monitor. (*B*) Execution of navigated surgical plan. An oscillating saw is used to make the distal femur cut at the planned resection level.

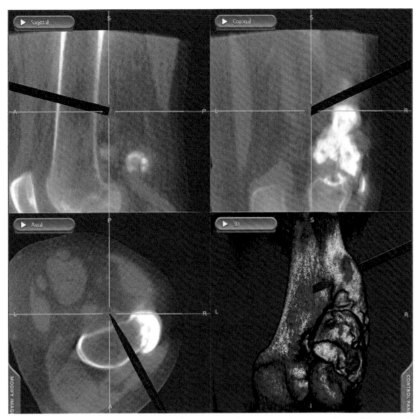

Fig. 6. Example of use intraoperative navigation for accurate, joint sparing resection of low grade surface osteosarcoma of the distal femur. Osteotome is represented on screen in blue in real time.

Table 1
Sources of Error when using CAOS

Step in Process of Navigation	Source of Error
Patient Imaging	• Patient movement while imaging in progress • Mismatch between patient orientation during imaging versus surgery • Image artifact from fiducial markers and/or implants
Preoperative Planning	• Video monitor resolution • Poorly distributed registration markers (best to place uniformly around the resection area in multiple planes) • Low number of registration markers (always use more than 4)
Surgical Set Up	• Equipment (camera, sensors) • Unstably fixed patient tracking elements that can move relative to the patient • Instrument calibration errors

Patient Registration	• Paired Point Regristration
	  ○ Mismatch between defined markers on imaging and the patient
	  ○ Inclusion of markers with high individual error
	• Surface Registration
	  ○ Pointer error due to not being in contact with bony surface
	  ○ Lack of spatial diversity in chosen surfaces (complex contours, nonlinear planes, and complex shapes are better)
	  ○ Too few points (at least 20 points should be chosen)

Table 2
Review of CAOS literature

Authors	Reference	Navigation System	Patient #	Case Type	Follow Up	Principle Observations
Hufner et al,[5] 2004	CORR, 426: 219-225; 2004	Surgigate CAS (Medivision, Oberdorf, Switzerland)	3	Sacrum and pelvis: recurrent malignant tumors	1 y, 3 y, 11 mo	1. CT and MRI for navigation 2. Navigated tools 3. Tumors excised accurately via histopathologic analysis
Krettek et al,[6] 2004	Injury, 35: SA79-SA83; 2004	Surgigate CAS (Medivision, Oberdorf, Switzerland)	2	Pelvis: malignant tumors	9 mo, 4 y	1. CT and MRI for navigation 2. Navigated tools 3. Complete tumor resection with negative margins
Wong et al,[7] 2007	JBJS (Br), 7: 943-947; 2007	Stryker Navigation (CT spine Version 1.60, modified by authors)	5	Sacrum, pelvis, femur, tibia: malignant tumors and metastatic disease	3.5-10 mo	1. CT and MRI for navigation 2. Registration via tracker attached to bone of interest 3. Navigated tools 4. Accuracy 0.36-0.44 mm 5. Negative margins in all cases
Wong et al,[8] 2008	CORR, 466: 2533-2541; 2008	Stryker Navigation (CT spine Version 1.60, modified by authors)	13	Sacrum, pelvis, femur, tibia: malignant tumors, benign bone tumor, metastatic disease	Mean 9.5 mo	1. CT and MRI for navigation 2. Resections validated by postoperative CT in 7 patients 3. Negative margins in all cases 4. Wound infections in 2 patients (1 deep)
So et al,[22] 2010	CORR, 468: 2985-2991; 2010	BrainLAB VectorVision Spine navigation (Hong Kong)	12	Sacrum, pelvis, humerus, radius, femur, tibia, fibula: malignant tumors, benign bone tumor	Mean 16 mo	1. Negative margins in all cases 2. Fluoro-CT intraoperative matching increased registration accuracy

Author, Year	Citation	Navigation System	N	Tumor Location	Follow-up	Results
Docquier et al,[23] 2010	Sarcoma, 1-8; 2010	Customized navigation software	1	Pelvis: malignant tumor	<1 mo	1. Negative margins by histologic examination 2. Navigation used to cut allograft 3. Transient femoral nerve paresis, hemostasis in corpus cavernosum requiring surgery
Wu et al,[24] 2011	Orthopedics, 34: 370-376; 2011	Medtronic O-arm navigation system (Minneapolis, MN)	5	Periarticular humerus, pelvis: benign tumors, metastatic disease	Mean 8.8 mo	1. Minimally invasive treatment of closed defects near joints 2. Curettage augmented with RFA 3. 1 patient had local recurrence treated with radiofrequency ablation
Cheong et al,[25] 2011	Cancer Control, 18: 171-176; 2011	Stryker Navigation (OrthoMap 3D, Mahwah, NJ)	20	Pelvis, femur, tibia: malignant tumors, metastatic disease	<24 mo	1. Negative surgical margins confirmed by pathology 2. Deep infection in 1 patient 3. Local recurrence in 1 patient 4. Limb length discrepancies less than 1.5 cm
Ieguchi et al,[26] 2012	CORR, 470: 275-283; 2012	StealthStation Treatment Guidance System (Medtronic-Sofamor Danek, Osaka, Japan)	16	Pelvis, humerus, femur, tibia, tarsus: malignant tumors (2 soft tissue), benign bone tumors	37 mo	1. 1 patient died of lung metastasis 2. Skip lesion on opposite side in one patient 3. Mean accuracy 0.93 mm

images.[12,13] For registration, the paired points are localized using a pointer on the patient, and matched with the image of the paired points. This approach provides the best accuracy possible. However, the risks include infection, pain, and the time associated with a separate procedure. A noninvasive variation of this technique can also be used, whereby the surgeon finds anatomic points that are precisely identifiable on the patient image. This technique is performed in the preoperative planning stage, and tends to be time-consuming. With both invasive and noninvasive PPM, the registration error decreases significantly when more than 4 pair points are used.

2. Intraoperative imaging: registration can also be performed using an intraoperative imaging device. A dynamic reference frame is fixed to the patient, imaging is performed, and the system completes the registration through matching intraoperative features with features from the preoperative patient images. The benefits of this method are improved accuracy, speed, and reduced patient morbidity from the surgical exposure required for PPM registration. The disadvantages include equipment costs, additional radiation exposure from radiographs, and the typical poorer quality of intraoperative images compared with preoperative images.[14–17]

In order to improve the accuracy of feature based registration, surface matching is routinely performed (**Fig. 4**). For this technique, the surgeon identifies 20 or more bone surface points using a pointer tracked by the navigation system. This "real" bone surface is then matched to the imaged bone surface.[14,16] Increased accuracy is achieved by matching a greater number of points, and if more complex surfaces are selected.[17–20] Some commercial navigation systems can bypass this step by using imaging data acquired intraoperatively (**Fig. 4**b). After successful patient registration and instrument calibration, the patient anatomy and movements of calibrated instruments in the region of interest are navigated in real time using a video monitor (**Figures. 5** and **6**).

VERIFICATION AND ERROR

The current navigation systems match the patient anatomy to the virtual image acquired from CT and/or MRI via the method of rigid body transformations.[4] This technique assumes that bone is rigid and nondeformable, and therefore spatial relationships between points are maintained on the patient and the virtual image. The rigid body

assumption (and thus the mathematical transformation) is no longer valid if the spatial arrangement of the bone is altered. Thus, only single bones are navigated and registered with current systems in use. Even with this constraint, errors can be introduced because of changes in the shape of the bone (eg, plasticity, tumor effects), image inaccuracy, and motion. **Table 1** shows a summary of error sources.

Phillips[15] noted that errors can occur at every stage of navigation, and that the errors are cumulative: they propagate as one progresses through the steps registration and navigation.[15] The standard currently accepted for accuracy is 2 to 4 mm for targeted points, and 1° to 3° for targeted trajectories. The true registration error is usually nonuniform over the patient volume, and is most dependent on the distribution of paired points used for anatomic feature–based registration. Error decreases when the distribution of paired points is close to the region of interest, and increases as one moves away from these regions.

To increase the accuracy of registration, several surface-matching techniques have also been introduced.[18–20] The surgeon identifies a defined number of points on the patient intraoperatively, and the computer algorithm locates the corresponding points. Nonetheless, a visual verification of the patient and image registration must always be performed as the final check before proceeding with navigation.

RESULTS (REVIEW OF CLINICAL LITERATURE)

The use of CAOS for tumor resection surgery is in its early stages. A review of the literature showed a limited number of studies reporting clinical outcomes after the use of CAOS for tumor resections (**Table 2**). All of the studies were case series with few patients and relatively short patient follow-up.

The first reports of using CAOS for tumor resections were in 2004, wherein 2 groups performed sacral tumor resections using navigation systems that were custom built through modifying systems available for spine surgery.[5,6] Krettek and colleagues[6] were the first to use navigated chisels for the resection.

Further modifications were introduced by Reijnders and colleagues[21] in 2007, who used implanted markers to improve registration accuracy. Wong and colleagues[8] modified the Stryker spine navigation system for use in tumor resections. They were among the first to report using navigation for resections from long bones, and for many years had the largest case series (13 patients in their 2008 study). The follow-up was short (mean, 9.5 months), but the series expanded on earlier expertise by the same group, who were the first to use MRI and CT image data to delineate the tumor margins beyond bone.[7] In their expanded study, the navigation software allowed visualization of CT, MRI, and PET scan data in a merged format or individually. The group believed that this allowed improvements in intraoperative accuracy and registration.[8] Their study was also the first to validate CAOS in determining the accuracy of the intended planned resection through comparing postoperative and preoperative CT images, and comparing the resection plane of resected specimens with that in surgical navigation.[8,10]

In 2010, So and colleagues[22] reported on 12 patients with a mean follow-up of 16 months. Tumors were resected from the sacrum, pelvis, and long bones. They were the first to evaluate and validate registration using intraoperative fluoroscopy, which was matched to preoperative CT scans. In another study from 2010, Docquier and colleagues[23] described the first case in which navigation was used for both tumor resection and subsequent reconstruction.

Most recently, CAOS techniques have been used to modify surgical treatment of benign tumors. Wu and colleagues[24] used navigation to plan and perform minimally invasive treatment of periarticular benign bone lesions.

The most recent case series have reported on larger numbers of patients for longer periods of follow-up (N = 16–20; follow-up, 24–37 months).[25,26] In one study, Cheong and colleagues[25] used the first navigation system specifically designed for tumor resection by commercial vendors. Some of the benefits reported included improved accuracy and precision of implant positioning, minimized leg length discrepancy, and improved implant rotational alignment. Ieguchi and colleagues[26] were the first to report on using CAOS for excising tumors that had a soft tissue extension. A mean accuracy of 0.93 mm was reported. No local recurrences were observed, although one patient subsequently died of lung metastases.

SUMMARY

Initial studies have shown that CAOS can be safely used for bone tumor resection surgery. The limitations of the technique have not been fully delineated, but it has the potential to improve surgical precision and accuracy, and to enable minimally invasive techniques for treating skeletal tumors. More study is needed to evaluate clinical outcomes for patients undergoing surgery when navigation is used, and to select appropriate patients in whom navigation will be of clinical benefit.

The more recent application that deserves further study is resection of soft tissue tumors. This application is more challenging, because the shape of soft tissues and relevant critical structures can change with factors such as patient position and breathing. Additional technological improvements that adapt to these shape changes will be needed to fully realize the application of CAOS for soft tissue tumor resection. Overall, the future of CAOS seems promising, and it will likely be increasingly used as efforts continue to improve surgical outcomes.

REFERENCES

1. Cartiaux O, Banse X, Paul L, et al. Computer-assisted planning and navigation improves cutting accuracy during simulated bone tumor surgery of the pelvis. Comput Aided Surg 2013;18:19–26.
2. Cartiaux O, Docquier PL, Paul L, et al. Surgical inaccuracy of tumor resection and reconstruction within the pelvis: an experimental study. Acta Orthop 2008;79:695–702.
3. Cartiaux O, Paul L, Docquier PL, et al. Computer-assisted and robot-assisted technologies to improve bone-cutting accuracy when integrated with a freehand process using an oscillating saw. J Bone Joint Surg Am 2010;92:2076–82.
4. Fehlberg S, Eulenstein S, Lange T, et al. Computer-assisted pelvic tumor resection: fields of application, limits, and perspectives. Recent Results Cancer Res 2009;179:169–82.
5. Hufner T, Kfuri M Jr, Galanski M, et al. New indications for computer-assisted surgery: tumor resection in the pelvis. Clin Orthop Relat Res 2004;(426):219–25.
6. Krettek C, Geerling J, Bastian L, et al. Computer aided tumor resection in the pelvis. Injury 2004; 35(Suppl 1):S-A79–83.
7. Wong KC, Kumta SM, Chiu KH, et al. Precision tumour resection and reconstruction using image-guided computer navigation. J Bone Joint Surg Br 2007;89:943–7.
8. Wong KC, Kumta SM, Antonio GE, et al. Image fusion for computer-assisted bone tumor surgery. Clin Orthop Relat Res 2008;466:2533–41.
9. Bowersox J, Bucholz R, Delp S. Excerpts from the final report for the second international workshop on robotics and computer assisted medical interventions. Comput Aided Surg 1997;2:69–101.
10. Saidi K. Potential use of computer navigation in the treatment of primary benign and malignant tumors in children. Curr Rev Musculoskelet Med 2012;5: 83–90.
11. Simon DA, Lavallee S. Medical imaging and registration in computer assisted surgery. Clin Orthop Relat Res 1998;(354):17–27.

12. Cho HS, Park IH, Jeon IH, et al. Direct application of MR images to computer-assisted bone tumor surgery. J Orthop Sci 2011;16:190–5.

13. Kim JH, Kang HG, Kim HS. MRI-guided navigation surgery with temporary implantable bone markers in limb salvage for sarcoma. Clin Orthop Relat Res 2010;468:2211–7.

14. Nolte LP, Beutler T. Basic principles of CAOS. Injury 2004;35(Suppl 1):S-A6–16.

15. Phillips R. The accuracy of surgical navigation for orthopaedic surgery. Curr Orthop 2007;21:180–92.

16. Zheng G. Effective incorporating spatial information in a mutual information based 3D-2D registration of a CT volume to X-ray images. Comput Med Imaging Graph 2010;34:553–62.

17. Zheng G. Personalized X-ray reconstruction of the proximal femur via intensity-based non-rigid 2D-3D registration. Med Image Comput Comput Assist Interv 2011;14:598–606.

18. Bachler R, Bunke H, Nolte LP. Restricted surface matching–numerical optimization and technical evaluation. Comput Aided Surg 2001;6:143–52.

19. Glozman D, Shoham M, Fischer A. A surface-matching technique for robot-assisted registration. Comput Aided Surg 2001;6:259–69.

20. Sugano N, Sasama T, Sato Y, et al. Accuracy evaluation of surface-based registration methods in a computer navigation system for hip surgery performed through a posterolateral approach. Comput Aided Surg 2001;6:195–203.

21. Reijnders K, Coppes MH, van Hulzen AL, et al. Image guided surgery: new technology for surgery of soft tissue and bone sarcomas. Eur J Surg Oncol 2007;33:390–8.

22. So TY, Lam YL, Mak KL. Computer-assisted navigation in bone tumor surgery: seamless workflow model and evolution of technique. Clin Orthop Relat Res 2010;468:2985–91.

23. Docquier PL, Paul L, Cartiaux O, et al. Computer-assisted resection and reconstruction of pelvic tumor sarcoma. Sarcoma 2010;2010:125162.

24. Wu K, Webber NP, Ward RA, et al. Intraoperative navigation for minimally invasive resection of periarticular and pelvic tumors. Orthopedics 2011;34:372.

25. Cheong D, Letson GD. Computer-assisted navigation and musculoskeletal sarcoma surgery. Cancer Control 2011;18:171–6.

26. Ieguchi M, Hoshi M, Takada J, et al. Navigation-assisted surgery for bone and soft tissue tumors with bony extension. Clin Orthop Relat Res 2012;470:275–83.

Malignant Soft Tissue Tumors in Children

Mihir M. Thacker, MD

KEYWORDS

- Pediatric • Sarcoma • Soft tissue mass • Lump • Extremity • Soft tissue tumor

KEY POINTS

- Soft tissue sarcomas (STS) in children are rare and may have overlapping clinical and imaging features with more common benign tumors and reactive processes, thus making them a diagnostic challenge.
- Soft tissue sarcomas, unlike bone sarcomas, often present as painless masses.
- Soft tissue sarcomas grow in a centrifugal fashion and usually have well defined margins, thus making the differentiation from benign soft tissue lesions challenging.
- Many STS have characteristic chromosomal abnormalities.
- Rhabdomyosarcomas (RMS) are the most common pediatric soft tissue sarcoma in the 0 to 14 age group and account for more than 50% of STS in this age group.
- Alveolar RMS and non-RMS STS are more common in the extremities.
- Treatment of RMS is a combination of chemotherapy, surgery, and radiation (as needed), whereas treatment of non-RMS STS is primarily surgery.

INTRODUCTION

Soft tissue masses in children include the more common reactive and benign soft tissue masses but also include the rare and much more serious soft tissue sarcomas (STS).[1,2] These sarcomas are a heterogeneous group of malignancies that arise from a mesenchymal cell of origin. Each year in the United States approximately 850 to 900 children and adolescents (age 20 years or less) are diagnosed with a STS. Of these, approximately 350 are rhabdomyosarcomas (RMS). The incidence of STS in this age group is 11 per million and these make up 7.4% of all cancers in this age group. Boys are affected slightly more frequently and in the adolescent population, African Americans are slightly more frequently affected.

Imaging findings in soft tissue masses are frequently nonspecific and biopsy, therefore, is an important component of the diagnostic workup of soft tissue tumors. Familiarity with the clinical and imaging appearance of STS may help the treating surgeon devise an appropriate evaluation and management strategy. Treatment of pediatric soft tissue sarcoma often involves chemotherapy and surgery. Radiation is used with caution in young children, especially for tumors close to growth plates. This review covers some of the essential concepts for making the diagnosis and understanding treatment principles of malignant soft tissue tumors in children. Also highlighted are some of the recent advances in imaging, diagnostic pathology.

DIAGNOSTIC STRATEGY

A primary care physician is often faced with the initial evaluation of a soft tissue mass in the child and they often send these children on to a general surgeon or an orthopedist for further evaluation. The differential diagnosis in this situation may be extremely broad. A complete history and the

Financial Disclosure: No financial disclosure to declare from National Institutes of Health (NIH); Wellcome Trust; Howard Hughes Medical Institute (HHMI); and other(s).
Conflict of Interests: No conflict of interests to declare.
Department of Orthopedic Surgery, Nemours - Alfred I duPont Hospital for Children, 1600 Rockland Road, Wilmington, DE 19803, USA
E-mail address: mihir.thacker@nemours.org

rapidly disappearing art of physical examination are extremely important in narrowing this down to a more appropriate list of differential diagnoses. **Pain is not a reliable indicator of malignant potential.** Solid (noncystic) lesions in children (and adults) need to be worked up further and this may include imaging (ultrasound for small superficial lesions and magnetic resonance imaging [MRI] for larger, deeper lesions). A high index of suspicion should be maintained in patients with premalignant conditions or cancer predisposition syndromes (**Table 1**). A biopsy is warranted in cases where the clinical and imaging findings are insufficient to clinch the diagnosis.

BIOPSY

With imaging being less specific in soft tissue compared with bone tumors, biopsy is an extremely important component to making the diagnosis. This biopsy may be excisional (typically for small, superficial lesions or those with characteristic clinical and imaging findings) or incisional (especially in masses close to neurovascular structures, such as in the popliteal fossa or axilla). Needle (core and fine-needle aspiration) biopsies are especially useful in deep soft tissue masses and are often used with image (ultrasound, computed tomography [CT], MR) guidance.[3,4] Obtaining adequate lesional tissue is paramount, as is a discussion of the clinical and radiographic information with the pathologist before the biopsy. This discussion helps to prepare for appropriate sample processing and further testing. Samples are best sent to the laboratory fresh on a moist nonadherent pad, so that the pathologist can obtain the appropriate tests, for example, flow cytometry cannot be performed on formalinized samples. Principles of biopsy of musculoskeletal lesions are detailed in **Box 1**.[5] The importance of an appropriately planned and performed biopsy cannot be overemphasized (**Fig. 1**). The hematoxylin and eosin appearance of the biopsied tissue is frequently diagnostic. With improving technology, pathologists now frequently use various adjuncts to confirm their diagnosis and also further subclassify tumors and give prognostic information. These include the following.

Immunohistochemistry

Immunohistochemistry is a technique that uses antibodies to identify specific molecules on different kinds of tissue. These molecules not only help to identify different histologic tissue types but may also help to understand how cells grow and differentiate, thereby helping to understand some of the pathways involved in pathogenesis of these tumors. There are more than 200 immunohistochemical stains available and this number is growing exponentially. Some of the commonly used immunohistochemical stains and the tissues that these are associated with are shown in **Table 2**.

Cytogenetics

The use of cytogenetics has resulted in increased recognition of chromosomal abnormalities associated with various tumors. Various cytogenetic techniques include karyotyping, fluorescent in situ hybridization, comparative genomic hybridization, and chromosome microdissection. The cytogenetic abnormalities associated with soft tissue tumors include a wide spectrum from gains to losses of chromosomal material (trisomies, deletions, translocations). **Translocation associated STS are commonly seen in the younger population (and frequently involve the *EWS* gene) compared with adults who frequently have nonspecific or complex aberrations.** Detection of these genetic changes has added another diagnostic weapon to our armamentarium, especially in borderline cases. Some of the more frequent cytogenetic changes are listed in **Table 3**.

Table 1		
Genetic disorders associated with increased risk of soft tissue sarcoma in young patients		
Beckwith Wiedemann syndrome	11p15	RMS, Wilms tumor
Noonan syndrome	12q24	RMS
Costello syndrome	12p12.1	RMS
Li-Fraumeni syndrome	17p13.1 (LFS 1); 1q23 (LFS3)	RMS, LPS
Hereditary retinoblastoma	13q14.2	LMS, Osteosarcoma
Neurofibromatosis type 1	17q11.2	MPNST
Adenomatous polyposis coli	5q21-q22	Desmoid tumors

Adapted from Coffin CM, Alaggio R, Dehner LP. Some general considerations about the clinicopathologic aspects of soft tissue tumors in children and adolescents. Pediatr Dev Pathol 2012;15(Suppl 1):11–25.

Box 1
Principles of biopsy of musculoskeletal tumors

1. Review the clinical and radiographic findings with the radiologist and pathologist before the biopsy.

2. The biopsy should be performed at the site of definitive treatment by appropriately trained personnel or in consultation with them, if the former not feasible.

3. Use a tourniquet whenever possible. Avoid expressive exsanguination (Eschmarck bandage).

4. Shortest possible incision, longitudinally placed, along the line of the eventual resection.

5. Minimum soft tissue dissection and contamination of tissue planes. Dissection through and not in between muscles to minimize contamination and need for eventual resection.

6. Choose the best site for the biopsy: usually the advancing edge of the tumor and not the central portion, which may often be necrotic. A thorough analysis of the MR images helps in planning this.

7. Obtain adequate amount of tissue for diagnosis and ancillary tests. Minimal distortion of the specimen and send it down fresh to the pathologist for appropriate tests.

8. Achieve hemostasis and use a drain (brought out in line with the incision and close to it), if needed.

9. Sutures placed close to the wound edges to minimize the amount of skin to be excised at the time of definitive resection.

Adapted from Thacker MM. Musculoskeletal oncology. In: Fischgrund J, editor. Orthopaedic knowledge update. 9th edition. Rosemont (IL): American Academy of Orthopaedic Surgoens; 2008. p. 197–220.

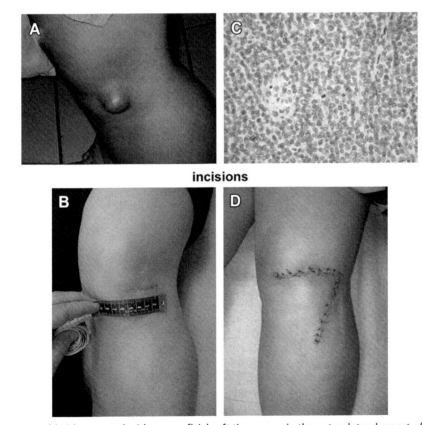

Fig. 1. (*A*) 14-year-old girl presented with a superficial soft tissue mass in the anterolateral aspect of the knee. (*B*) This mass was excised using a transverse incision. (*C*) Pathology from the excision revealed an extraskeletal Ewing sarcoma. (*D*) Surgery for tumor bed excision necessitated excision of the prior incision and track followed by a local transposition flap.

Table 2
Commonly used immunohistochemical markers and the tissues/tumors with which they are commonly associated

Marker	Tumor Type
S-100	Neurogenic tumors mostly, but fairly nonspecific
Cytokeratin, epithelial membrane antigen	Carcinomas, synovial sarcoma, epithelioid sarcoma, myoepithelial tumors
CD 31, CD 34	Vascular lesions, CD 34 also in DFSP, spindle cell lipoma
Myogenin (more specific) and MyoD1	Skeletal muscle, rhabdomyosarcoma
Smooth muscle actin	Leiomyosarcoma, myofibroblastic lesions
Caldesmon	Smooth muscles, GIST, glomus tumor
Podoplanin 2	Lymphatic malformations, Kaposi sarcoma
TLE1 (transducin-like enhancer of split 1)	Synovial sarcoma
Ki-67	Marker of proliferation

Abbreviations: DFSP, Dermatofibrosarcoma protruberans; GIST, Gastro-intestinal stromal tumor.

CLASSIFICATION AND STAGING SYSTEMS

The World Health Organization classification of soft tissue tumors is shown in **Box 2**.[6]

RMS is the most common pediatric STS and is staged using the Intergroup Rhabdmyosarcoma Study Group staging system. This staging system incorporates site-based TNM staging as well as the extent of resection and extent of disease.[7] STS other than RMS are staged using the American Joint Committee on Cancer system, although this system is not validated for pediatric STS. The International Classification of Childhood Cancer divides STS into RMS: embryonal and alveolar subgroups; fibrosarcoma (fibrous lesions and malignant peripheral nerve sheath tumors [MPNSTs]); Kaposi sarcoma; other defined types—including liposarcoma, Ewing sarcoma, and so on; and undefined.

TREATMENT PRINCIPLES

Treatment begins with establishing the appropriate diagnosis. The natural history and presence of symptoms guide the aggressiveness of treatment. The gold standard for treatment of most symptomatic STS is wide surgical excision. With improvement in the understanding of the pathogenetic processes involved, less invasive and less morbid treatment options are being used and improved on. Nonsurgical treatment options including targeted therapies continue to evolve.

STS need a multidisciplinary team approach and are often treated with a combination of

Table 3
Cytogenetic abnormalities in some common tumors

Tumor	Cytogenetic Abnormality
Myxoid LPS	t(12;16)(q13;11) and t(2;22)(q13;q12)
Infantile fibrosarcoma	t(12;15)(p13;q25)
Embryonal rhabdomyosarcoma	Loss of heterozygosity at 11p15
Alveolar rhabdomyosarcoma	t(2;13)(q35;q14) or t(1;13)(q36;q14) or 25%–40% cases without either
Angiomatoid fibrous histiocytoma	t(12;16)(q13;11) or t(2;22)(q13;12)
Synovial sarcoma	t(X;18)(p11;q11)
Epithelioid sarcoma-proximal	22q11.2 alterations
Alveolar soft part sarcoma	der(17)t(x;17)(p11.2;q25)
Extraskeletal myxoid chondrosarcoma	t(9;22)(q22;q12) or t(9;17)(q22;q12) or t(9;15)(q22;q21)
Extraskeletal EWS	t(11;22)(q24;q12) and other less common variants

Box 2
World Health Organization classification of soft tissue tumors (abbreviated)

Adipocytic tumors

Benign: includes lipoma and its variants, lipomatosis, lipoblastoma, lipoblastomatosis

Intermediate: atypical lipomatous tumor/well-differentiated liposarcoma (LPS)

Malignant: liposarcomas: myxoid/round cell, pleomorphic, mixed, dedifferentiated

Fibroblastic/myofibroblastic tumors

Benign: includes nodular fasciitis and not modular fasciitis, fibrous hamartoma of infancy, myofibroma/myofibromatosis, fibroma of tendon sheath, calcifying aponeurotic fibroma, etc

Intermediate (locally aggressive): superficial fibromatoses—palmar, plantar, Desmoid-type fibromatosis, lipofibromatosis

Intermediate (rarely metastasizing): hemangiopericytoma/solitary fibrous tumor, inflammatory myofibroblastic tumor, infantile fibrosarcoma

Malignant: adult fibrosarcoma, myxofibrosarcoma, low-grade fibromyxoid sarcoma, sclerosing epithelioid fibrosarcoma.

"Fibrohistiocytic" tumors:

Benign: includes giant cell tumor of tendon sheath, diffuse giant cell tumor, benign fibrous histiocytoma

Intermediate (rarely metastasizing): plexiform fibrohistiocytic tumor

Malignant: malignant fibrous histiocytoma/undifferentiated pleomorphic sarcoma and its variants

Smooth muscle tumors:

Benign: deep leiomyoma, angioleiomyoma

Malignant: leiomyosarcoma, excluding skin

Skeletal muscle tumors:

Benign: includes rhabdomyoma-adult/fetal/genital

Malignant: rhabdomyosarcoma-embryonal/alveolar/pleomorphic

Vascular tumors:

Benign: includes hemangioma, angiomatosis, lymphangioma

Intermediate (locally aggressive): Kaposiform hemangioendothelioma

Intermediate (rarely metastasizing): Retiform hemangioendothelioma, composite hemangioendothelioma, Kaposi sarcoma

Malignant: epithelioid hemangioendothelioma, angiosarcoma

Pericytic (perivascular) tumors:

Glomus tumor and its variants, including malignant glomus tumor, myopericytoma

Chondro-osseous tumors:

Benign: soft tissue chondromas

Malignant: mesenchymal chondrosarcoma, extraskeletal osteosarcoma

Tumors of uncertain differentiation:

Benign: includes intramuscular myxoma, pleomorphic hyalanizing angiectatic tumor

Intermediate (rarely metastasizing): angiomatoid fibrous histiocytoma, ossifying fibromyxoid tumor, parachordoma

Malignant: synovial sarcoma, epithelioid sarcoma, alveolar soft parts sarcoma, clear cell sarcoma of soft tissue, extraskeletal myxoid chondrosarcoma, primitive neuroectodermal tumor, extraskeletal Ewing sarcoma, neoplasms of perivascular cell differentiation (PEComa, clear cell melanocytic tumor)

chemotherapy and/or surgery and/or radiation therapy, which is discussed in more detail below.

Some of the common malignant soft tissue tumors seen in children are discussed below.

STS
RMS

RMS is the most common soft tissue sarcoma in children and accounts for 3.5% of cancers in the 0- to 14-year age group. The incidence is approximately 4.5 per million children with half the cases seen in the first decade. Increased risk may be seen in the cancer predisposition syndromes (see **Table 1**).

This mesenchymal tumor is traditionally thought to arise from primitive myoblasts, but is often seen in locations devoid of skeletal muscle (urinary bladder, bile ducts, and others). The two common subtypes seen in children are alvelolar and embryonal (**Fig. 2**). Pleomorphic RMS is seen mostly in

adults and is not discussed here. The features of alveolar and embryonal subtypes are shown in **Table 4**. The staging workup includes CT chest, bone scan, bilateral bone marrow aspirates and biopsies, and selective lymph node sampling. F-Fluorodeoxyglucose positron emission tomography (PET)[8] and, more recently, full-body MRI is being increasingly used in staging. The role of PET response to neoadjuvant chemotherapy is being evaluated for prognostic and therapeutic implications.[9] Treatment, as with most other sarcomas, is a multidisciplinary approach. Treatment stratified based on tumor site (favorable, orbit, urogenital, and biliary tracts, vs unfavorable, other sites), size (<5 cm vs >5 cm), histology (alveolar, unfavorable), completeness of the resection before chemotherapy (group I, complete resection; group II, microscopic residual disease; group III, gross residual disease; group IV, metastases), lymph node status, and metastatic disease.

Rhabdomyosarcoma

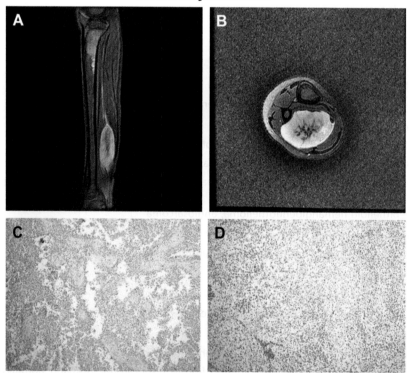

Fig. 2. A 7-year-old boy presented with a mass in the distal portion of the calf. An MRI (short TI inversion recovery) sagittal profile (*A*) and a T2 fat-saturated axial view (*B*) demonstrate a large soft tissue mass in the deep posterior compartment of the leg. There is also hyperintense signal in the proximal tibial metaphysis (metastatic disease). This child was treated with chemotherapy and then surgery. Histomicrographs (×10, Hematoxylin and Eosin) showing the changes in alveolar (*C*) and embryonal RMS (*D*). In alveolar RMS there is an attempt at the cells being grouped with areas of central clearing resembling alveoli. The cells in embryonal RMS lack this feature and are often arranged in sheets.

Table 4
Characteristics of alveolar and embryonal rhabdomyosarcoma

Rhabdomyosarcoma Subtype	Alveolar (>50% Alveolar Element)	Embryonal
Incidence	Less common (approximately 25% of RMS in children)	More common, approximately 75% of RMS in children
Gender	Equal	Males more common (1.5 times)
Extremity involvement	More frequent	More in genitourinary and biliary tract
Myogenin expression	Patchy	Diffuse
Prognosis	Worse, especially if PAX3 mutation Translocation negative alveolar RMS prognosis similar to embryonal RMS	Better

Chemotherapy with vincristine, adriamycin, and cyclophosphamide is the mainstay of treatment. Local control is with nonmutilating surgery and radiation for residual disease. Prognosis of the embryonal RMS and nontranslocation associated RMS is better than the translocation-associated alveolar RMS. Also, the PAX3-FOXO1 subgroup of the alveolar RMS does somewhat worse than the PAX7-FOXO1 patients.[10] Prognosis is worse for children less than 1 year of age and in the 10- to 19-year-old age group, compared with the 1- to 9-year-old group.

Synovial Sarcoma

Synovial sarcoma is the second most common soft tissue sarcoma in children and young adults. The name is misleading because the cell of origin is not a synovial cell, and the joint is involved in only 0.5% to 5% cases. **It, however, is frequently seen close to joints (Fig. 3)**. Its peak incidence is in the third and fourth decades but can often be seen in children in the second decade. The lower extremity is the most common location (especially knee and ankle), but upper extremities such as head, neck, and even solid organs may be involved. It usually arises as a painless soft tissue mass with a variable growth rate.

Histologically, the tumor may be monophasic with spindle cells (fibrous) or epithelial variants, or biphasic with epithelial and spindled areas. These tumors often have the characteristic X:18 translocation with fusion of the *SYT gene* on Chr 18 to the *SSX* genes on the X chromosome. Prognosis in SYNSA is influenced by size of the primary tumor and depth; upper extremity location is better than the lower extremity, p53 overexpression, high Ki-67 reactivity, nuclear beta-catenin, and cyclin D1 expression (metastasis), and high nuclear and cytoplasmic survivin expression (all poor prognostic factors). Treatment is primarily surgery,

with radiation also useful in decreasing local recurrence. The role of chemotherapy is still unclear.[11,12] Targeted therapy may become an option in the future. Late recurrences are relatively common and follow-up should be a minimum of 10 years.

MPNST

MPNSTs are one of the more common non-RMS pediatric sarcomas. Ten to 20% of MPNSTs are diagnosed in the first 2 decades. Lifetime risk of MPNST in patients with NF-1 is 2% to 10% higher in patients less than 30 years old. In contrast to adults, less than 50% of MPNSTs in children arise in the setting of NF-1. Radiation is also a risk factor for the development of MPNST. The clinical presentation is a progressively enlarging soft tissue mass, frequently with absence of pain or neurologic symptoms. The large spinal nerves in the trunk, retroperitoneum, and proximal extremities are more frequently involved. These sarcomas may arise in pre-existent plexiform neurofibromas or may arise de novo. Intratumoral heterogeneity, peritumoral edema, infiltrative margins, absence of split fat, or target signs on imaging raise the suspicion of MPNST. PET scan may be useful in this setting and seems to have higher sensitivity than MRI in making the distinction between benign and MPNST.[13] Histologic features suggesting malignancy include infiltrative growth pattern; hyperchromatic, enlarged nuclei; increased cellularity; and mitotic activity in a neurofbormatous lesion. S-100 immunoreactivity is usually weak. Treatment is primarily wide surgical excision, because chemotherapy and radiation have limited efficacy. Prognosis is poor, with a 38% to 51% 5-year survival rate.

Infantile Fibrosarcoma

Infantile fibrosarcoma is the second most common soft tissue sarcoma (after RMS) in children younger

synovial sarcoma

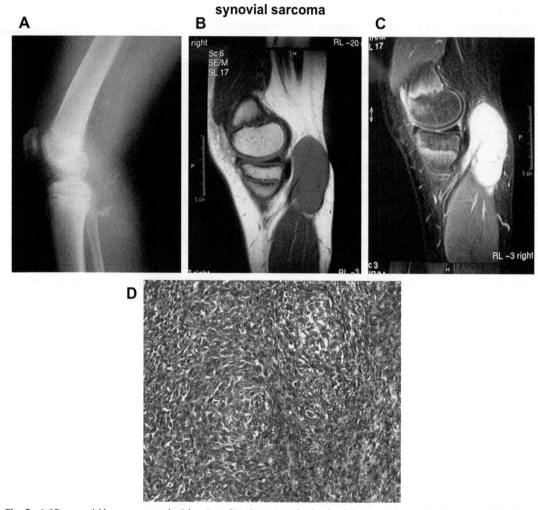

Fig. 3. A 13-year-old boy presented with a "popliteal cyst" at the back of the knee. Lateral radiograph of the knee (*A*) demonstrated a soft tissue mass in the popliteal fossa with calcifications within it, making the diagnosis of a "popliteal cyst" suspect. An MRI was obtained with sagittal T1-weighted sequences (*B*) showing a well-defined hypointense to iso-intense mass in the popliteal fossa, which on the T2 fat-saturated sequences (*C*) was hyperintense to skeletal muscle. A biopsy was performed, which demonstrated (*D*) a monophasic synovial sarcoma.

than 1 year of age. It is an intermediate grade malignant tumor seen mostly in the first 2 years of life, with half of them diagnosed antenatally or at birth. Soft tissues of the trunk and distal extremities are frequently involved. The clinical course is characterized by a rapidly growing large soft tissue mass that rarely metastasizes. The overlying skin may be red, tense, and even ulcerated with enlarged veins, causing it to be mistaken for a vascular lesion. It occasionally may be associated with disseminated intravascular coagulopathy, which may be confused with the Kasaback-Merritt phenomenon seen with kaposiform hemangioendotheliomas. Imaging reveals a poorly circumscribed mass with isointense signal on T1-weighted and inhomogenously hyperintense signal on T2-weighted sequences and heterogeneous enhancement with contrast. There may be scattered areas of low signal on all pulse sequences, suggesting fibrous tissue foci. Histologically, it demonstrates a widely variable morphology and is characterized by t(12;15)(p13;q25) translocation with *ETV6-NTRK3* gene fusion. Differential diagnoses include desmoid tumor, lipofibromatosis, myofibromatosis, RMS, and hemangiopericytoma. Treatment is mostly surgical with chemotherapy used for large unresectable lesions. Overall prognosis is good with approximately 80% 5-year survival in contrast to the poorer prognosis of adolescent/adult fibrosarcoma.[14]

Other Non-RMS STS

Other non-RMS STS include myxoid liposarcoma,[15] alveolar soft part sarcoma (ASPS),[16] epithelioid sarcoma (ES),[17] and extraskeletal Ewing sarcoma (see **Fig. 1**).[18] All of these sarcomas are fairly rare in the pediatric population. Some characteristic genetic changes are listed in **Table 3**.

Alveolar Soft Part Sarcoma

ASPS is another sarcoma of uncertain lineage. It is seen in adolescence and early adulthood, with girls and women more commonly affected. The deep tissues of the thigh (**Fig. 4**) or buttock are the most common site of involvement (around 40% of cases).[16] Approximately 20% are metastatic at presentation, and metastatic disease may develop late; therefore, long-term surveillance is recommended. These tumors are characterized by an unbalanced der(17)t(X;17)(p11;q25) translocation that results in fusion of the TFE3

transcription factor gene to ASPL gene. This results in upregulation of mesenchymal epithelial transition receptor tyrosine kinase gene and may be a potential therapeutic target. Treatment is complete local excision. The role of vascular endothelial growth factor inhibitors as adjuvants is being investigated. Five-year survival of localized ASPS is close to 90% but drops to 20% for patients with metastases at presentation.

Epithelioid Sarcoma

ES accounts for 4% to 8% of non-RMS STS in children. It is a slow-growing tumor that is often mistaken for a reactive process and presents as a painless dermal or subcutaneous nodule. Deeper lesions can extend along tendon sheaths or aponeuroses. ES is the most common soft tissue sarcoma in the hand. The "proximal"-type ES is a much more aggressive variant and represents as high as 37% of the pediatric ES. The differential diagnosis of ES includes a broad spectrum of

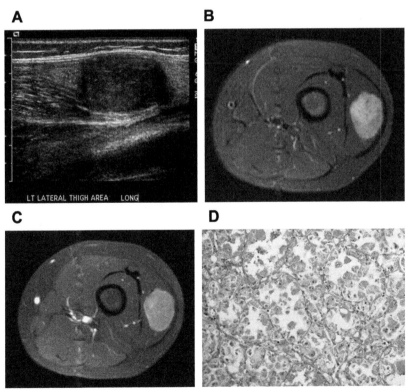

Fig. 4. An 8-year-old boy presented with a mass in the lateral distal thigh. An ultrasound was performed (*A*), which demonstrated a solid intramuscular mass. He then underwent an MRI, which demonstrated a well-defined hyperintense intramuscular soft tissue tumor within the vastus lateralis on T2 fat-saturated axial sequences (*B*) and postcontrast images (*C*) demonstrated enhancement with contrast compared to precontrast T1 fat-saturated images (not shown). A needle biopsy was performed, which demonstrated changes suggestive of an alveolar soft parts sarcoma (*D*). The patient underwent a wide resection of the tumor and remains tumor-free.

pathology, including rheumatoid nodules, granuloma annulare, necrobiosis lipoidica, granulomatous infections, superficial fibromatosis, and rhabdoid tumor. Treatment is primarily surgical, and a high index of suspicion is essential to avoid mistaking it for any of the above listed entities. Lymph node metastases in children are less common than in adults.[17]

Extraskeletal Ewing Sarcoma

This rare soft tissue sarcoma characterized by a nonrandom translocation, t(11;22), mostly presents in the second decade, with boys more commonly affected than girls. Extraskeletal Ewing sarcoma (EWS) accounts for approximately 30% of EWS and is most frequently seen in the soft tissues of the trunk and extremities. Axial locations, but not the pelvis, are more frequently involved in extraskeletal EWS versus skeletal EWS.[18] These sarcomas often present as painful soft tissue masses within the subcutaneous or deeper tissues (see **Fig. 1**) and occasionally with metastases without a known primary site. Imaging findings are nonspecific, and histology is similar to skeletal EWS with sheets of uniform round to oval cells with round nuclei, finely dispersed chromatin, finely vacuolated or amphophilic cytoplasm, and pseudorosette formation. S-100 and CD99 immunoreactivity are characteristic but not specific. Fluorescent in situ hybridization to detect the *EWS* gene break is useful in equivocal cases. Treatment is similar to skeletal EWS with surgery and/or radiation for local control and chemotherapy for systemic treatment. Outcomes for localized disease are slightly better for extraskeletal EWS versus skeletal EWS but similar for patients presenting with metastatic disease.[18]

ADVANCES
Imaging

Role of PET
The role of PET scans continues to evolve. Their use is standard for melanoma and lymphoma staging but use is increasing in the pediatric population, especially in staging for RMS, assessment of response to chemotherapy,[9] and prediction of local control in RMS.[19] PET seems to be especially useful in detecting regional lymph node metastases and bone involvement, although it is inferior to standard CT for the detection of pulmonary metastases.[20] The use of PET-CT is therefore being recommended with increasing frequency. PET scans are also useful in the setting of neurofibromatosis to detect malignant change in plexiform neurofibromas (uptake more than that of the liver is often used as a diagnostic cutoff).

They have high sensitivity but lower specificity in detection of MPNSTs in the setting of plexiform neurofibromas.[21]

Role of the whole body MR imaging
Whole body MRI for staging of malignant soft tissue tumors is now becoming more common. Siegel and colleagues[22] reported the results of the American College of Radiology Imaging Network 6660 Trial. They found that there was improved accuracy in nonlymphomatous tumors and in the detection of skeletal metastases, but it was inferior to conventional imaging for detection of pulmonary metastases.

Pathology

The increased use of immunohistochemistry, as well as flow cytometry and cytogenetic studies, has resulted in improved diagnosis and classification of tumors. It has also helped in understanding some of the pathways leading to tumorigenesis. This understanding will likely only improve with increasing use of genomics and proteonomics. A better understanding of the pathways involved should then allow the identification of appropriate targets for therapy.

Treatment

With an improved understanding of the pathways involved in the pathogenesis of malignant soft tissue tumors, there are numerous phase I and II trials using targeted therapies. Their efficacy, however, remains limited for now. Collaborative efforts are needed to get enough numbers of these rare tumors so as to be able to make progress in finding newer and more effective treatments.

ACKNOWLEDGMENTS

I would like to acknowledge Katrina Conard, MD, Chief of Pathology at the AIDHC, for some of the histology pictures and Kenneth Rogers, PhD, ATC for his help in preparing the article.

REFERENCES

1. Kransdorf MJ. Benign soft-tissue tumors in a large referral population: distribution of specific diagnoses by age, sex, and location. AJR Am J Roentgenol 1995;164(2):395–402.
2. Kransdorf MJ. Malignant soft-tissue tumors in a large referral population: distribution of diagnoses by age, sex, and location. AJR Am J Roentgenol 1995;164(1):129–34.
3. Carrino JA, Blanco R. Magnetic resonance–guided musculoskeletal interventional radiology. Semin Musculoskelet Radiol 2006;10(2):159–74.

4. Genant JW, Vandevenne JE, Bergman AG, et al. Interventional musculoskeletal procedures performed by using MR imaging guidance with a vertically open MR unit: assessment of techniques and applicability. Radiology 2002;223(1):127–36.

5. Thacker MM. Musculoskeletal oncology. In: Fischgrund J, editor. Orthopaedic knowledge update. 9th edition. Rosemont (IL): American Academy of Orthopaedic Surgoens; 2008. p. 197–220.

6. World Health Organization Classification of Tumors. Pathology and genetics of tumors of soft tissue and bone. Lyon (France): IARC Press; 2002.

7. Maurer HM, Beltangady M, Gehan EA, et al. The Intergroup Rhabdomyosarcoma Study-I. A final report. Cancer 1988;61(2):209–20.

8. Federico SM, Spunt SL, Krasin MJ, et al. Comparison of PET-CT and conventional imaging in staging pediatric rhabdomyosarcoma. Pediatr Blood Cancer 2013;60(7):1128–34.

9. Eugene T, Corradini N, Carlier T, et al. (1)(8)F-FDG-PET/CT in initial staging and assessment of early response to chemotherapy of pediatric rhabdomyosarcomas. Nucl Med Commun 2012;33(10):1089–95.

10. Skapek SX, Anderson J, Barr FG, et al. PAX-FOXO1 fusion status drives unfavorable outcome for children with rhabdomyosarcoma: a children's oncology group report. Pediatr Blood Cancer 2013;60(9):1411–7.

11. Stanelle EJ, Christison-Lagay ER, Healey JH, et al. Pediatric and adolescent synovial sarcoma: multivariate analysis of prognostic factors and survival outcomes. Ann Surg Oncol 2013;20(1):73–9.

12. Ferrari A, De Salvo GL, Dall'Igna P, et al. Salvage rates and prognostic factors after relapse in children and adolescents with initially localised synovial sarcoma. Eur J Cancer 2012;48(18):3448–55.

13. Derlin T, Tornquist K, Münster S, et al. Comparative effectiveness of 18F-FDG PET/CT versus whole-body MRI for detection of malignant peripheral nerve sheath tumors in neurofibromatosis type 1. Clin Nucl Med 2013;38(1):e19–25.

14. Orbach D, Rey A, Cecchetto G, et al. Infantile fibrosarcoma: management based on the European experience. J Clin Oncol 2010;28(2):318–23.

15. Alaggio R, Coffin CM, Weiss SW, et al. Liposarcomas in young patients: a study of 82 cases occurring in patients younger than 22 years of age. Am J Surg Pathol 2009;33(5):645–58.

16. Viry F, Orbach D, Klijanienko J, et al. Alveolar soft part sarcoma-radiologic patterns in children and adolescents. Pediatr Radiol 2013;43(9):1174–81.

17. Casanova M, Ferrari A, Collini P, et al. Epithelioid sarcoma in children and adolescents: a report from the Italian Soft Tissue Sarcoma Committee. Cancer 2006;106(3):708–17.

18. Applebaum MA, Worch J, Matthay KK, et al. Clinical features and outcomes in patients with extraskeletal Ewing sarcoma. Cancer 2011;117(13):3027–32.

19. Dharmarajan KV, Wexler LH, Gavane S, et al. Positron emission tomography (PET) evaluation after initial chemotherapy and radiation therapy predicts local control in rhabdomyosarcoma. Int J Radiat Oncol Biol Phys 2012;84(4):996–1002.

20. Benz MR, Tchekmedyian N, Eilber FC, et al. Utilization of positron emission tomography in the management of patients with sarcoma. Curr Opin Oncol 2009;21(4):345–51.

21. Treglia G, Taralli S, Bertagna F, et al. Usefulness of whole-body fluorine-18-fluorodeoxyglucose positron emission tomography in patients with neurofibromatosis type 1: a systematic review. Radiol Res Pract 2012;2012:431029.

22. Siegel MJ, Acharyya S, Hoffer FA, et al. Whole-body MR imaging for staging of malignant tumors in pediatric patients: results of the American College of Radiology Imaging Network 6660 Trial. Radiology 2013;266(2):599–609.

Index

Note: Page numbers of article titles are in **boldface** type.

Orthop Clin N Am 44 (2013) 669–675
http://dx.doi.org/10.1016/S0030-5898(13)00136-3
0030-5898/13/$ – see front matter © 2013 Elsevier Inc. All rights reserved.

orthopedic.theclinics.com

United States Postal Service

Statement of Ownership, Management, and Circulation
(All Periodicals Publications Except Requestor Publications)

1. Publication Title — Orthopedic Clinics of North America

2. Publication Number — 9 5 0 - 9 2 0

3. Filing Date — 9/14/13

4. Issue Frequency — Jan, Apr, Jul, Oct

5. Number of Issues Published Annually — 4

6. Annual Subscription Price — $293.00

7. Complete Mailing Address of Known Office of Publication (Not printer) (Street, city, county, state, and ZIP+4®)

Elsevier Inc.
360 Park Avenue South
New York, NY 10010-1710

Contact Person — Stephen R. Bushing

Telephone (Include area code) — 215-239-3688

8. Complete Mailing Address of Headquarters or General Business Office of Publisher (Not printer)

Elsevier Inc., 360 Park Avenue South, New York, NY 10010-1710

9. Full Names and Complete Mailing Addresses of Publisher, Editor, and Managing Editor (Do not leave blank)

Publisher (Name and complete mailing address)

Linda Belfus, Elsevier, Inc., 1600 John F. Kennedy Blvd. Suite 1800, Philadelphia, PA 19103-2899

Editor (Name and complete mailing address)

Jennifer Flynn-Briggs, Elsevier, Inc., 1600 John F. Kennedy Blvd. Suite 1800, Philadelphia, PA 19103-2899

Managing Editor (Name and complete mailing address)

Adrianne Brigido, Elsevier, Inc., 1600 John F. Kennedy Blvd. Suite 1800, Philadelphia, PA 19103-2899

10. Owner (Do not leave blank. If the publication is owned by a corporation, give the name and address of the corporation immediately followed by the names and addresses of all stockholders owning or holding 1 percent or more of the total amount of stock. If not owned by a corporation, give the names and addresses of the individual owners. If owned by a partnership or other unincorporated firm, give its name and address as well as those of each individual owner. If the publication is published by a nonprofit organization, give its name and address.)

Full Name	Complete Mailing Address
Wholly owned subsidiary of	1600 John F. Kennedy Blvd., Ste. 1800
Reed/Elsevier, US holdings	Philadelphia, PA 19103-2899

11. Known Bondholders, Mortgagees, and Other Security Holders Owning or Holding 1 Percent or More of Total Amount of Bonds, Mortgages, or Other Securities. If none, check box ☐ None

Full Name	Complete Mailing Address
N/A	

12. Tax Status (For completion by nonprofit organizations authorized to mail at nonprofit rates) (Check one)
The purpose, function, and nonprofit status of this organization and the exempt status for federal income tax purposes:
☐ Has Not Changed During Preceding 12 Months
☐ Has Changed During Preceding 12 Months (Publisher must submit explanation of change with this statement)

PS Form 3526, September 2007 (Page 1 of 3 (Instructions Page 3)) PSN 7530-01-000-9931 PRIVACY NOTICE. See our Privacy policy in www.usps.com

13. Publication Title — Orthopedic Clinics of North America

14. Issue Date for Circulation Data Below — July 2013

15. Extent and Nature of Circulation

		Average No. Copies Each Issue During Preceding 12 Months	No. Copies of Single Issue Published Nearest to Filing Date
a. Total Number of Copies (Net press run)		1215	1103
b. Paid Circulation (By Mail and Outside the Mail)	(1) Mailed Outside-County Paid Subscriptions Stated on PS Form 3541. (Include paid distribution above nominal rate, advertiser's proof copies, and exchange copies)	412	357
	(2) Mailed In-County Paid Subscriptions Stated on PS Form 3541 (Include paid distribution above nominal rate, advertiser's proof copies, and exchange copies)		
	(3) Paid Distribution Outside the Mails Including Sales Through Dealers and Carriers, Street Vendors, Counter Sales, and Other Paid Distribution Outside USPS®	373	384
	(4) Paid Distribution by Other Classes Mailed Through the USPS (e.g. First-Class Mail®)		
c. Total Paid Distribution (Sum of 15b (1), (2), (3), and (4))		785	741
d. Free or Nominal Rate Distribution (By Mail and Outside the Mail)	(1) Free or Nominal Rate Outside-County Copies Included on PS Form 3541	97	102
	(2) Free or Nominal Rate In-County Copies Included on PS Form 3541		
	(3) Free or Nominal Rate Copies Mailed at Other Classes Through the USPS (e.g. First-Class Mail)		
	(4) Free or Nominal Rate Distribution Outside the Mail (Carriers or other means)		
e. Total Free or Nominal Rate Distribution (Sum of 15d (1), (2), (3) and (4))		97	102
f. Total Distribution (Sum of 15c and 15e)		882	843
g. Copies not Distributed (See instructions to publishers #4 (page #3))		333	260
h. Total (Sum of 15f and g)		1215	1103
i. Percent Paid (15c divided by 15f times 100)		89.00%	87.90%

16. Publication of Statement of Ownership
☐ If the publication is a general publication, publication of this statement is required. Will be printed in the **October 2013** issue of this publication. ☐ Publication not required

17. Signature and Title of Editor, Publisher, Business Manager, or Owner

Stephen R. Bushing – Inventory/Distribution Coordinator

Stephen R. Bushing

Date — September 14, 2013

I certify that all information furnished on this form is true and complete. I understand that anyone who furnishes false or misleading information on this form or who omits material or information requested on the form may be subject to criminal sanctions (including fines and imprisonment) and/or civil sanctions (including civil penalties).

PS Form 3526, September 2007 (Page 2 of 3)

Moving?

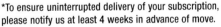

Make sure your subscription moves with you!

To notify us of your new address, find your **Clinics Account Number** (located on your mailing label above your name), and contact customer service at:

Email: journalscustomerservice-usa@elsevier.com

800-654-2452 (subscribers in the U.S. & Canada)
314-447-8871 (subscribers outside of the U.S. & Canada)

Fax number: 314-447-8029

Elsevier Health Sciences Division
Subscription Customer Service
3251 Riverport Lane
Maryland Heights, MO 63043

Printed and bound by CPI Group (UK) Ltd, Croydon, CR0 4YY

03/10/2024

01040378-0005